ONE WORLD

Jimmy Carter, C. Everett Koop, Sir Michael
Atiyah, Sir Gordon Wolstenholme, Lonnie
Bristow, Donna E. Shalala, Priscilla
Kincaid-Smith, Alexander "Sandy"
Macara, Robert Gallo, Suresh
Arya, Victor Villalobos, Duane
Alexander, M.D., Jonathan
Mann, Luc Montagnier,
Jonas Salk, Linus Pauling,
Christiaan Barnard, T.
Adeoye Lambo, Oladipo
Akinkugbe, Sadako
Ogata, Jean-Claude
Mulli, Federico Mayor,
Carl Sagan, James
Hansen, Thomas
Lovejoy, Paul Johnston,
Ruth Stringer, David
Santillo, Lynn Goldman,
Maurice Strong, Nafis Sadik,
W. Harding le Riche,
Francisco Ayala, Audrey
Chapman, Thomas Kempf,
Sir David Plastow, Sir Dai Rees,
Hiroshi Nakajima, Carmen Lawrence,
Adib Domingos Jatene, Diane Marleau,
Simone Veil, C. Silvera, Shoichi Ide, Edward
Nechaev, Virginia Bottomley, Boutros
Boutros-Ghali

ONE WORLD

The Health and Survival of the Human Species in the 21st Century

Robert Lanza, M.D.

Health Press

Santa Fe, New Mexico

Published by Health Press
P.O. Drawer 1388
Santa Fe, NM 87504

Printed in the United States of America.

10 9 8 7 6 5 4 3 2

Library of Congress Cataloging in Publication Data

Edited by Harriet Slavitz
Design by Jim Mafchir

TABLE OF CONTENTS

**An Open Letter From the
Former President of the United States**   xi
by Jimmy Carter

Introductory Statement   xv
by C. Everett Koop,
Former Surgeon General of the United States

Foreword   xix
by Sir Michael Atiyah,
President of the Royal Society

1 Introduction
Robert Lanza, M.D., Editor   3

2 Health on Earth: Goodwill Towards Men   9
Sir Gordon Wolstenholme, Founder of Action in
International Medicine and Former President of
the Royal Society of Medicine

3 The Winds of Change   19
Lonnie Bristow, President of the
American Medical Association

4 The Challenge of Our Times   25
Donna E. Shalala,
U.S. Secretary of Health and Human Services

5 Changes in Modern Medicine   31
Priscilla Kincaid-Smith, President of the World
Medical Association and President of the
Royal Australasian College of Physicians

6 Medicine in the Next Century   39
Alexander "Sandy" Macara, Chairman of the
Council of the British Medical Association

7 Advances in Genetics: Gene Therapy   49
Robert Gallo, Chief of of Tumor Cell
Biology National Cancer Institute and Adjunct
Professor of Genetics at George Washington University

8 Advances in Genetics:
Food and Agricultural Products   59
Victor Villalobos, Senior Officer of the
United Nations Food and Agriculture Organization

9 Advances in Reproductive Medicine   67
Duane Alexander, M.D., Director of the U.S.
National Institute of Child Health and Human
Development

10 AIDS   75
Jonathan Mann, Director of the International
AIDS Center; Director of the Francois-Xavier
Bagnoud Center for Health and Human Rights at
Harvard University; and Founding Director of the
World Health Organization's Program on AIDS

11 The Future of AIDS Research:
What to Do?   81
Luc Montagnier, Discoverer of the AIDS Virus

12 Vaccines: What the Future Has in Store   89
Jonas Salk, Founder of the Salk Institute for
Biological Studies; Developed the Polio Vaccine

13 Problems Introducing a New Medical Field   93
Linus Pauling, Awarded the Nobel Peace Prize,
and the Nobel Prize in Chemistry

14 Medicine Negated   103
Christiaan Barnard, Emeritus Professor of
Surgical Science at the University of Cape
Town; Performed the World's First Human
Heart Transplant

**15 Constraints on World Medical and
Health Progress**   111
T. Adeoye Lambo, Deputy Director-
General of the World Health Organization

**16 Adapt, Adopt, or Quo Vadis? A Dilemma in
the Developing World**   129
Oladipo Akinkugbe, Professor and Former
Dean of Medicine at the University of Ibadan, Nigeria

**17 Refugee Emergencies: New Challenges
for Humanitarian Action**   137
Sadako Ogata, United Nations High
Commissioner for Refugees

18 War and Health   149
Jean-Claude Mulli, International
Committee of the Red Cross

**19 The End of the Cold War:
A Culture of Peace**   161
Federico Mayor, Director-General of the
United Nations Educational, Scientific, and
Cultural Organization

**20 Between Enemies: Reconstruction of
Civilization Away from Weapons of
Mass Destruction**   169
Carl Sagan, David Duncan Professor of
Astronomy and Space Sciences at Cornell
University

21 Climatic Changes: Understanding Global Warming   173
James Hansen, Director of the NASA Goddard
Institute for Space Studies

22 Preserving the Earth's Biological Resources   191
Thomas Lovejoy, Counselor to the Secretary of
the Smithsonian Institution

23 The Tilting Balance   195
Paul Johnston, Ruth Stringer, and
David Santillo for Greenpeace International

**24 Toxic Exposure and Health: Perspective of
the U.S. Environmental Protection Agency**   205
Lynn Goldman, U.S. Environmental
Protection Agency

25 Environment and Development   215
The Honorable Maurice Strong, Secretary-General
of the 1992 U.N. Conference on Environment
and Development

26 Population and Development   221
Nafis Sadik, Secretary-General of the United Nations
International Conference on Population and
Development and Executive Director of the U.N.
Population Fund

27 The Bottom Line   231
W. Harding le Riche, Emeritus Professor
of Epidemiology at the University of Toronto

**28 The Way Forward:
Health and Human Rights**   247
Francisco Ayala, Retiring President of the
American Association for the Advancement of
Science; Audrey Chapman, Director of the Science
and Human Rights Program of the American
Association for the Advancement of Science

29 Science and the Humanities   255
Thomas Kempf, Secretary of the Conference of
German Academies of Sciences and Humanities

**30 Goals for the Next Century: Science,
Health, and the Impacts of Population,
Environmental, and Social Change**   261
Sir David Plastow, Chairman of the U.K. Medical
Research Council; Sir Dai Rees, Chief
Executive of the U.K. Medical Research Council,
President of the European Science Foundation

**31 Charting the Future:
Health Goals for the Next Century**   269
Hiroshi Nakajima, Director-General of the
World Health Organization

STATEMENTS FROM THE MINISTRIES OF HEALTH

32 Australia   273
The Honorable Carmen Lawrence

33 Brazil   283
The Honorable Adib Domingos Jatene

34 Canada   293
The Honorable Diane Marleau

35 France   297
The Honorable Simone Veil

36 India   303
The Honorable C. Silvera

37 Japan   309
The Honorable Shoichi Ide

38 Russia   311
The Honorable Edward Nechaev

39 United Kingdom   317
The Honorable Virginia Bottomley

Concluding Statement by Boutros Boutros-Ghali   323
Secretary-General of the United Nations

About the Editor   325

A Salute to Jimmy Carter and to C. Everett Koop

THE EDITOR DEDICATES THIS BOOK to James Earl Carter, Jr., thirty-ninth president of the United States, and to C. Everett Koop, former surgeon general of the U.S. Public Health Service. Together with the other contributors in this volume, their generosity, wisdom, and creativity have done much to improve the human condition.

Jimmy Carter left an indelible mark on history during the four years of his 1977 to 1981, presidency. In addition to improving human rights and negotiating the Mideast peace agreement, he achieved passage of the Alaska National Interest Lands Conservation Act, the largest land-conservation legislation in U.S. history. In the 14 years since he left office, his Carter Center has established programs in sustainable agriculture in a number of sub-Saharan African nations as well as health-related development programs in more than 20 countries. These programs not only improve health and prevent disease in some of the poorest countries of the world but help slow deforestation, encourage the protection of land, the control of erosion, the increased production of food grains, and the prevention of siltation of streams. The former president was also very involved in the 1992 United Nations Earth Summit and again in the 1994 population conference in Cairo. His book *Talking Peace* was devoted to an analysis of how environmental degradation contributes to the rise of violence and violent confrontation and civil wars and to the massive movement of people into already overcrowded–and sometimes starving–urban centers.

C. Everett Koop was surgeon general of the United States from 1981 to 1989. During these years his independence made him one of America's most trusted figures and a champion of issues of public health–including smoking, diet, nutrition, immunization, and AIDS. He became known for his down-to-earth programs for many of the medical/social ills of the country. Since returning to private life he has continued to promote health reform and to extol high-tech communications to link primary care doctors with major medical centers. In 1992 he set up the C. Everett Koop Institute at Dartmouth to foster reforms in medical education, teaching students about sensitivity toward patients and preventive medicine: "We're trying not only to turn out a humanitarian physician who is a good listener and communicator, but one who entwines prevention and ethics in every decision he makes."

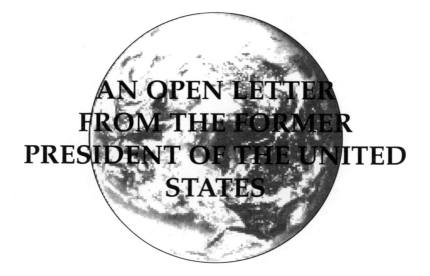

AN OPEN LETTER FROM THE FORMER PRESIDENT OF THE UNITED STATES

JIMMY CARTER

FOR MANY PEOPLE, our global interdependence became clear, at least for a short period of time, only after pictures of Earth were taken from outer space. For some, such as Polybius more than 2000 year ago or Gandhi in more recent times, this idea of interdependence permeated their thinking. The current and future quality of this world depends on more than just a few wise people understanding the concept or many feeling only momentarily connected. The hope for a quality world in the future depends on large proportions of the population incorporating such ideas into their everyday life-style.

Unfortunately, the evidence in this country and the world is that instead of joining hands to share both the benefits and the burdens of the world, the gap continues to grow between the rich and the poor, with the rich consuming ever larger proportions of the resources while the poor struggle to divide what remains. UNICEF's *State of the World's Children* report, issued in December, 1994, demonstrates that while the average wealth of the world continues to improve, the gap in wealth between the rich and the poor is actually increasing. In the United States, the richest 1 percent of the population now owns almost 40 percent of the total wealth. The richest 20 percent of our population accounted for the total increase of wealth in the U.S. in the 1980s.

If this is to be reversed, it will be because those with the wealth, the science, the knowledge, the power, and the influence take deliberate action instead of relying on things to "work out." Three mind-sets are particularly important in planning such deliberate action. First, the understanding that each of us is truly part of an extended family that includes all people everyplace and also extends in time to include all who will ever be born. We have a responsibility to those family members separated from us by centuries. Second, that equity is more than just important . . . it is indeed the basis for the Golden Rule. We can't allow ourselves to enjoy the benefits of the world with the poverty of the poor actually subsidizing our enjoyment. Third, it is important to understand that interdependence goes beyond the human race. Everything affects everything, and just as hairspray used in Atlanta has had effects on the ozone layer and health throughout the world, so does the health in Sudan have direct impact on the gross national product of Atlanta.

This book contains a remarkable wealth of information to be used in formulating such a deliberate plan. It makes clear the importance of each person believing every day that they are writing history...because you are.

–President Jimmy Carter

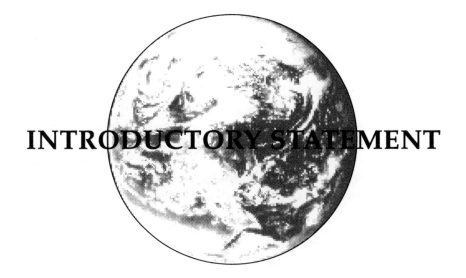

INTRODUCTORY STATEMENT

C. EVERETT KOOP
Former Surgeon General of the United States

MY LIFE HAS BEEN FULL, rewarding, and varied. Almost everything that I have done in my professional life has some bearing on the repeated themes that are stated by the multiple contributors to this book. For the longest period of my professional life, I was a pediatric surgeon and also a professor of pediatric surgery. Then, I had the opportunity to serve the United States as its surgeon general for eight years. During that time, I also served the Department of Health and Human Services as the Director of International Health and often assumed the role of chief delegate to the annual World Health Assembly of the World Health Organization. Since leaving the government, I have been deeply concerned with preventive medicine and the reform of the health-care system in the United States, and I have maintained my abiding interest in health-care delivery in developing countries.

As you read this remarkable collection of essays, I am sure that you will ponder the juxtaposition of opposing philosophies in three general areas:

> **Treatment/Prevention:** The history of the healing arts has always been heavily weighed in favor of treatment rather than prevention. That might have been acceptable when we did not know as much about preventive medicine as we now do; today it is inexcusable. The high technologies that have brought us modern medical miracles have simply become too costly. We need to reduce our emphasis on rehabilitative and reparative medicine and surgery, focusing instead on prevention because an ounce of prevention is worth a pound of cure in the health-care economy.

> Paradoxically, modern medicine decreases mortality while increasing morbidity. In other words, we have more people living longer, but many of them are living sicker. Many of these people, while not fully cured, live productive lives; for others, we merely prolong their process of dying. An active philosophy of disease prevention and health promotion can postpone up to 70 percent of all premature deaths, whereas the traditional curative and reparative approach can postpone no more than 10 to 15 percent of such deaths. The best way to reduce the demand for health care (and, therefore, make it affordable) is for each of us to take charge of his or her health so that we need to use the health care system less often.

Ethics/Economics: Health-care reform in nations around the globe is usually driven by the need to control costs. The debates usually focus on the economic and political feasibility of health-care reform. That puts the cart before the horse.

More important than either politics or economics is the ethical imperative for health-care reform. Any nation determined to enact effective health-care reform must first agree on the basic values and ethics upon which its health-care system and, indeed, its society is based. If an ethical consensus could be reached, many of the economic and political problems of health-care reform would be easily solved.

Health-care reform poses the greatest political challenge to a democratic republic such as the United States because each of us is being asked to do something for all of us. Many of us feel that what might be best for all of us is not best for each of us. It is just that simple. It is just that complex.

Personal Responsibility/Greed: Many of the problems faced by health systems, in rich and poor countries alike, stem from one of humanity's greatest afflictions–greed. The pernicious effect of greed in health-care systems is the fault not only of those who provide health care. Patients who expect limitless care and results can be as greedy as health-care providers or third-party payers who allow greed to dictate medical decisions.

The abrogation of personal responsibility has weakened the structure of modern society. In health care and prevention, personal responsibility could reduce the demand for health-care services and also lead to more equitable costing for the delivery of such services.

When I have decisions to make, in reference to health, medicine and health care, I find that keeping these three areas of opposing philosophies in mind leads to a sense of balance in an ever-changing world where the principles must remain the constant.

—*C. Everett Koop, M.D.*

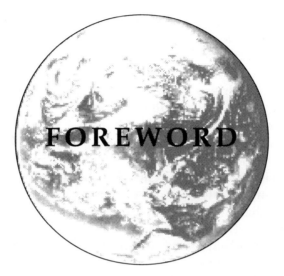

FOREWORD

SIR MICHAEL ATIYAH
President of the Royal Society

IT IS A GREAT PLEASURE FOR ME, as a representative of the world's scientific community, to contribute a foreword to this volume. The future health of the world, interpreted in its broadest sense to include medical, social, and economic factors that determine our well-being, should be the central concern of all of us. The rapid pace of change, driven by technological advances on an enormous scale, means that the twenty-first century will bring crucial challenges to our whole civilization. The problems of population growth, resource limitation, environmental pollution, and widespread poverty are already upon us and have to be grappled with as a matter of urgency.

Fortunately, there is increasing evidence that the conscience of the world community has been aroused. International conferences, under the auspices of the United Nations and other bodies, are constantly acknowledging the problems and pointing the way forward. This book, *One World*, focusing on health, is another indicator of world concern–but the process must continue. Inertia and vested interests have to be overcome and there has to be increasing recognition that the widespread inequalities in the world have to be redressed.

In the years ahead the scientific community has a special responsibility to lead the way. Science is fundamentally a universal endeavor that should aim at benefiting mankind, and scientists by tradition work across political and cultural barriers. In addition, many of the problems we face, such as overpopulation or industrial pollution, are the side effects of benefits produced by science. Since there is no way the clock can be turned back, scientists of the future will have to help to devise solutions for the problems of the past.

The range of contributions in this volume shows the wide spectrum of problems that we face, but it also indicates the degree of concern that is felt and the positive steps that are being taken. The message that emerges is of the urgent need for continuing efforts by all of us.

—*Sir Michael Atiyah*

ONE WORLD

1
INTRODUCTION

ROBERT LANZA, M.D.
Editor

THIS BOOK WAS INSPIRED by a twofold interest: my love for medicine and science and my concern about environmental issues and the ultimate fate of mankind. I believe that a closer correlation should exist between these two aspects: that medicine and science should perhaps take another look at their aims and accomplishments as they relate to humanity on a global basis; and that, on the other hand, the governing powers-that-be should use to a greater extent the available medical and scientific achievements and know-how in their efforts to improve the human condition in large parts of the world. Medical researchers report ever newer discoveries in their fight against disease, while at the same time appalling health conditions prevail in large parts of the world.

As we approach the threshold of a new century, indeed, a new millennium, the idea struck me: Why not compile a book with contributions not only by leading scientists but by educators, statesmen, and experts from various other areas of accomplishment, indicating facts and possibly thoughts and suggestions for necessary changes for the new century, thus offering a multifaceted picture of where we stand and where we intend to go.

To choose among the many possible contributors was not easy, and I was not sure what their reaction would be to my request. The response was overwhelming and gratifying, dispelling any doubt I may have had about the need and relevance of such an assessment and/or commentary as this book represents. The positive response also indicated that the leaders of our time, from scientists to politicians, recognize that much remains to be done to improve the health and well-being of humanity, not only by further advancement of medicine and science but even more so by promoting growing awareness of the problems and their possible solution among society at large and policy makers in particular and by overcoming apathy, prejudice, and superstition, which stand in the way of reaching this goal. The contributors in this book work in Australia, Brazil, Canada, Egypt, France, Germany, India, Italy, Japan, Nigeria, Russia, South Africa, Switzerland, the Netherlands, the United Kingdom, and the United States, among other countries. By cooperating in this way, they may inspire others to take a world view of the health of humanity.

Medicine has scored tremendous successes that have demonstrated the splendor of science and the human mind, and its achievements have spared millions of fellow humans from catastrophic diseases. It has, for example, virtually eradicated smallpox from the face of the earth and has halted the advance of some of the most devastating diseases mankind has known. In less than a century, our life expectancy has more than doubled, from around 36 to 76 years of age.

However, many of today's brilliant victories have taken place in an atmosphere of global distrust, at a time when, according to Sir Gordon Wolstenholme in chapter 2, "most people live in daily dread of the willful or accidental explosion of nuclear weapons; when conventional fighting between feuding factions and the bombs of terrorist fanatics increasingly claim a toll of innocent victims; when a social revolution is needed in regard to the ethics and economics of employment; when AIDS brings its innumerable personal tragedies and threatens to decimate at least one generation on which the economic viability of some nations depends; when climatic and environmental changes may soon affect the world's capacity to sustain its population, and alter the geographic distribution both of agricultural productivity and also of epidemics affecting plant, animal, and human life; and when, over the whole planet, inequalities and injustices abound."

Although modern medicine and science can hardly be blamed for all of our present ills, they may be in danger of accepting the mechanical worldview and losing touch with the basic needs of humanity. Have they fully lived up to their broader global obligations? Medical resources are sparsest there where death and disease are most widespread. In today's cold human climate, at least 500-1,000 million people are suffering from malnutrition and disease. So disastrous is the picture that in many regions of the developing world one in four infants will not live to see a first birthday. Meanwhile, people are multiplying at a frightening rate; our land, air, and water are being poisoned by chemicals and carcinogens; and large areas of the world's agricultural land are being destroyed. Is it beyond our combined human capacity to alter this intolerable situation? And the emphasis in this question should be on "combined." Medicine's objective is and should be the improvement of the health and well-being of the human species, but it must be supported by a responsive populace and governing agencies who will recognize the value of medical discoveries and apply them indiscriminately where they are needed to ease the life of human beings.

As Christiaan Barnard comments in chapter 14: "[It] is a bit like cleaning the Augean stables. We keep on wiping the floor without turning off the tap. Ideologies, social systems, and economic theories–all of which we consider to be beyond our legitimate ken–produce the disease processes we are fighting."

Medical and scientific research, of course, is fundamental to the conquest of diseases. It must continue to unearth new facts and expand the boundaries of its knowledge. Scientific history has demonstrated the immense value of acquiring knowledge for its own sake–it is impossible, not to say arrogant, for society to determine the cost-benefit of an increment of human knowledge. The public must share in the intrinsic exhilaration of understanding and recognize that without "pure" science medicine will be crippled in its fight to eliminate disease and preserve health. Young scientists must be encouraged, rather than hindered or confined, to follow their intellectual curiosity, spurred by youthful idealism and a genuine desire to seek fundamental paradoxes in nature and to find means to free mankind from unnecessary suffering.

Medicine and science still have a long way to go before they solve the remaining problems of biological existence. New horizons promise to prevent genetic diseases and to overcome many of the problems of old age. International research efforts have to be stepped up to find better birth control methods, assess natural and industrial toxicants, and to treat, or better yet prevent or forestall, the disabilities of old age in a populace that should enjoy, but often suffers from, the years added to our prolonged life span. Advances in tissue engineering and cellular medicine will soon allow doctors to grow and replace damaged body tissues and organs. In the field of molecular biology and genetic engineering advances may soon lead to new drugs and vaccines that, we hope, will prevent disabling and killing diseases, such as AIDS and multiple sclerosis; that will improve world health by means that were inconceivable just a few years ago; and that will possibly conquer leading causes of death, such as cancer and heart disease.

What is vitally needed for these endeavors is not just more money, research, and education but a one-world concept of humanity. "The health of the world," concludes Jonathan Mann in chapter 10, "is bound together. The photograph of Earth from space, that image of our entire world, blue, green, and brown against a black immensity, must guide and usher in a new era of understanding about the true meaning of global health." Society, from scientist to politician to media representative to the man in the street, must displace its apathy, overcome resistance to new concepts of healing, and lay aside its religious taboos. It must arouse public concern and stimulate the political will to attack problems based on an assessment of their damaging effects on humanity and the environment, rather than on nationalistic and sectarian politics. Medicine and science have found the means to alleviate or remove much of human suffering from diseases, but their progress is often hindered by the lack of or wrong motivations of society at large. Concerted international action, ever greater research efforts and global exploration and application of our increasing fund of knowledge in areas of medicine and public health are urgently needed.

Knowledge alone does not necessarily subserve the welfare of humanity, for without an ethical dimension and base it can harbor the seeds of cruelty and destruction. As many of the contributors to this book passionately point out, some of civilization's greatest scientific discoveries have damaged our environment, often beyond repair, and have led us to the brink of nuclear and biological extinction. Considering the immense and growing power of the sciences over life, it becomes imperative that a concerted, cooperative, global effort is made by governments, scientists, educators, and the media to ensure that this power is used not for the destruction, but for the benefit and progress of man.

The editor wishes to express his indebtedness and gratitude to all the contributors, who generously gave of their time and knowledge in the preparation of this book. He also thanks **Scott Randall** and **Barbara O'Donnell** for their valuable assistance and encouragement throughout.

2

HEALTH ON EARTH: GOODWILL TOWARD MEN

SIR GORDON WOLSTENHOLME
is President and Founder of Action in International Medicine,
a worldwide alliance of health professionals acting through
their universities, academies, and associations to strengthen and improve
the health-care system. Sir Gordon was formerly Harveian Librarian of the
Royal College of Physicians, London; Director of the CIBA Foundation; and
President of the Royal Society of Medicine.

"Homines ad deos nulla re proprius accedunt quam salutem hominibus dando." (In nothing do men more nearly approach the gods than in giving health to men.)

–Cicero
Pro Ligario, 12

THE PURPOSES OF THIS CHAPTER are threefold: to outline the slow, erratic, and limited development of international cooperation in health; to draw attention to the apathy of governments and most people, including physicians, to the absence of health from some two billion fellow humans; and to suggest that, for political and economic as well as for the obvious humanitarian reasons, a vast improvement should be attempted in regard to this intolerable situation. Our world sorely needs a global, concerted demonstration of active goodwill.

EARLY INTERNATIONAL HEALTH MEASURES

In the centuries before medicine became, partly, a science, governments could be excused for having no central policy for the protection of their people from disease or for the promotion of their health. The Romans were quick to realize the benefits of sanitation, and in the sixth century the Emperor Justinian issued edicts to isolate travelers coming from areas of known pestilence, releasing them with a certificate of health when they were considered to pose no threat to his people.

In the 14th century, the island of Rhodes, the city of Ragusa (Dubrovnik), and the State of Venice introduced policies of quarantine for vessels arriving from ports known to be affected by epidemics of plague or cholera. Fear and greed rapidly induced most other trading nations to adopt similar measures, both on land and sea; fear because of the devastating nature of the epidemics that swept across Europe from the East and greed because it was soon realized how easily quarantine could be exploited to harass and hinder the trade of commercially competing nations. Savage measures were taken against individuals who tried to break out of a quarantine area. For example, when the English Court moved from London to Windsor in 1625 to escape an epidemic of plague, orders were given that anyone arriving from London should immediately be hanged. Ships and cargos could be burned and their crews and passengers held in isolation hospitals where those in need of treatment might expect to receive care, at a cautious distance, from doctors who protected themselves by copiously drinking wine.

The system lent itself at the best to bureaucratic obstruction–the authorities at Marseilles wanted to shoot Napoleon for landing from Egypt without permission–and at the worst to bribery, corruption, and murder. The extreme severity of the epidemics often disorganized whatever cooperative resistance there might have been. The Black Death, which killed nearly a third of the population of Europe in the 14th century, so broke up central administration in England that during the great plagues that followed in the next three hundred years measures taken locally in London did not apply elsewhere; each English port was left to its own medical defenses.

Eventually demands began to be heard for international agreement on quarantine regulations, and France led the way in organizing a series of international sanitary conferences, which started in 1851 and continued up to World War II.

SCIENTIFIC AWAKENING IN HEALTH

So long as it was not known what caused the epidemics or how the diseases were transmitted, the sanitary conferences were little more than confrontations where the protagonists of different theories could assert their unfounded authority. The British government, in particular, wanted the least possible interference with trade and travel, drawing the comment from a Spanish expert that "[the] British say time is money, but public health is gold."

When Snow and Hassall in London and Pacini in Florence demonstrated the existence of cholera vibrio and its spread through contaminated water, even its mode of action in the intestine, this news failed to penetrate the noise of debate by those who thought they knew better; it remained for Robert Koch, some thirty years later, to produce undeniable, incontrovertible evidence of the specific microorganisms, the realization of which caused von Pettenkofer, the chief German official of the old school of thought, to kill himself. Treatment of affected patients could at last begin to be carried out on a rational basis, and quarantine could be largely discontinued in favor of the careful supervision of immediate contacts.

PUBLIC HEALTH CONCERNS

The international sanitary conferences that began in 1851 succeeded from the beginning, however, in establishing that there were advantages in multinational cooperation in matters of health. Interestingly, at the first International Sanitary Conference in Paris in 1851, each of the eleven participating nations was represented by one statesman and one doctor. (They were given independent votes and did not always agree with each other.) From the second conference, in 1859, doctors were excluded; the "scientific facts" were though to have been established and the necessary conventions could now be drafted by the diplomats.

Doctors, and some notable non-medical individuals, had begun before that time to expand the horizons of the doctor–single patient relationship. At the end of the 18th century, Johann Peter Frank (1745-1821) set out in six volumes his principles for health administration, including medical education, the collection of vital statistics, health education, urban sanitation, good housing, safe food and drink, seasonable clothing, regulation of conditions at work, and marriage hygiene. He pointed out the absurdity of allowing horses but not peasant women to rest before and after parturition. He also addressed such matters as the rearing of children, care of the needy and dying, prevention of epidemics, and a well-ordered public health system. Frank did most of this in the interest of absolutist monarchs in Germany and Austria, but he was not himself seeking to aid them in the provision of cannon-fodder. He observed that "saving one single life must come to be regarded as a deed loftier than the bloody conquest of a province."

WAR AND COMPASSION

On 24 June 1859, at the Battle of Solferino in Italy, the young Swiss bible-scholar and colonial farmer, Henri Dunant, witnessed not only the appalling massacre of nearly 40,000 French and Austrian troops in one fateful day but also the willful neglect and ill-treatment of the wounded of the one side by the medical personnel of the other in the following days. This led him to establish, with a few private friends in Geneva in 1864, the International Red Cross, for the future treatment of wounded irrespective of nationality. Few acts in history can have done so much to awaken a sense of a common humanity. Also from the horrors of war came the great work of Florence Nightingale on the British side and of N. I. Pirogov on the Russian in the Crimean War, leading to the creation of an educated profession of nursing (and much else).

MEDICAL SOCIETIES

Writing in 1902, William Osler commented that "The great republic of medicine knows and has known no national boundaries." Throughout the second half of the 19th century in particular, doctors were busy forming association and societies both on a national and an international basis. International medical congresses were organized every two or three years beginning in 1867. In the early days there was a wide selection of chosen subjects for discussion: for example, marsh miasma, gunshot wounds, venereal diseases, cancer, hospital hygiene, the effect of railways on health, and relations between doctors and governments. Soon the division of subjects became formalized under the headings of medicine, surgery, obstetrics and gynecology, biology, public health, ophthalmology, otology, and pharmacology. But from an early stage people with special interests, such as chemistry, physiology, dermatology, ophthalmology, otology, hygiene and demography, public health, mental medicine, and various organizations concerned with alcohol abuse began to arrange international gatherings at regular two to five-year intervals. Similar conferences were started on a regional, pan-American, and Australasian basis.

In Europe, French was the dominant language of communications, but the British medical journal *The Lancet* deplored the fact that Latin was no longer the international language of science and medicine. When women qualified as doctors, they were excluded from the congresses on the grounds that their presence would inhibit free and open discussion; but by 1899 they had their own international congress of women. Warring nations had to be avoided as congress centers, the meetings being removed by common consent to neutral alternatives.

Soon it was being said that congresses were "as plentiful as blackberries." In Paris in 1900, in connection with a world exhibition, no less than 128 international meetings took place, of which 12 were of direct interest to medicine and at least another 12 partly covered medical ground. Since that time specialization, however divisive it may be to medical practice, led to the formation internationally and regionally of many hundreds of active specialist societies. Although the people taking part in them might not see themselves in this light, they may be regarded as defying or ignoring the narrow and competitive nationalism of the political world.

Doctors have always readily accepted that a Pasteur or a Koch or a Lister can all remain good patriots while their work is done for the whole world, their nationality being of no more consequence than that of a great composer. But the many international gatherings of medical men, however valuably they may cement friendships and increase the sum total of knowledge, rarely go as far as extending an expression of care to the millions of people outside the Western world who can never hope to experience the enjoyment of good health or normal energy.

On the occasion of the 11th Medical Congress in Rome in 1894, a leading article in *The Lancet* noted that it was in Rome, according to Setonius, that professors and practitioners of healing were first given the rank of citizens by Julius Caesar: "It is in Rome that the profession is marking another stage on its path to that still higher citizenship–the brotherhood of the nations, the citizenship of the world."

INTERNATIONAL COOPERATION

This human and pious hope moved a little toward realization at the eleventh

International Sanitary Conference held in Paris in 1903. An international convention called for the creating in Paris of an Office International d'Hygiene Publique (OIHP) "to collect and disseminate facts and documents of general public health interest, and especially those relating to infectious diseases, notably cholera, plague and yellow fever." Started by nine countries in 1908, OIHP soon had 60 member nations and extended its range of competence to biological standardization, brucellosis, leprosy, human and bovine tuberculosis, typhoid, venereal diseases, and water purification.

When the United States decided not to join the League of Nations in 1920, and therefore also remained outside its Health Organization, American membership of OIHP kept it in coexistence with the League's organization until both were taken up after World War II into the World Health Organization (WHO). Expert members of OIHP played an active and leading role in the Health Organization of the League of Nations. The latter was set up under a clause of the Treaty of Versailles to bring health authorities of different countries into a closer working relationship, to achieve more rapid transmission of information about epidemics, and to unify the appropriate international action to be taken to control them. This entailed liaison with the International Labour Office, to coordinate measures for the protection of industrial workers from injury and disease; cooperation with the International Red Cross and similar bodies; and the organization of missions to any part of the world to provide medical advice "with the concurrence of the countries affected."

THE LEAGUE OF NATIONS

It is generally agreed that the one successful achievement of the ill-fated League of Nations was its Health Organization. It began its international work at a time when major countries were starting to create their own ministries and departments of health. The organization gave impetus to this tendency, and leading members of the national ministries soon took on the role of international health experts. It is significant that they opened their own channels of communication with each other, without recourse to normal diplomatic channels. The organization's work was of course limited by the amount of money and attention that governments and public opinion were prepared to grant it, and it has been estimated that its total budget over twenty years was equivalent to the cost of one battleship of that time.

Sadly, too, the national ministries and departments of health were conceived in narrow medical and sanitary terms, from which they have never escaped. Poverty, housing and town planning, water supplies, nutrition, education in biology and health, the state of the environment, and other factors of major significance to health have usually been the responsibility of other and often more powerful departments of government. Similarly, the ministers and secretaries of health have almost always been of only two kinds: the respected old warhorses put harmlessly out to grass, or the young and ambitious party politicians already looking to the next stepping stone to power. If this has been the concept by government on the priority of health at the national level, small wonder that the imagination of statesmen has stopped short of recognizing what an offense it is to humanity that there should continue to exist such a vast store of largely preventable misery among so many of the world's people.

Despite the success of the League's Health Organization, when preliminary steps were taken after World War II to create the United Nations Organization, incredibly–but significantly–health was at first overlooked, only later being included at the insistence of a few individuals.

At the end of World War I there had been other activities of significance to world health. The League of Red Cross Societies had been founded principally by Henry Pomeroy Davison, who had been a brilliantly successful leader of the American Red Cross Society during the war. Davison thought that voluntary subscriptions would continue to flood in and that with such support a world health program could be devised to anticipate, diminish, and relieve the misery produced by disease and calamity. Unhappily, all too few shared his vision, and contributions fell off even as society became more affluent. The League became a valuable institution, but of secondary international importance. And mention must be made of the significance of private philanthropic organizations active in support of national and international health, of which the Rockefeller Foundation offers the supreme example, striving since 1913 "to promote the well-being of mankind throughout the world."

RELIEF AND REHABILITATION

In 1943, during World War II, Roosevelt conceived the idea of the United Nations Relief and Rehabilitation Administration (UNRRA), which, in the chaos of war and the immediate post-war period, not only carried out the reestablishment of millions of displaced people but also for a time (January 1945 to December 1946) constituted the temporary world center for information on epidemics. Its work has been described as "the greatest act of charity the world has ever seen." But many who wished to attack Roosevelt politically did not hesitate to denigrate its work.

WORLD HEALTH ORGANIZATION

After the unprecedented slaughter and maiming of tens of millions of people in World War II, a visitor from another planet might well have thought that the surviving members of the human species would have turned eagerly toward measures, comparatively simple and inexpensive in themselves, that would enable them never again to suffer unnecessarily from disabling and killing diseases and disasters. Instead, as earlier remarked, world health was almost overlooked among the potential benefits of the creation of a community of nations. The United States was so fearful of "socialized medicine" that it delayed for two years its ratification of the agreement to WHO, although its representatives attended the meetings. The one American physician with the longest experience of international health work described those who were trying to create WHO as "star-gazers and political and social uplifters . . . advanced internationalists"–none of which was intended as complimentary or constructive. Within six months of the establishment of WHO in 1948, Russia and the Cominform countries withdrew from cooperation in world health on political grounds and remained aloof for seven years while China held back for five years, giving as an excuse the impossibility of recognizing the membership of Taiwan. These, and similar difficulties from time to time concerning the membership of countries such as Vietnam, South Africa, the German Democratic Republic, Israel, and Zimbabwe, have emphasized the drawbacks of the intergovernmental structure of U.N. agencies. Too often this means that a problem is tackled not on an assessment of the injury it is doing to humanity, but rather as a trade-off between nations whose almost exclusively chauvinistic concern is with problems within their own frontiers.

The principles guiding the work of WHO are often derided as hopeless ideals, and ideals they certainly are. Health, which is defined by WHO as the state of complete physical, mental, and social well-being, is considered to be the right of every individual without distinction of race, religion, political belief, or economic or social condition; the health of all peoples is fundamental to peace; improvement of the health of citizens of any state is of value to all but unequal development of health endangers all; the health of children is particularly vital; and governments and peoples are to be encouraged to take more responsibility for more healthful living.

Although WHO has had some major failures over the 47 years of its activity, its successes have affected a wide range of human health, most spectacularly in the eradication of smallpox. WHO suffers not only from intergovernmental bargaining over where its resources are to be directed but also from multigovernmental representation on its staff, more or less irrespective of qualifications for the job. Most of all, it suffers from budget limitations. For this least controversial of all global objections, less than $900 million a year is allocated, compared with a world armament expenditure of $900 billion a year to defend us from each other. Such a cynical and contemptuous opinion, expressed financially, of the importance of human well-being reveals the near-total lack of any one-world concept of humanity. It betrays a general indifference, for example, to the family tragedies involved in the avoidable deaths of some 14 million children every year and to the hundreds of millions of people suffering from malnutrition, infections and infestations, who barely have the energy to survive and certainly not enough energy to be self-reliant and self-supportive.

There are, indeed, grounds for suspicion that this attitude is worse than indifference. The governments of developed nations appear to feel that they have more than enough problems within their own borders and that the miseries of countless multitudes can be conveniently ignored until some other generation. No one would pretend that the answers lie wholly or mainly in what is normally and inadequately understood as the health field; food and water alone would transform the situation for the better. But medical science, which has made possible the brilliant successes of which the privileged countries can take full advantage, needs far more support and much more concerted international effort in order to turn a greater part of its research effort in the direction where its successes would do the most good to the most people. Banting, the codiscoverer of insulin, reminds us that "medical research is the most wholly international commodity we possess. It knows no protective tariff, no embargo, no boundary line to prevent its free disseminations for the good of all."

THE FUTURE

On the administrative side, nations could start by upgrading and expanding the health departments of their governments to enable them to take more comprehensive responsibility for the many aspects of people's lives which contribute to health, which Disraeli described as "the foundation on which all their happiness and all their powers as a State depend."

On the world stage, what is vitally necessary is a new spirit of determination that the avoidable sickness of the multitudes has endured too long; that what affects any part of the human race affects us all; and that health for all constitutes the one positive step on which people of every race, nation, and religion can for once agree.

GOODWILL

This is the time for such a move, when most people live in daily dread of the willful or accidental explosion of nuclear weapons; when conventional fighting between feuding factions and the bombs of terrorist fanatics increasingly claim a toll of innocent victims; when a social revolution is needed in regard to the ethics and economics of employment; when AIDS brings its innumerable personal tragedies and threatens to decimate at least one generation on which the economic viability of some nations depends; when climatic and environmental changes may soon affect the world's capacity to sustain its population and alter the geographical distribution both of agricultural productivity and also of epidemics affecting plant, animal, and human life; and when, over the whole planet, inequalities and injustices abound. Health for the world is one campaign which could be taken up by all, would be wholly constructive, and most likely to lead to early demonstrable benefits. Lewis Thomas has recently commented that "when we gather in very large numbers, as in the modern nation-states, we seem capable of levels of folly and self-destruction to be found nowhere else in Nature." Is it possible that wisdom, kindness, tolerance, and survival are not beyond our combined human capacity?

HEALTH AND HUMANITY

The group of people that bears the greatest responsibility and that also has the greatest opportunity to arouse this new spirit of global concern is physicians and, indeed, all health-care professionals. They have to convince others, especially politicians, that the present conditions under which about one-third of the human species suffers are no longer tolerable. A determination that "Health for all by 2000" is attainable, if not all at least for untold millions; that nothing less than global equality of access to factors favoring health is humanly acceptable; and that research, knowledge, skill, and service shall be combined as never before to that end, could assure one generation at least of a unique place in the history of mankind. It is a practical possibility. If it can be done, why not do it? Other benefits, even peace, might well follow such an exercise in human cooperation. I call on all to awake and combine and to arouse others from their apathy, ignorance, and inability to comprehend what heartening developments are possible. Could this volume, *One World*, help vitally to re-create the necessary political will for health in human societies?

3

WINDS OF CHANGE

LONNIE BRISTOW
is President of the American Medical Association.
The AMA is the largest organization of physicians in the United States.
It was organized in 1847 to promote the science and art of medicine
and the betterment of public health.

THERE IS A SAYING that "change is the only constant," perhaps implying that only the foolhardy attempt to thwart change while the wise try to guide it to the best of their ability. Just during the last decade, the world has seen enormous geopolitical upheaval, much of which seemed unpredictable even six months before it occurred. Out of many possible examples, three are particularly meaningful: the collapse of the Berlin Wall in November 1989, the dissolution of the USSR in December 1991; and the peaceful transfer of government in South Africa from de Klerk to Mandela in 1994. These historic moments uniquely signal humanity's willingness to ultimately place human values above material values, often in the face of insurmountable odds. That capacity may soon be sorely tested in the arena of health-care, where material considerations already are overrunning human concerns.

Here, at the end of the twentieth century, the profession of medicine finds itself enveloped in numerous changes that, with one singular exception, seem almost dwarfed by the past decade's more colossal geopolitical upheavals. That singular exception is the explosion of medicine-related information.

Against other events, the changes in health-care may seem small by comparison, but that would be an inaccurate assessment if one looks into the near future. Many of the changes buffeting health-care today result from the blowing winds of the development, organization, and flow of information. And where information is concerned, it was never more true that "in the land of the blind, the one-eyed man is king."

Health care in America is experiencing its most profound changes in modern memory; more is yet to come. The tension between humanity's health needs and the finite limitations of health resources around the globe means that what happens in the U.S. has a ripple effect on the rest of the world–an effect that is more a question of timing than of certainty.

Many recent American health-care changes are information-driven. When that information is translated into technology, it impacts not only the outcomes of care but also the types and numbers of health-caregivers, the location of patient interactions with those caregivers, and the design of organized caregiving systems. Even the underlying philosophy that defines where the allegiance of the profession lies is under siege by change.

Our ability to collect and analyze enormous quantities of data rapidly and to convert that analysis into meaningful action is responsible for breathtaking advances in pharmacologic agents, diagnostic tools, and procedural techniques. The results are readily evident: in just 10 years we have seen death rates from heart disease fall 30 percent and from stroke 50 percent. Ten years ago, a manual laborer who needed gallbladder surgery could expect, as the standard of care, a hospital stay of eight to 10 days, with another five weeks of recuperation. Today, thanks to technologic improvements, the standards are different. Now you can expect to spend only a day-and-a-half in the hospital, and you will be back to work eight to 10 days after that. Physicians know this means increased productivity and enhanced quality of life for their patients, but we also are chagrined that those aspects never seem to be added into the quadratic equation that is used to calculate today's "cost" of medical services as compared to a decade ago. Nonetheless, cost is another extremely powerful engine pushing change.

As we become technically more proficient, there is a correspondingly increasing need in the work force for individuals with more specialized skills and knowledge. On the other hand, as hospital stays shorten, they also become more intensive and more expensive; and university medical centers, largely by the very nature of their mission, frequently attract patients with the most intensive and expensive problems. Still, concerns about escalating costs, accompanied by a desire for assurance of the value received, are rising steadily.

This concern is prompting an enthusiastic examination of efficiencies of the systems from which patients get their care. Prepaid health-care was first introduced in the Pacific Northwest over seven decades ago. Since then, it has grown as a viable alternative to pure indemnity (or a classic fee-for-service) health insurance. Some commentators simplistically thought these two approaches were driven by conflicting motivations, that is, the potential for underservice versus overservice of patient needs; but knowledgeable physicians recognize that ethical physicians always offer–to the best of their professional ability–the right amount of care. Actually, the prepaid approach is simply a natural evolution (by the addition of insurance) of the group practice style of practice. It is an alternative to the cottage industry approach of long tradition. The point is: Businesslike concerns may quite properly be brought to the practice of medicine, but they must never supplant it.

Initially, these continued to be physician organized and directed, but almost a decade ago, seeking to enhance the attraction of prepaid health-care, containing cost by controlling utilization became such a dominant motivation for some enterprises that they renamed themselves "managed care." Within the last six years or so, some of these entities became "for-profit" corporations, with the prospect of going public and trading as a stockholder company. Essentially, they became investor owned and directed. With this very substantive modification, their priorities changed to earning maximum yearly dividends for stockholders while competitively increasing their equity value in comparison to other offerings in the open market. These companies, to assure creation of a healthy bottom line, asserted a right to fire or discharge physicians without cause or due process. The individual physician, trying to practice medicine under that hammer, is vulnerable to being intimidated in his traditional role of advocating only that which is honestly believed to be in the best interests of the individual patient. Business concerns begin to supplant patient concerns. The public policy question for society becomes obvious: Which comes first–profits or patients?

Meanwhile, technology now brings within reach the power to share data and information across continents and around the globe. The ability to transmit digitalized, high-resolution imagery inexpensively is but a very few years away. The last decade has seen the transformation of a great deal of traditional surgery by new laparoscopic and endoscopic procedures. The emergence of artificially created environments of virtual reality along with tools which provide realistic force feedback to the operator as additional components of telemedicine will expand the potential universe enormously. Projects are already in development to combine virtual reality with robotics capable of replicating the movements of the surgeon's hand while simultaneously conveying back realistic tactile sensation. The possibility is obvious for surgeons to practice a difficult procedure many times without utilizing actual patients or even experimental animals, as are the possibilities for the training of future students. Also under development are digital sensor-implanted "tactile" gloves which could transmit sensations experienced by the hand of one examiner to a consultant at a remote site, even thousands of miles away.

Carlos Pellegrini, M.D., Professor and Chair of Surgery at the University of Washington Medical Center, predicts that within five to 10 years, 40 to 60 percent of all surgeries will be performed using video endoscopic and video laparoscopic techniques.

The implications for delivering high-quality care to rural and inner-city America are easily recognized and exciting. While the immediate health needs of many nations differ from those of the United States, many of those differences relate to the lack of technology in less advantaged countries. That gap cannot last long, as technology becomes less expensive and as satellite hookups become more available. I believe that we will close that gap in the next 20 years.

The likelihood then is that telemedicine will reach around the world in less than a generation. A failure to start the adaptive process now, in the mid-1990s, could well cause catastrophic medical work force problems in the first and second decades of the new century. The adjustments we must make in our medical education system are profound if that transition is to be both rational and responsible. We must make adjustments in our thinking for the role of the international medical education community. What licensing changes will be necessary to adequately protect the public? How many specialists will we need? How many limited-license practitioners? How are distribution problems best resolved? The questions go on and on.

As difficult as the answers may be, I submit that the single most important issue is whether the underlying philosophy of the allegiance of the medical profession is to change or not. If we are to transit through these veritable typhoon-like winds of change, while still placing human values above all else, then the philosophic commitment of physicians to place the needs of the individual patient first must be defended with all our heart and soul. That ethical imperative must never be lost. The challenge must be recognized and met. The credo of the medical profession must continue to be "patients first, profits second." If we lose that moral compass, we will lose our direction and be destroyed by the winds of change.

However, if we can preserve that core value, with appropriate strategic planning for modification of the system of medical education, the future is brilliant with promise. Better and more affordable care will be available for more people because we will be more effective and more efficient. Whether medicine will continue to bring the added quality of "compassion" to the bedside will hinge on how deeply commercialism erodes the profession's very reason for existence.

Telemedicine is a revolutionary tool that will not be denied. It is the technological key to keeping alive the human and humane precepts of the Hippocratic oath–the ethical guidepost for medicine since antiquity, by which we can still channel today's ferocious winds of change.

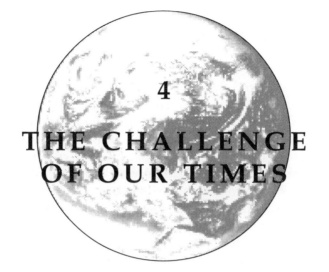

4

THE CHALLENGE
OF OUR TIMES

DONNA E. SHALALA
is U.S. Secretary of Health and Human Services.
In addition to the Agencies of the Public Health Service, Dr. Shalala oversees
the National Institutes of Health (NIH), the Food and Drug Administration
(FDA), and the Centers for Disease Control (CDC).

TODAY, PEOPLE ARE LIVING longer and they are living better. The average life expectancy in the U.S. at birth has increased from 47 at the turn of the 20th century to 76 in 1993. Infant mortality is down from more than 100 deaths per 1,000 live births in 1915 to 8.3 per 1,000 in 1993. Medical and pharmaceutical advances have allowed many people to spend their later years without the constraints of disability; and thanks to programs like Medicare and Social Security, many of our parents and grandparents enjoy their retirement without living in poverty. Yet, at the same time, there are millions who do continue to live in poverty, struggling to pay for food, shelter, and medical care. More than 40 million people in the U.S. have no health insurance to protect them against the very high cost of medical care, and millions more have less insurance than they need.

So, the challenge of our times is to continue to improve health while assuring that those benefits reach everyone, regardless of age, race, class, or income. This is not a simple task, and no single action can achieve it.

To continue and sustain improvements in health, it is first necessary to identify the major current causes of morbidity, mortality, and disability and those that are likely to persist into the twenty-first century. These include: chronic illness; newly emerging infectious disease; diseases caused by environmental agents; diseases related to such high-risk behavior as cigarette smoking, alcohol abuse, sexual activity without the proper use of contraceptives and prophylactics, and use of illicit drugs; and suicide, homicide, and other forms of violence.

There is not one easy solution to the complex set of factors that contributes to these problems. The broad-based approach required draws on the work of a number of public health and medical scholars who have contributed to the modern understanding of health and disease. Of particular interest are concepts about the determinants of health and the relative importance of behavior, socioeconomic status, human biology, the environment, and medical care in determining health status.

The Centers for Disease Control and Prevention used an epidemiological model for health policy to define factors contributing to mortality in the U.S. for the 10 leading causes of death in 1990. The results indicate that risk factors due to lifestyle contributed to approximately 46.8 percent of mortality; human biology contributed 27.1 percent; environmental factors contributed to 16.6 percent; and inadequacies in the health-care system contributed to 10.8 percent of mortality.

Based on the 1990 data, when the leading causes of death were examined in terms of years of potential life lost per 100,000 population before the age 65 years, life-style was even more important (52.3 percent), followed by environment (19.8 percent), human biology (18.6 percent), and health care (9.8 percent).

In another analysis of U.S. mortality data for 1990, the following prominent contributors to mortality were identified: tobacco (an estimated 400,000 deaths), diet and activity patterns (300,000), alcohol (100,000), microbial agents (90,000), toxic agents (60,000), firearms (35,000), sexual behavior (30,000), motor vehicles (25,000), and use of illicit drugs (20,000). Approximately half of all deaths in 1990 could be attributed to these factors.

These studies tell us that a greater emphasis should be placed on population-based approaches to improving health, particularly those related to behavior and the environment. A rather different conclusion is reached by another study that measured the effects of medical care (curative medicine) and clinical preventive measures on extending life expectancy and the quality of life. Among the clinical preventive services examined were screening, immunization, hormone replacement for postmenopausal women, and aspirin prophylaxis for heart attack in men over 40 years of age. Among the clinical curative services examined were those for colorectal cancer, diabetes mellitus, heart disease, cerebrovascular disease, kidney failure, tuberculosis, and maternal mortality. It was observed that "the current effects of preventive measures on life expectancy (roughly 18-19 months) are less than half as great as the prolongation of life from curative measures (roughly 44-45 months)."

The conclusion to be drawn from these analyses is that both personal medical care and population-based protection and prevention programs play important and complementary roles in improving health. A useful case in point is the dramatic decline in mortality from stroke (50 percent) and heart disease (40 percent) in the past 20 years. This resulted from the application of advances in biomedical, behavioral, and epidemiological research to public health practice and individual medical care. In particular, the decline in mortality from cardiovascular disease began in the early 1970s with a broad-based cooperative approach among investigators at the National Institutes of Health (NIH) and universities, clinicians in a variety of practice settings, and public health practitioners. The strategy involved both public health approaches (e.g., efforts to reduce cigarette smoking, public education about hypertension, and screening) and the widespread application of improved treatment for individual patients.

To deal effectively with the threats to health in the twenty-first century, there needs to be continued support for research. The links between research and improvement in personal health-care and public health practice need to be made abundantly clear. For example, the survival time of people with AIDS has doubled in the last decade, largely due to scientific advances in the treatment and prevention of opportunistic infections.

One of the most important advances in HIV prevention research resulted from an NIH clinical trial testing the efficacy of AZT in preventing transmission of HIV infection from mothers to their babies. The study showed a 67.5 percent reduction in the risk of HIV transmission with AZT therapy. Research in the biomedical sciences, behavioral and social sciences, epidemiology, and in health services/systems and health policy will be the engine that drives future advances in health.

To be more effective in applying research findings and achieving improvements in the health status of a population, public health programs and personal health care services must collaborate. A number of managed-care organizations have recognized that strong public health programs contribute to the high quality and success of their health plans. For example, HealthPartners, the parent company of a family of health plans and health-related companies, is implementing a program called "Partners for Better Health." It shifts the focus of health care from medical intervention and treatment of disease to prevention of disease. This program plans to bring providers, members, and the community together to prevent illness and improve the health status of people who are at a high risk of incurring targeted diseases. Examples of the initial goals set for HealthPartners members include reducing heart disease by 25 percent and increasing from 75 to 95 percent the number of children who are fully immunized by age two. By providing a framework to coordinate population-based prevention and protection services and personal health care services, HealthPartners is positioning itself to maximize consumer satisfaction and benefits. The gain will be a healthier population.

The idea that public health programs and personal health-care services can be more effectively integrated to achieve public health objectives is not a new one. The 1990 report, *Healthy People 2000: National Disease Prevention and Health Promotion Objectives,* outlines 300 measurable, achievable objectives for the United States. It also details the roles and responsibilities of public health, personal health-care service,s and other sectors of society that are essential to achieving the objectives. In addition to individuals doing their part, to achieve the goals in *Healthy People 2000* there is a need to adopt social policies that can affect the broader social and economic factors that influence health.

Differences in mortality by social class have been documented for years. In the United Kingdom and the United States, studies have illustrated a causal link between socioeconomic status and health status. It has been noted that: countries that have universal health insurance show the same socioeconomic status and health gradient as that found in the United States, where such insurance is not provided; socioeconomic differences can be found between levels at the upper range of the socioeconomic hierarchy; and socioeconomic differences appear in a wide range of diseases, both those that are amenable to treatment and those that are not.

In fact, for virtually all of the chronic diseases that lead the list of killers, low income is a special risk factor. For example, the risk of death from heart disease is more than 25 percent higher for low-income people than for the overall population. The incidence of cancer increases as family income decreases, and survival rates are lower for low-income cancer patients. Infectious diseases, such as HIV/AIDS and tuberculosis, are also often found disproportionately among the poor. Just as poor health is more likely among persons of low income, so are some, but not all, of the major risk factors for poor health. Higher-than-average rates of obesity and high blood pressure, which are major risks for heart disease and stroke, have been linked directly with low-income status. Tobacco use, which has declined dramatically in the past two decades for the population as a whole, has remained virtually constant since 1966 for those who completed less than 12 years of schooling.

For the future, perhaps no challenge is more compelling than that of equity. The disparities experienced by people who are born and live their lives in poverty define the dimensions of that challenge. The relationship between poverty and health are complex and cannot be reduced to a simple one-to-one relationship between dollars available and level of health. Low income may, in fact, be a product of poor health, just as poor health may be caused by environmental exposures, material deficiencies, and lack of access to health services that adequate income might correct or improve. While, from a public health perspective, the leverage available to effect improvements is limited largely to the availability and quality of health services, improvements in education, job training, and other social services are necessary to erase the health effects of current income disparities.

Obviously, maintaining health involves more than medical care. Other factors include human biology, the environment, behavior, and socioeconomic status. To address these very real concerns, the Clinton administration has begun a number of actions in the U.S. that will sustain and continue to improve health. The first accomplishment toward this end was restoring steady economic growth and creating jobs.

To extend these benefits to communities in the U.S. that are often left behind, the president proposed the Community Empowerment Initiative. It advances the creation of new employment and business opportunities in selected communities and promotes integration of social and human development as important components of a complete economic and community development agenda. Investment in human capital to create trained, functional, and healthy people is clearly as important to economic regeneration and growth as are tax credits, loan funds, and technical business assistance. The Community Empowerment Initiative together with the administration's Reinventing Government Initiative are about building a federal government that is responsive to state and community needs through a comprehensive, coordinated, integrated approach.

With economic growth, community empowerment, and reinventing government supporting the dramatic changes occurring in the health-care system through the shift from traditional solo practice and indemnity, fee-for-service payment to managed care based on integrated delivery systems with capitated payments, the U.S. has an unprecedented opportunity to improve the healthy life span of its citizens and to reduce the health disparities among social classes and different ethnic groups.

However, as long as significant portions of society are excluded from the health insurance system, the promise of better health is but a cruel hoax for millions of people, many of whom work hard every day, pay their taxes, and play by the rules. President Clinton tried to address these needs by elevating health-care reform on the national agenda. While efforts to enact comprehensive reform ultimately failed, the goals expressed in the effort–universal coverage, affordable insurance, high-quality care, expanded choice, and simplification–remain in place. As the U.S. moves forward in a more gradual manner, we must keep these goals in mind and take effective steps toward achieving them. Such steps should include: reform of insurance rules to eliminate blatant discrimination; creation of voluntary insurance pools to allow small businesses and their workers to have access to the same affordable rates given to large companies; assistance for low-income workers, the self-employed, and the unemployed to purchase coverage; help with the cost of long-term care for the elderly and the disabled; and finding ways to provide coverage to the many millions of children who are uninsured.

The challenge of our times, then, is to combine the knowledge and the skill of the public health profession with the brilliance of the medical profession to create the maximum opportunity for all to enjoy lives of good health and longevity.

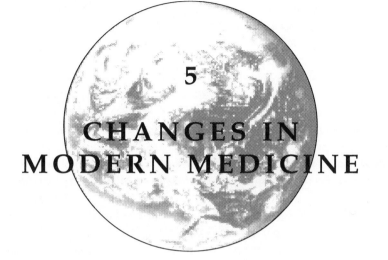

5
CHANGES IN
MODERN MEDICINE

PRISCILLA KINCAID-SMITH
is President of the World Medical Association and President of
the Royal Australasian College of Physicians. Professor Kincaid-Smith
holds her Chair at the University of Melbourne and
is Director of Nephrology at Epworth Hospital in Australia.

AFTER A PERIOD of relative stability for the best part of this century, profound structural changes are occurring in health-care delivery in the developed world.

The pattern in which the doctor-patient relationship was sacrosanct, and in which the doctor's word was law both in the hospital and the consulting room, is rapidly being replaced by a system in which many other influences intrude into the decision-making process, even in the consulting room. I was recently in a consulting room with a friend, who is probably the most respected specialist in his field in the U.S., while he waited for what seemed a ridiculously long time to get permission to perform a procedure that was clearly necessary. The person who granted permission was a clerk in an insurance office!

Doctors naturally resent this type of intrusion into the doctor-patient relationship, which they cherish as a pivotal element of the art and science of medicine. James Spence best described this relationship in 1960 when he said that "the essential unit of medical practice is the occasion when, in the intimacy of the consulting room, a person who is ill, or believes himself to be ill, seeks the advice of a doctor whom he trusts. This is the consultation and all else in medicine derives from it."

While doctors and medical associations fight to retain the important elements of this process, many forces are combining to intervene between doctor and patient and are eroding the doctor-patient relationship. Managed-care organizations use a variety of approaches to alter doctors' decisions. The common element is that the organization or institution limits choices that have traditionally been made exclusively within the patient-physician relationship.

One current trend influencing decision-making by doctors is welcomed by many but resented by some, and this is the sharing of responsibility with the patient. Patients are better educated and informed and are more willing to discuss options with the doctor. The AIDS epidemic, and the demands of those infected with this devastating virus to be involved in decisions about their management, provides a good example of this recent empowerment of patients. Many patients with AIDS are indeed better informed than their medical practitioners about treatment options for AIDS. In general, the profession has come to terms with the legitimate interest that patients have in their illness. Most doctors now readily accept the need for fully informed consent for treatment of all patients.

Doctors are far more resentful about the change in the power structure and the control being exerted over medical decisions in hospitals. Governments and insurance companies, through their managers, are intruding even into essential features of medical practice, such as which drugs may be prescribed for a particular illness. This would have been unheard of a decade or more ago but is now a commonplace practice under the cost-containment umbrella.

Governments, aware that health is usually the most costly portfolio and one in which costs are rapidly escalating, are putting major efforts into containing costs. However, a more serious threat to the quality of medical care comes from health corporations and their managed-care plans. Governments must respond to pressure from the electorate when standards are eroded, but companies are responsible to their shareholders. The major objective of these large powerful "for-profit" corporations is to channel as much of the health dollar as possible to their shareholders, who in turn vote huge salaries for their chief executive officers if dividends increase sufficiently. A greater proportion of funds for the shareholder and manager means that there is less for the patient. This diversion of the health dollar away from services to patients surely poses one of the greatest threats to medical practice at this time.

These market changes create a considerable threat to the professional integrity of doctors. From recent columns of *The Lancet*, we learn that California's doctors regard themselves as "guppies in a tank of sharks who already control the market." More disturbingly, it is reported that the numerous health maintenance organizations (HMOs) in California pick and choose doctors and determine which services will be provided. "Gag" clauses in contracts prevent doctors from criticizing HMOs, and those who do not toe the line find their contracts summarily terminated.

Medical practice also is being altered by the demands of the "purchasers," namely, governments and health corporations, for more cost-effective medicine. This has the potential to improve standards of practice but will inevitably bring about other changes. There are considerable difficulties in assessing benefits and weighing them against costs, and the methodology for doing so is far from perfect.

Modern medicine is based on a system, developed over the past century, in which the doctor had the power to decide the method of treatment. Consider this together with the fact that the majority of medical and surgical procedures in use at this time have not been subjected to rigorous controlled studies to demonstrate their efficacy. Inevitably, the slow evolution of methods of treatment over a period before controlled trial methodology existed has led under many circumstances to arbitrary selection of treatment. Clinical trials of drugs have been carried out regularly only in the past thirty years, and controlled evaluation of surgical procedures is a much more recent and patchy phenomenon. Lack of clear-cut data about many therapeutic options or procedures has led to the so-called "variation phenomenon," which means that patients with similar conditions are treated differently in different health-care settings. This variation phenomenon tends to undermine the claim by the medical profession that their treatment is based on scientific method and has been a major factor causing managers to challenge the professional autonomy of doctors.

Governments and managers will continue to demand that doctors justify their selection of treatment by data from controlled trials, but they need to recognize that much of the collection of data will need to be prospective. They must also appreciate that many valuable treatments have not been subjected to evaluation by controlled trials and that it is often unethical to do so–for example, in the use of penicillin for pneumonia or in the drug treatment of malignant hypertension. The profession, on the other hand, needs to recognize the potential for good in scientific evaluation of methods of treatment. Cost-effective treatment that has been scientifically evaluated is highly desirable and has great potential for improving health-care delivery.

Even where a technology is of unquestioned benefit, as, for example, dialysis for renal failure, doctors have been free to choose the method of dialysis and to decide the staff and equipment requirements. This has resulted in very significant differences in costs in different centers. In a recent study in Australia, the lowest cost of dialysis was $14,000 per patient per year, whereas some costs were as high as $50,000 per patient per year. The powerful purchasers of health-care will no longer tolerate such differences in cost nor indeed can they be justified in a health-care system in which there is never enough money to go around. Unfortunately, as fast as efficiency is improved in one area, another demand arises to absorb the potential savings. In dialysis, even if all patients were dialyzing at the relatively low cost of $14,000 per annum, patients' recent demands for ready access to genetically engineered erythropoietin could almost double this annual cost. Because this drug corrects anaemia, patients have a legitimate claim to access to erythropoietin; but providing access to each expensive new drug or technological advance is a major factor in continually spiraling health costs. Situations of this nature are occurring in all other areas of medicine. The AIDS lobby has taught government that they ignore such demands at their peril. Nevertheless, the cost of health-care must rise as demands escalate.

Treatment methods vary not only among doctors and health-care centers but also among health-care systems in different countries. A recent publication in the *New England Journal of Medicine* demonstrates that not only do Canadians have lower rates of access to cardiac investigation and treatment of coronary artery disease than U.S. citizens but that they also have poorer outcomes in this most common form of heart disease. If this data is substantiated, it has the potential to provoke a public outcry in Canada. Demand for appropriate expansion of cardiac services would be a very costly exercise for the Canadian government. This information has been published at a time when Canada's health-care system is under threat from initiatives in most provinces demanding commensurate services and at a lower cost. These initiatives include closures, mergers, and restructuring of hospitals, with some shift in funding to community-based facilities–a scenario that is similar to that in most Western countries.

The implication of cost-containment by purchasers of health-care services, and the opposing influences of a rapidly expanding range of costly new drugs and technologies to which our informed patients are demanding access, has created stresses within the health-care systems of all developed countries. The doctor is caught between the demands of the patient and the cost constraints placed on him by governments and health corporations, which inevitably leads to rationing of health-care.

Rationing of health-care is occurring at this time, in one form or another, in all developed countries. It is obvious at a much more basic level in the developing world. Rationing reduces patient access and provokes constant political debate.

For doctors, rationing of health-care poses special difficulties. As the patient's advocate, the doctor must always try to ensure that the individual patient has access to the best available treatment. He is ethically committed to this, and serious conflicts arise for the medical practitioner who is under pressure to restrict access to investigations and treatment. The enormous expansion in managed care in the U.S. has seen fee-for-service medicine falling from 85 to 15 percent in the past decade, and the percentage of the population covered by managed-care plans has risen from 11 to 85 percent over the same period. This has driven many doctors into salaried positions in health corporations, where they are expected to restrict patient access to costly investigation and treatment. Where a medical practitioner is rewarded for depriving his patients of appropriate access to health-care, as happens in some managed-care programs, an extreme conflict of interest arises.

While the doctor should never deprive the individual patient of access to appropriate investigation and treatment and must strive to provide this, he must be prepared to participate, and indeed, to lead in discussions and in making decisions at another level of rationing, for example, in decisions about rationalization of expensive facilities, such as magnetic resonance imaging (MRI). The professional expertise of the doctor is a very necessary element in these situations. It is clearly impossible for each institution to have MRI equipment, but there must be a balance that takes account of geography and the length of waiting lists to plan carefully for the location of new MRI units. The distribution of CT Scanners, the forerunner of the MRI, seemingly was uncontrolled in some countries, so that Japan has 30 per million persons compared with 2 or 3 per million in most European countries where there is no perceived shortage. In the U.S., with a fee-for-service structure, there are 15 CT scanners per million population and in Australia, which also has fee-for-service, there are 8 per million. Clearly, there are too many CT scanners in some countries and certainly too few in some, but surely the medical profession is best equipped to decide on necessary numbers and their distribution. Those who stand to gain financially from purchasing this expensive equipment should not participate in making such decisions.

Interesting anomalies exist between the services provided in different countries. I have already alluded to the differences between the U.S. and Canada in investigation and treatment of coronary artery disease. In this same discipline, ten times as many coronary artery bypass procedures are carried out in the U.S. as in Sweden. At first sight this might be assumed to relate to the fact that the U.S. spends 14 percent of gross domestic product on health services compared to 8.6 percent in Sweden. However, when one compares this to an even more costly high technology, that of bone marrow transplantation for chronic myeloid leukemia, Sweden performs much better than the U.S. and, indeed, better than ten other Western countries.

The probable explanation as to why the U.S. leads the world in certain expensive high-technology procedures, such as coronary artery surgery and dialysis, but lags sadly behind in others may well relate to government funding available through Medicare for certain categories, such as dialysis, and for all patients over 65. This age-group would automatically be excluded from bone marrow transplantation, the $140,000 price tag of which would certainly ensure that only those either with government funding or full private cover would receive it. Both dialysis, which is covered by Medicare for all patients, and coronary artery bypass surgery, which is most frequently carried out in persons over 65, are paid for by the bottomless purse of the U.S. government. By comparison, some degree of rationing probably occurs in Canada and in many other Western countries.

In addition to the high cost of new technologies and drugs demanded by our more sophisticated patients, the aging of the population will exert a major influence on increasing health-care costs into the next millennium. The postwar baby-boomer population group is approaching old age. This undoubtedly will increase spending on health-care particularly in the U.S., where those over 65 are funded through Medicare. Only 4 percent of the Australian population are over the age of 75, but 25 percent of the health dollar is spent on this group and the percentage is rapidly rising.

The influence that the revolution in information technology will have on the practice of medicine has been understated. Internet currently connects 2 to 3 million host computers. New technology contains computer, telephone, compact disc, and video in one instrument, and fiberoptics will make telemedicine widely available. Consumers of health-care are already accessing medical information databases to help them make medical decisions and may well become better informed about their complaints than their doctors.

Ethical issues will arise as medicine adapts to cost-containment and new technologies. The relative freedom that the profession has hitherto enjoyed in developing new technologies, such as *in vitro* fertilization, will not continue, as public pressure exerts more control over techniques in this controversial area. In other areas, such as genetic engineering, the public will undoubtedly demand a voice based on religious and moral considerations.

Public attitudes in areas such as euthanasia or, more correctly, assisted suicide, will create pressure for the profession to review its conservative stance. Already the majority of the public believes that a doctor should be able to end the life of a patient who is suffering from an incurable condition and who requests this. In the Netherlands and the state of Oregon, legislation permits medically assisted suicide, and it is likely that other states and countries will move in the same direction. AIDS patients have taken a lead in this area, providing themselves with the means to end life when it becomes unbearable, and the profession will have to decide whether or not to participate in this process.

From a global perspective, the major influence on the future of health-care in the developing world will be the population explosion, 90 percent of which is occurring in developing countries. Every second the world population increases by three, with five births and two deaths. If predictions of a population of 14 billion by 2100 are fulfilled, this will create a threat to the very survival of the human race. The Cairo conference placed a major emphasis on the empowerment of women to control their own fertility as a potential solution to the population explosion. Surely our profession must support the rights of Third World women to control their own fertility, particularly when we consider the huge burden of misery, illness, and death that results from unwanted pregnancies.

Provision of access to adequate contraception, and in particular the education of women, in developing countries would rapidly reduce population growth and prevent the disasters that we have observed in Ethiopia, Somalia and Rwanda, where women and children have carried the major burden of the suffering and death and where water is becoming more precious than oil.

6
MEDICINE IN
THE NEXT CENTURY

ALEXANDER "SANDY" MACARA
is Chairman of the Council of the British Medical Association.
The BMA is the largest professional association and trade union
of doctors in the United Kingdom.

IN THIS CHAPTER I propose to look at the medical profession and the challenges that face it as we move into the twenty-first century.

I will use as a case study the medical profession in the United Kingdom and the National Health Service (NHS) in which it works and examine the factors exerting pressure on the profession. The challenges it faces are not unique to the U.K., and I hope that this discussion of these challenges and the changing context of the practice of medicine will be of interest to readers in both the developed and developing world.

REFORMS

The NHS in the U.K. is unusual, if not unique, in several respects: historically, having been conceived in a wartime union of faith in a pacific future, married to the vision of a welfare state fit for heroes; economically, in acceptance of corporate responsibility for the health of all the people; ethically, in enshrining the principles of the Judeo-Christian and utilitarian traditions; and politically, in achieving a broad consensus among the people, their government, and the professions who care for them. This remarkable phenomenon, tailored to a national need and a national creed, inadvertently but inevitably nurtures a comforting mythology of self-sufficiency of philosophy if not always of practice.

This illusion has been shattered by two simultaneous forces, both originating from outside the United Kingdom. One is the *Health of the Nation* policy, commendably if belatedly introduced in 1992 to implement the 1985 targeting strategy of the European Regional Office of the World Health Organization (WHO). This strategy derived in turn from the global Alma Ata Declaration of 1978, in which the WHO and UNICEF (United Nations International Children's Emergency Fund) joined forces in the call for health for all. This involved a drive for healthy lifestyles, priority for health promotion and disease prevention, and the reorientation of health-care systems toward primary health care.

The other force for change has been the massive reform of the U.K. NHS, implemented in 1991, which has resulted in major changes in the organization of the service and, some would argue, has lead to a deterioration in the service.

When examining these changes it is important to understand the nature of the NHS prior to the reforms. We have already noted that the health service– "the envy of the world"–is seen as part of the national fabric of society in the U.K.. The development of a health service free at the point of use, and built on the principles of equality of entitlement and access to services, has been a great achievement. The system has traditionally been a centrally planned and funded bureaucracy and monopoly provider intended to meet all reasonable health-care needs. The various sectors of care, such as hospital and primary care, have been the responsibility of different authorities; but, essentially, the NHS was conceived as a single unified organization with collective aims and objectives held by all levels and sectors of the service.

During the late 1970s and early 1980s, governments were under increasing economic pressure to curb rising expenditures for public services. At first this was done through efficiency drives–which led to public concerns about "health service cuts"–and also through the strengthening of management of the service. Then, in 1989, Margaret Thatcher's government found an ideologically appealing solution to the "problem" of expenditure by introducing a market system into the NHS. This was not to be a true market, as services remain free at the point of use and patients are not shopping around individually for health-care. What it did do, was to separate the NHS into "purchasers" (authorities who would purchase health services on behalf of local people) and "providers." Providers could be existing local NHS hospitals or private hospitals, thus introducing an element of competition into the service and, in theory, improving quality, efficiency, and value for money by doing so.

Citizens of nations where personal health insurance and competition for the insurer's business are the norm may well be wondering why there should be a problem with the concept and workings of a market for health-care. However, I hope I have given some indication of why the introduction of the reforms was a culture shock to the general public in the U.K. and to those working in the service.

There are those, not least the U.K. government, who argue that the NHS reforms are working well and have effected real improvements in the service. Still, my concern here is with the medical profession, many members of which are convinced that despite the service remaining a publicly funded one, a market system is not appropriate for the delivery of health-care.

Let me sketch briefly these concerns. Firstly, this massive experiment was not subject to a pilot trial of any kind, and its effectiveness is not subject to comprehensive independent monitoring. Secondly, the ability of the system to deliver central, strategically planned objectives has been weakened because of the divisions in the functions of the service and the notion of competition between some elements. Thirdly, the service is becoming a federal rather than unified structure, and there is a very real risk that one of the founding principles of the service–namely, that of equality of access regardless of where people live–will be lost. Fourthly, power is vested in the managers of the service rather than in those who use it and, the health professionals who work in it. Finally, despite market mechanisms, the basic problem of underfunding will remain.

No health-care system is free of problems. Much recent publicity has focused upon the United States, where per capita spending on health is more than double that in the United Kingdom but where 15 percent of the population are without basic health coverage. Last year the Alberta government announced a 20 percent cut in health spending phased over four years, mirroring a similar announcement by the Australian government in 1991. Similarly, the Germans have introduced severe controls on prescribing costs, and the Danes have placed restrictions on referrals. The health reforms in the U.K. were also introduced in response to apparent financial crisis. Rather than seeking to rationalize through an open process of service cuts, the U.K. government chose to apply a radical and, some would argue, inappropriate ideological solution.

HEALTH-CARE SYSTEMS: "THE EXTERNAL TRIANGLE"

In addition to the above changes associated with the NHS reforms, the NHS is also subject to pressure from three underlying international trends in health-care.

All health-care systems manifest evidence of a three-sided health-care problem. The first element of this problem is the need to secure reasonable resources for health-care. With economic recession, health-care has to compete with education, industry, transport, and defense for a share of the gross national product. That share is determined by political forces and by the perception of governments of the electoral value or otherwise of investment in health-care. We are fortunate in the United Kingdom that the NHS is still viewed politically as a valuable national resource. Ultimately, however, the public and the health professions are distanced from the discussions that lead to the announcement of the annual NHS expenditure proposals.

The second element of the health-care problem is the issue of priorities. No government or nation can hope to afford all the technologies that modern medical science can offer. Public tolerance of personal suffering is probably at an all time low, encouraged by emphasis on consumer rights and individual choice as enshrined in the patients' charter. As Kierkegaard observed, in every choice there is a sacrifice. If sacrifices are not to be borne by those least able to articulate their need, there must be rational debate about "posteriorities" as well as priorities. This principle holds whatever the level of funding. It is not an accident that the most publicized experiment in seeking an explicit set of health-care priorities has been conducted in Oregon, one of the United States' richer states. The conference held by the British Medical Association, the *British Medical Journal*, and the King's Fund in March 1993 on priorities and health-care for the U.K. health service showed how essential it is to forge a consensus of patients, caregivers, professionals, the public as a whole, and government. If the essential values of equity and justice are to be served, consensus is vital. Recently in the U.K., a House of Commons (parliamentary) health committee reported on priority setting in the NHS, stressing the need for an honest and realistic set of explicit, well-understood, ethical principles at the national level to guide the NHS into the next century. The committee stressed that these should be based on the principles of equity, public choice, and the effective use of health service resources.

The third element of consideration is the quality of the outcome of health-care. Having decided how much to spend and what to spend it on, everyone concerned has an interest in ensuring that the outcome is what is required by the purchaser. To achieve this, we must meet two conditions. Firstly, as in priority setting, we need mechanisms for reaching a consensus about the issues. Secondly, we need a substantial investment of commitment and energy in developing appropriate outcome measures, supported by acceptable clinical guidelines, routine audit, and peer performance review. This is primarily a task for the health professions, supported by management. There exists in the U.K. a Clinical Standards Advisory Group, in which leading professionals and managers are working together to assess the quality of alternative approaches to important areas of diagnosis and treatment.

The preceding sets the context of a changed NHS, which has become a devolved service with locally rather than nationally determined priorities; and of the universal pressures on health care, that is, the need for priorities to be assessed and treatments examined for their relative effectiveness. But what are the other factors in this changing environment of medical practice?

NEW TECHNOLOGIES

It is difficult to assess what the impact of new medical technology will be over the next 25 years. There is nothing new in new technology as an influence for far-reaching change in the practice of medicine. The introduction of the stethoscope transformed the physician's ability to adequately examine a patient's chest and abdomen. More than a century ago, microscopy and radiology transformed the diagnosis and treatment of communicable disease.

The significance of modern medical technology is in the pace of change and development and in its cost. We now also have a media and public hungry for news of and the benefit of new medical technology. In addition, the patient is now an educated consumer whose rights as a consumer of health-care are covered by such initiatives as the U.K. patient's charter, which sets basic minimum standards for the service delivered by the NHS.

Information technology certainly will have an impact on medical practice and raises the need for new approaches to safeguarding patient confidentiality. Information links will also mean that in future treatment may take place in new settings, leading to a move away from hospital-based care and a possible reassessment of the roles of specialist and generalist as currently defined in the U.K. health system.

The most exciting advances are in general surgery, with the development of minimally invasive techniques; an increase in early intervention in cases of myocardial infarction (angioplasty and coronary artery bypass grafts); the increasing number of liver transplants using splitting; and the use of stenting for aortic aneurysms. The provision of hip transplants as a standard procedure is being followed by knee replacement, and bone marrow transplantation is becoming a common procedure. Medical developments include the increased use of cytokines in rheumatoid arthritis and of beta-interferon in multiple sclerosis. Improved techniques are making the treatment of mental illness more effective and expensive, and crisis intervention is becoming routine. Diagnosis is being enhanced by the expansion in endovascular surgical techniques, the availability of bone densitometry equipment to investigate osteoporosis, the development of automated immunoassay in microbiology, and constant refinements in imaging techniques.

The development of genetic screening and fertility treatments gives the medical profession and society a new range of ethical dilemmas to wrestle with. In its 1992 report, "Our Genetic Future: The Science and Ethics of Genetic Technology," the British Medical Association concluded that "The techniques of genetic modification have the potential through application in agriculture, medicine and technology to increase the well-being of people and to promote the health of the population by disease prevention. Wrongly used they have the potential to cause harm . . . . Care must be taken to optimise the benefits and minimise the risks it offers . . . . Those developing the techniques and applications of new technology have a duty to consider the consequences of their activities."

The profession and society need also to ask: Do we need and can we afford, both financially and ecologically, to pursue all these advances? Effective technology need not be expensive or complicated, however. Countless lives are being saved in the developing world through the universal application of oral rehydration fluids. Smallpox has been eradicated throughout the world, thanks to a combination of improved technology in the form of freeze-dried vaccines and rigorous management of the program. Equity dictates, however, that the developed world should continue to transfer technology to the developing world with the help of agencies such as UNICEF and WHO.

We cannot rely on technology alone but have also to maintain our traditional defenses against disease. These are the promotion of health in the individual and communities, for example, through healthy environments, good housing, good nutrition and child care and personal hygiene. The reemergence of tuberculosis and resurgence of viral hepatitis in menacing new forms are testimony to this need.

CULTURAL CHANGES

The cultural and societal contexts in which doctors practice also are changing. The demographic makeup of our society is changing. The proportion of older people in the population is increasing and the numbers of the very old will continue to increase. There are more single-parent families. Society is more ethnically and culturally diverse. More women work, and patterns of childbearing and childrearing are altering.

Social attitudes also are changing. As already noted, the public has higher expectations and altered perspectives on the rights and responsibilities of the individual. They expect more information about their illnesses and possible treatments and a greater part in making choices and decisions about their care.

The culture of the U.K. health service itself also is changing. As we have seen, much responsibility has been transferred to the local level. The role of managers has been enhanced, care is now being orientated toward communities, and institutional beds are being cut. The balance of power in the service is shifting, therefore, from hospital to primary/community care and between managers and health professionals. Within health-care professions, there is also a greater emphasis on teamwork and a re-appraisal of roles within the team. These changes in the traditional emphasis of the service are a relatively recent phenomenon, and the tensions that they are creating need to be tackled and worked through.

WHAT SHOULD THE PROFESSION DO?

So far, this chapter has perhaps painted a picture of a beleaguered profession. Of course, doctors are continuing to practice with caring and compassion and trying to do their best for their patients. However, there is a need for the profession to act to meet the challenges it faces and begin to set its own agenda again.

Many of these challenges would have arisen regardless of the NHS reforms, as the trends are international, as are changes in society's attitudes. The profession cannot hope for a return to unquestioning acceptance of the profession's wisdom. It needs, therefore, to examine its professional attitudes and practices and change them where necessary to meet the changing times. This is not to say that the profession should be blown by the winds of change but that their forces should be recognized.

In the U.K. the profession has begun the process of examining its practice and, most importantly, its core values as a profession. A report of a conference of 70 leading members of the profession in November 1994, which examined the future role of doctors, has been circulated for consultation not only within but also outside the profession. It raised questions as to how the profession can balance the freedom of doctors to use their clinical judgment for the good of individual patients with the obligation to practice effectively and how to make the doctor/patient relationship into a partnership based on mutual trust. The report also began the process of reminding the profession and society that the profession still upholds core professional values and caring and that these values should remain at the heart of medical practice, however technologies and society may change in future decades. In brief, the report concludes that:

- The patient/doctor relationship should be a partnership of mutual trust, with the personal consultation remaining the bedrock of medical practice. This will continue to be so despite the rapidly changing context, content, and nature of medical practice, with its startling advances in clinical and scientific research and technology.

- The profession's core values include:
  - Commitment
  - Caring/Compassion
  - Integrity
  - Competence
  - Spirit of Enquiry
  - Confidentiality
  - Responsibility
  - Advocacy

- The exercise of these ideals and self-regulation of the profession's standards and performance show doctors' commitment to high-quality medical services.

- Doctors have an essential role in maintaining and restoring the health of individuals, but health is not just health-care: it depends on action by society to improve housing, education, nutrition, and life-styles.

- Doctors have a responsibility to the community, with whom they should also work in partnership.

- Doctors should advise on priorities for health-care, but should not be the individual arbiters of rationing decisions.

- An effective working relationship at the interface of primary and secondary care is necessary for the provision of good quality services, with teamwork among health professionals a crucial ingredient.

• Doctors will need to link up with colleagues, other health-care professions, managers, their patients, and the public to influence the development of health services in the coming decades.

CONCLUSION

In conclusion, there is much in the practice of medicine that is changing and will continue to change. The profession needs to evolve, as it always has, to ensure that the practice of medicine remains of relevance to the society it serves. However, despite these changes, core values such as caring and compassion remain central to the practice of medicine and are the profession's greatest asset. Whatever changes may occur, the relationship between doctors and society, whether collectively or as individual patients, must be informed by these values and must remain at the heart of medical practice.

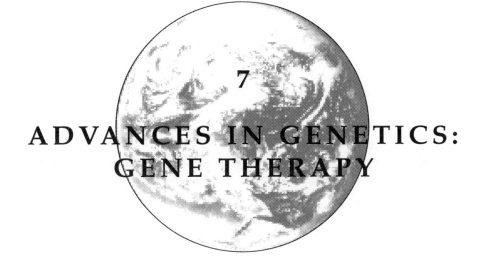

7

ADVANCES IN GENETICS: GENE THERAPY

ROBERT GALLO

is the most referenced scientist in the world according to the U.S. Institute for Scientific Information (1980s). He is the Chief of the Laboratory of Tumor Cell Biology at the National Cancer Institute, Adjunct Professor of Genetics at George Washington University, and Adjunct Professor of Biology at Johns Hopkins University. Dr. Gallo and his co-workers discovered the first human retrovirus (which was subsequently linked to human leukemia), interleukin 2 (a major advance in cellular immunology and a tool in cancer therapy), and (with scientists at the Pasteur Institute) that AIDS was caused by a human retrovirus (HIV). Uniquely, he has been awarded the prestigious Albert Lasker Award in Medicine twice, for basic medical research in 1982 and for clinical medical research in 1986. Suresh Arya is a Senior Investigator in Dr. Gallo's laboratory and has made numerous contributions to HIV gene regulation and AIDS research, including molecular cloning and characterization of the *tat* gene.

GENE THERAPY, the art and science of gene transfer in the pursuit of disease treatment and prevention, holds great promise for ameliorating human suffering in the coming decades. In a sense, gene therapy is the crown jewel of the genetic revolution that began with the recognition that genes were discrete elements and that observable characteristics of an organism were dependent on these genetic elements. Though nature plays its role, nurture provides the substance. It was the elaboration of the recombinant DNA technology that brought gene therapy into the realm of feasibility. From its infancy only a few years ago, gene therapy is now entering its vigorous youthful phase and, like all youth, insists upon marching toward its adulthood in a hurry. Also like all youth, it is full of optimism, sometimes even irreverent disregard for some lessons of human history, but it is also experiencing growing pains tinged with anxiety and anticipation. Indeed, the aim of gene therapy is truly lofty–to cure human diseases that have so far remained intractable. The previous great breakthrough of medicine, that is, the discovery of penicillin and the use of antibiotics to control infectious diseases, may in the end pale before the hoped for accomplishments of gene therapy.

The ability to practice gene therapy is, of course, contingent upon the knowledge of the constitution and functioning of the genes and molecular definition of genetic disorders. Our genes, like the genes of all organisms, consist of DNA, the so-called master molecule of life. It is the genes that determine what an organism will be–from as small a creature as a virus to as impressive a presence as an elephant. Fundamentally, it is genes that endow us, the humans, with the ability to embark on flights of imagination and inquire into the mysteries of life and nature, but they also can be a source of sorrow when they do not function in the manner in which they were designed to do. The malfunctioning of the genes underlies inherited as well as acquired genetic diseases. We can inherit defective genes from our parents or our genes can malfunction after we are born, perhaps as a result of an environmentally induced insult. Cancer, a collection of deadly diseases of perhaps of all times, in all cases probably is a result of a malfunctioning gene or genes, or the acquisition of new ones with cancer-causing potential. The ability to correct this malfunction requires identification of the gene and knowledge of its specific function. As nature would have it, our genome possesses both kinds of genes: oncogenes, that can cause cancer and tumor suppressor genes or antioncogenes, that can prevent the development of cancer. Our genes, like those of other organisms, are strung together like beads on a string on structures called chromosomes. They function by synthesizing their gene products, called proteins, the workhorses of the cells. The information imprinted in the gene is thus translated into a protein by way of an intermediate molecule called RNA (ribonucleic acid). Our total genetic makeup is collected together in a compound we call the genome. To be able to identify the genes and know their function in health and diseases, it is necessary to decipher the language of the human genome and be able to read it intelligently. Great strides have been made in this endeavor in recent years. With the implementation of the human genome project, more rapid progress is expected in identifying genes that underlie genetic disorders.

In addition to the diseases resulting from malfunctioning of the genes within us, we are subject to invasion by other organisms. These foreign organisms are not always harmful to us as host but are harmful often enough to give rise to many infectious diseases. These organisms introduce their own genes, which, of course, are designed for their survival and multiplication. In the process, however, they can cause great injury to their host. The control of infectious diseases has been one of the heartening success stories of our times, but this success has been achieved largely against bacterial diseases. It has not been significantly effective in combating human maladies caused by viruses, the tiniest of organisms lying at the boundary of living and nonliving. Among these is the virus called human immunodeficiency virus (HIV), the cause of acquired immunodeficiency syndrome (AIDS). Controlling the diseases caused by the viruses, including AIDS, is the great challenge and opportunity for gene therapy. Gene therapy is expected to bring into effective application the heretofore theoretical concept of intracellular immunization, whereby a cell, and hence an organism, is protected from the onslaught of an infectious agent.

Of necessity, gene therapy entails two different approaches: gene replacement therapy and gene insertion therapy. In gene replacement therapy, the objective is to exchange a defective or undesired gene with a normal or desired gene. The idea is to physically excise the defective gene copy and insert a nondefective copy in its place. The intention of this substitution could be to achieve a positive or a negative outcome. A gene could undergo changes or mutations resulting in the expression or readout of an aberrant gene product or protein. This gene then could be replaced with a copy that expresses normal protein. Alternatively, a gene normally could be silent but begin to express at an inappropriate time or in excessive amounts, thus requiring silencing by replacement with an inactive or appropriately regulated gene. Gene replacement therapy depends upon the technology called homologous recombination, where segments of otherwise identical DNA molecules pair with and replace each other in the chromosome. At present this entails growing or culturing the cells *in vitro* in the laboratory; introducing a good copy of the gene into the cultured cells; allowing this copy to exchange itself with the undesired copy during cell division and chromosomal reassortment; and transplanting the modified or transduced cells back into the body. The technology of homologous recombinant, which achieves targeted insertion as compared with random insertion, is yet in its infancy and not ready to be clinically implemented.

Gene insertion therapy aims to insert a good copy of the gene or the desired gene without regard to the presence of the deleterious gene. It does not attempt to eliminate or delete the bad gene. The objective here is to insert the nondefective or desired gene in such a way that it makes enough product to compensate for the inability of the defective resident gene to produce such a product. The celebrated cases of the first human gene therapy trial involving adenosine deaminase deficiency is an example of this approach. The current attempts to control ravages of cystic fibrosis is another. The inserted gene could also function to supplement the gene product being produced in insufficient quantity by the resident gene. Such shortcomings as growth hormone deficiency are amenable to this kind of approach. Further, a gene, for example, a viral gene, could be inserted to counteract the action of a foreign gene that might have invaded the host cells. In this case, the inserted gene would be a therapeutic or protective gene–not a native gene or its relative but a gene custom designed to target the foreign gene. It could directly interfere with the functioning of the foreign gene or boost host defense mechanisms to accomplish this task. Most infectious diseases would be amenable to attack by this approach.

The nature of the gene to be inserted by gene therapy can be as varied as our knowledge and our imagination will allow. In addition to exchanging gene for gene, there have been some newer conceptional developments in the field. One is the concept of employing a genetically engineered gene that produces molecular decoys. As the name implies, the inserted gene produces molecules that fool the products elaborated by the deleterious or injurious gene into believing that they are the target of the latter, thus subverting the deleterious gene molecules from performing their original function. The other concept has been the recognition of transdominant negative mutant genes. These genes are almost identical to the gene they imitate but for a small but strategically located change. Rather than acting like the genes they resemble, they counteract by molecular mimicry of the action of those genes. However, the slightly altered gene cannot perform the harmful function of the gene it imitates.

There are other gene therapeutic modalities with more general and wider scope than those targeted to specific defects. For example, we could use toxin genes to kill cells we want to eliminate, such as cancer cells. Conversely, there may be cells we may want to protect from the toxic effects of chemotherapeutic agents used in the treatments of certain cancers, such as breast cancer. These cells could be equipped with a gene, called multiple drug resistant, which confers on the recipient cell the ability to get rid of the agent before it has had the chance to do harm

Once the target of gene therapy has been identified, there remains the matter of ferrying in the desired gene. Several devices, called vectors, are being developed for this purpose. These vectors are expected to deliver the gene to a specific target cell and generally allow a high-level expression of the gene, ensure its persistent long-term expression (usually by integrating or making the introduced gene a part of the host chromosomes), and provide for its regulation. Not all of these properties may be desirable in every case. There may be instances where we may want to express the introduced gene for a limited period of time and then eliminate the gene, or, failing that, eliminate the cell carrying the gene. It is in this latter situation that the concept of the use of the suicide gene comes into play. This entails not only the introduction of the desired gene but also, along with it, a gene that can be ordered from outside to kill the cell on demand.

Two broad categories of vectors, viral and nonviral, are being developed. Each of these vectors has its strengths and weaknesses. Viral vectors are an interesting twist on the nature of things. Viruses infect human cells to reproduce themselves and bring in their own genes for this purpose. Viral vectors utilize the ability of the virus to bring in the genes–not its own gene but the genes we desire. These vectors retain that part of the viral genetic apparatus that is essential for ferrying in the gene and its efficient expression but excise that part that allows viral reproduction and harm to the host cells. Viral vectors include those based on such DNA viruses as adenovirus, adeno-associated virus and herpes virus, and those based on RNA viruses such as retroviruses, a group that includes HIV. Adenoviruses–some members of this group cause respiratory infections in man–are able to infect a variety of human cells, dividing and non-dividing cells, and express large amounts of gene products. However, their genes or the genes they ferry in do not integrate or become part of host cell chromosomes. These vectors are thus useful for short-term or transient expression of the introduced gene. They are being considered specifically for *in vivo* delivery of desired genes to the cells of the respiratory track, such as those to combat cystic fibrosis. Adeno-associated virus, a virus much smaller than the adenovirus but usually isolated with adenovirus as that virus needed for the reproduction of adeno-associated virus, can also infect human cells, and its genes are integrated into the host cell chromosome, therefore allowing for the long-term, stable expression of the gene. Normally, adeno-associated virus genes are integrated at a specific chromosome (number 19) and are therefore potentially a vehicle for targeted delivery. Herpesvirus, with some members causing cold sores in humans, has the proclivity to infect cells of the nervous system and therefore may provide the vehicle to deliver desired genes to this otherwise generally inaccessible system. Other herpesviruses preferentially infect human cells in the blood, and vectors based on them could be utilized to deliver genes to the immune cells. Retroviruses are able to infect a number of cells, but only those cells that are dividing. Genes are integrated into the host chromosomes in these cells. Much about the life cycle of these viruses is known. This fact, coupled with their ability to integrate and therefore produce a long-term effect, provides an incentive to develop and use them as vectors for gene therapy. Still, their genes and genes they carry integrate randomly in the host chromosome, thus raising the concern about the possibility, rare though it may be, that they may integrate next to a normal gene and alter its function in unpredictable ways.

Nonviral vectors for gene transfer include adenovirus DNA-ligand complexes, liposomes, particle bombardment, and naked DNA itself. The adenovirus DNA-ligand complex consists of viral DNA coated with a protective molecule of polylysine and conjugated to a molecule of ligand, which has the property of binding to a cell surface molecule called a receptor. This complex is a trafficking device, and when attached to the DNA of the desired gene it directs that gene to specific cells. Liposomes are composed of a complex of special bipolar lipid molecules that adopt a spherical shape and entrap the added DNA, containing the gene on their surface or inside their shell. The liposomes have the property to fuse with the cell membrane and deliver their contents to the inside of the cell. The particle bombardment technique is still in its infancy. The gold metal particles coated, with a film of DNA containing the gene, are forced into the host cell by ballistic bombardment with a specifically designed apparatus. The simplest of the gene delivery vehicles is, of course, no vehicle at all; that is, direct delivery of DNA, itself containing the gene, is a recently developed approach. The goal in this case is to treat the gene just like any other drug. The utility of this technique is problematic at this time, although successful local expression of directly infected DNA has been demonstrated.

A special case of gene therapy strategy is the use of biological molecules called ribosomes. Until recently it was thought that the molecules called enzymes, that catalyze or speed up biochemical reactions, were all proteins. Then came the discovery that some RNA molecules from plant viruses possess catalytic properties. These molecules were named ribosomes (*ribo*, from ribonucleic acid and *zyme*, from enzymes). They are thought to be the remnants of the ancient RNA world (in contrast to our modern world, where the master molecule of life is DNA). The ribosomes possess the ability to cleave or break down RNA molecules, to which they attach by a specific pairing mechanism. The ribosomes can be engineered to carry with them information that directs them to bind specific RNA molecules and thus break them down. This allows the targeting for destruction of RNA molecules with undesirable characteristics.

Two different procedures are available for delivering desired genes or genetic information to the host cells. One is the *in vivo* procedure, where the gene placed in a suitable context or a vector can be directly administered to the animal, including man. This could be done by any one of the routes conventionally used to administer other drugs, such as injection into the bloodstream or muscle. The other procedure, called *ex vivo*, is special to gene therapy. This involves removing the cells from the body, growing them or keeping them alive in the laboratory, genetically altering them by delivering into them the desired gene by any of the available techniques, and returning them to the body. The act of genetically modifying cells in this manner is termed transduction.

HIV infection and AIDS provide suitable models and a challenge to evaluate gene therapy approaches. AIDS is among the most dreaded diseases currently extant. It starts with an infection with HIV, a retrovirus, that attacks the cells of the immune system in the body, undermining the capacity to fight back. As the immune system deteriorates, opportunistic infections take hold and cause the syndrome we call AIDS. These generally are not esoteric infections but the sort of infection that the body normally is able to overcome, but because of the deficiencies of the immune system caused by HIV, the infected person succumbs. Despite considerable commitment of human effort and intellect, the cure for AIDS so far has remained elusive. However, it is readily agreed that tremendous progress has been made in our understanding of HIV in the past decade or so. It is not easy to imagine a period in the history of medicine when such extraordinary progress in understanding was made in such a short period of time, most particularly in the years 1983 to 1985. Admittedly, much remains to be known: The gaps in our knowledge about the manners by which HIV causes the immunodeficiency remain to be filled. Because of the intensive effort and resource commitment of the past decade or so, sufficient information about the biology and genetics of HIV has been obtained to mount a concerted attack on the virus's ability to reproduce and cause damage. Gene therapy approaches hold the promise of instituting intracellular immunization against HIV, by which the host cell would become refractory to HIV infection or altered in a way that will not support the viruses' reproduction. In the latter case, the virus would be entering a dead-end road.

HIV, like other organisms, employs a series of processes to reproduce itself. Being a virus, it is unable to reproduce without the help of the host cell's biosynthetic machinery, which it subverts for its own purposes. The virus is composed of two major components–the outer shell, called the envelope, and the inner core, which contains the viral genes in the form of an RNA and a special enzyme called reverse transcriptase. (The discovery of reverse transcriptase provided the first exception to the then prevailing central dogma of molecular biology; that is, that genetic information flows from DNA to RNA to protein. Reverse transcriptase reverses the first step to RNA to DNA. The second major exception was the discovery of ribosomes mentioned above). After attaching to the host cell by specific molecular interactions involving virus envelope and the cellular receptor molecule called CD4, the virus enters the outer part of the cell (the cytoplasm). Here, the viral genes are copied into DNA by reverse transcriptase and polymerization, and this DNA form of the viral genes enters the inner sanctum of the cell (the nucleus). The viral DNA then integrates into and becomes part of the host cell DNA contained in the chromosomes. The DNA form of viral genes are then copied into RNA by the process of transcription; some viral RNA molecules undergo modification by the process of splicing and after leaving the nucleus are translated into viral proteins. The viral proteins and viral RNA assemble into a core that leaves the cell by budding through the cellular membrane and carrying the outer shell of envelope already inserted into the cell membrane.

Although the virus uses the basic biosynthetic machinery of the cells, there are processes in the virus life cycle that are more specific to it than to the life processes of the host cell. These processes then provide the targets for gene therapy approaches using RNA-based or protein-based strategies. Nearly every step of the virus replication cycle provides a target for intervention. Among the more promising of these steps is the reverse transcription. The enzyme reverse transcriptase is unique to HIV (and other retroviruses); it is not a constituent of the host cell but is brought in with the infecting virus. This enzyme is the target of current conventional chemotherapy treatment of AIDS, using azidothymidine (AZT) and other nucleoside analogs. It is also a promising target for gene therapy. Some progress has been made in developing a class of molecules called antibodies that, when directed at this enzyme, would bind with the enzyme and render it nonfunctional. Other relatively novel approaches of gene therapy to combat AIDS include the use of molecular decoys and transdominant mutants. Genes-encoding molecular decoys and transdominant mutants, aimed at specific genes and functional proteins of HIV, are being explored. These include entities called poly-TAR and poly-RRE decoys, which are aimed at two genes of HIV, named *tat* and *rev,* that are essential for virus reproduction. Transdominant mutant genes that work against these two essential genes also are being developed. These latter mutant genes produce an altered form of the product that inhibits the function of the normal gene product.

As mentioned above, there is the special case of the use of ribosomes for gene therapy. Specific ribosomes have been engineered to carry information that allows them to bind to the HIV viral RNA and degrade it. These and other strategies are at various stages of development, some at the laboratory investigation stage and others in clinical trials with humans. The future looks promising. However, prudence requires that the possible limitations of current gene therapy approaches to AIDS be appreciated. For the therapy to be truly effective, hematopoietic stem cells or precursors of various blood cell types will need to be transduced with the protective gene. The technology to grow stem cells is still under development. The efficiency of transduction of target cells with presently available methodologies leaves something to be desired. To make a real impact on the epidemic of AIDS, possible direct *in vivo* techniques that are simple and cost-effective will need to be developed. This factor is especially important for achieving success in the developing countries of the world.

Like other human endeavors that take us into the unknown, gene therapy raises some ethical issues. The current focus of gene therapy, duly approved by the regulatory agencies, is the somatic cell therapy, whereby the cells of an adult individual are genetically altered and these genetic alterations are not transmitted to the offspring. There appears to be no outstanding objection to somatic cell gene therapy. As presently conceived, it can be seen as a logical extension of conventional drug therapy. For example, an individual with insulin deficiency diabetes receives a daily injection of insulin, the product of the insulin gene. Transplantation of a tissue or organ producing insulin to this individual would be accepted without much objection. Transplantation of the insulin gene as a part of a modified somatic cell would then also seem acceptable. Like medical intervention, somatic cell gene therapy must meet commonly accepted standards, such as informed consent and confidentiality, benefit-risk analysis, nondiscriminatory practice, and judicious use of the available resources. Fetal application of somatic cell gene therapy, where the cells of the fetus are genetically modified, is a special case, posing a dilemma of informed consent. Germ line gene therapy, on the other hand, raises some serious issues. It entails the modification of the reproductive cells, which modifications will be passed on to offspring and future generations. For reasons of safety and predictability, this therapy will require gene replacement therapy in contrast to the gene insertion therapy envisioned for somatic cells. Though the technology to achieve this end is not in hand, the ethical issues it raises must continue to be debated across cultural and religious traditions. It is a matter for debate whether we have the intelligence, let alone the wisdom, to institute measures that will affect future generations. The issues become more critical when we consider the use of germ line gene therapy not for therapeutic or corrective purposes but to enhance some traits we find useful or desirable. Can we assume that we have enough insight into the nature of man to be able to predict what will be desirable in times to come? Do we want this responsibility? Will we have the luxury to decide, or will the events take over? While the history of human failings cannot be denied, the ability to make judicious decisions is also a part of our heritage. There is no need to doubt that we will rise to the occasion.

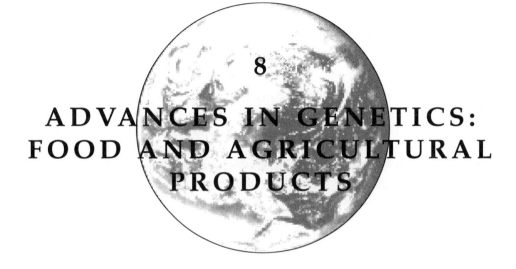

8

ADVANCES IN GENETICS: FOOD AND AGRICULTURAL PRODUCTS

VICTOR VILLALOBOS
is Senior Officer of the Food and Agriculture Organization of the United
Nations. In addition to its efforts to raise the levels of nutrition and standards
of living of the world's people, the objectives of the FAO are to improve
the efficiency of the production and distribution of food and other agricultural
products; to improve the conditions of the farm populations; and, by coordinating,
on an international basis, programs in the entire range of food and agriculture, to
contribute toward an expanding world economy. It has also launched extended
campaigns to arouse public support for a mass attack against hunger by creating
a general awareness of the food problem and the possibilities for solving it.

EARLY HUMAN POPULATIONS made an empirical selection of agricultural products to satisfy their need for food, clothing and fibers, medicine, and construction materials. For millennia, human tribes hunted wild animals, fished and collected wild products. Later, increased population forced an intensification of food supply and the establishment of villages where food availability was guaranteed and climatic conditions were not too harsh. Agriculture became a principal anthropocentric activity, and over centuries empirical selection of plants and animals created a collection of desirable products, mainly food plants selected from the wild stock.

Further progress gradually took place, associated with the need for guaranteed food supply, health, and shelter. Many developments, such as astronomy, botany, engineering, and irrigation, were related to agriculture. In this way, early humans were part of the environment and ecological systems, living in harmony with it in a way that is now identified as sustainable. This equilibrium was maintained until essentially extractive agricultural systems could no longer support the increased demands of a growing human population and the needs for sociocultural development.

POPULATION GROWTH AND AGRICULTURE PRODUCTION

Agricultural systems, empirical or specialized, have met the constantly increasing demand for food since the earliest human times. Increasing demographic and market needs required new developments in agriculture practices and technology. Thus, technology was developed for extensive agriculture, involving the use of genetically uniform varieties, mechanization, postharvest technology, processing, and development of the plant protection industry. Although these improvements increased total yield crops, as has been demonstrated during the present century, and more recently by the Green Revolution during the 1970s and 1980s, there is concern that excessive uniformity could involve plant vulnerability and result in unsustainable agricultural production. Crop uniformity might foster genetic erosion, reduction of the genetic base of plant populations, and enhance the vulnerability of cultivated plants to pests, diseases, and adverse environmental factors, such as salinity and drought stress. Also, extensive agriculture reduces food diversification, due to concentration on a limited number of crops. At present, 94 percent of human food comes from no more than 30 plants, eight of which comprise three-quarters of the plant kingdom's contribution to human energy. Three crops–wheat, rice, and maize–account for over 75 percent of human cereal consumption.

With the intensification of agricultural technology, the use of pesticides expanded rapidly, with an increased demand, particularly in developing countries, that in 1990 accounted for 26 percent of the world's pesticide market, valued at $4 billion per year. Successful breeding greatly increased yield potentials of major field crops, that is, rice, maize, sunflower, and wheat. Yields were several times higher after selection processes and the recombination of genes through crossing with wild relatives to improve resistance to diseases and environmental factors.

An important factor influencing agriculture was undoubtedly the dramatic increase in human population. Only 30 years ago, the world population was 3 billion. In 1990 it was 5.3 billion and is expected to grow to 7.2 billion by the year 2010. This represents an increase of 1.9 billion (36 percent) in 20 years. Some 94 percent (1.8 billion) of the total increase in world population will be in the developing countries, which have the highest incidence of poverty and malnutrition.

How has agriculture responded to these increases in human world population? Until now, production has grown faster than population. Per capita production is today about 20 percent above that of 30 years ago. World food consumption directly by human beings is today equivalent to some 2,700 kilocalories per person per day, up from 2,300 calories 30 years ago.

With the addition of about 640 million tons of cereals for livestock, per capita food availability is some 3,000 calories in the net sense. The present level of per capita food availability is, therefore, sufficient for everyone on the planet to have adequate nutrition, if it were distributed equally. Food is not, however, distributed equitably. At one extreme, Western Europe's per capita food availability is some 3,500 calories and in North America some 3,600 calories. At the other extreme they are only 2,100 calories in sub-Saharan Africa and 2,200 calories in India and Bangladesh. Thus, for much of the developing world, food availability is far from being adequate for all people to have access to sufficient food to give them food security at all times. So long as this situation persists, a human food problem will continue, notwithstanding adequate production at the global level.

THE ROLE OF BIOTECHNOLOGY IN FOOD SECURITY

In recent years, biotechnologies applied to plants have been considered a set of tools with a great potential to benefit agriculture. Research has produced important breakthroughs in agriculture. Biotechnologies have provided new approaches to overcome the problems of plants in marginal environments, abiotic stresses, pests, and diseases and also to achieve agricultural development by the production of unique gene combinations through genetic engineering, the production of pest resistant genotypes, and germ plasm conservation.

Thanks primarily to conventional methods of genetic improvement (interchange of genetic material between sexually compatible species), there has been a significant increase in food availability in recent years. World grain production increased by 4.2 percent (1,959 million tons). World tuber and root production has increased by 3.5 percent over the 1991 level. However, despite these achievements, many countries are gravely affected by limited food supplies and are dependent on international aid. In addition, it is predicted that crop increase from conventional methods will not continue at the same rate. Therefore, the incorporation of genetic engineering techniques, which greatly reduce the time needed to produce new varieties, will become necessary. Some agricultural problems directly related to food security are those of: monoculture, high salinity of crop lands, erosion and decertification, and the abuse of fertilizers and pesticides.

Recent discoveries in plant biotechnology point to practical solutions to these problems. Since 1983, when the first experiment in transformation was accomplished, more than 50 food crops have successfully been transformed (by bypassing the natural barriers of sexual compatibility) and the number is growing constantly. Recipient plants can accept the isolated genes of other organisms that give desirable agronomic characteristics, in addition to the ones already mentioned, such as improved nutritional properties by means of modified protein, fat, and carbohydrate levels and postharvest processing capacity. An example of the last is the "FlavrSavr" tomato, with a longer storage life, which was commercialized in the United States in the second half of 1994. Recently, there has been increased interest in using plants as vehicles for synthesizing enzymes needed for the food industry, for industrial oils, and for polymers.

Agricultural productivity, and consequently food availability in general, is expected to increase through the direct use of biotechnology and genetic improvement. The path that this science is taking, though, is oriented almost exclusively toward crops of high economic importance, such as wheat, maize, soybean, and cotton. Other species, of great socioeconomic importance to developing countries but of little to international markets, do not appear on the priority list of the leading biotechnology companies–for example, cassava, sweet potato, banana, and plantain. Under these circumstances, any research on the biotechnological improvement of these and other species will have to take place locally within the interested countries. One serious limiting factor, though, is that research levels and the use of biotechnology in developing countries are generally far below the necessary standards.

If the benefits of biotechnology are to reach developing countries, particularly those with food deficits, it will be necessary to employ a strategy that will gradually give them access to the appropriate biotechnologies, and that can be defined as those techniques that contribute to sustained development, which are technically feasible, environmentally safe, and culturally and socioeconomically acceptable.

THE BIOTECHNOLOGIES AVAILABLE

Biotechnology applied to plants comprises two major groups of tools, which are, to a certain extent, complementary: tissue culture and genetic engineering. Biotechnologies in crop production are primarily for:

- Micropropagation of plants, especially when combined with culture for virus-free plant production, and disease indexing to produce large quantities of clean planting material. More than 50 different plant species have been successfully freed from virus infection using this technique;

- diagnoses based on the use of immunological methods and nucleic hybridization for the identification of plant diseases;

- plant genetic improvement using different tissue culture techniques;

- genetic engineering of individual species to introduce novel traits for plant improvement, plant protection, and to enhance quality of agricultural products;

- genetic mapping technologies as an aid to conventional plant breeding programs; and

- the use of tissue culture and cryoconservation techniques for plant germ plasm conservation and exchange.

POTENTIAL NEGATIVE EFFECT OF BIOTECHNOLOGY

The possibility of a negative impact of biotechnology in developing countries has been much discussed. The threat of the biotechnological substitution of products such as vanilla and cocoa butter is frequently mentioned, as is the substitution of certain pharmaceutical compounds, scents, flavorings, and spices. Although it is true that biotechnologically derived substitutes for these products are subjects of research, the higher production cost of this methodology is a limiting factor. If, in addition, we consider society's tendency to prefer natural products, the significance of this threat is greatly diminished. A good example of this is the case of the vanilla industry: the use of a very simple biotechnology tool, such as a tissue culture techniques for cloning superior (more resistant to disease and high yielding) individuals, could be a strategy to reduce the risk of vanilla from Madagascar being replaced by that of large-scale fermenters producing vanillin, the synthetic form.

There is another type of risk that should be taken more seriously in developing countries in particular: lack of knowledge of the scope and the limitations of biotechnology. Countries seeking the benefits of such technologies should be able to identify those that can and cannot be useful to them. They should also recognize that the development of biotechnology is a long and costly process and that its benefits may not be perceivable in the short term. Governments mostly rely on chosen teams of scientists, who serve as intermediaries between science and policymakers throughout the process. Above all, it must be realized that biotechnology is desirable only as a tool for the betterment of agriculture and not as an end in and of itself.

A STRATEGY FOR APPLICATION OF BIOTECHNOLOGY IN DEVELOPING COUNTRIES

Biotechnology applied to agriculture has hitherto been transferred to developing countries mainly through universities with scientific interests and, often, with educational objectives. More recently, the international centers of the Consultative Group on International Agricultural Research have also participated actively in the transfer of biotechnology to their counterparts, the national programs, for practical applications. In some countries, such as Brazil, China, India, Mexico, Singapore, and Thailand, biotechnology companies have been established in recent years; in this way, the necessary elements for biotechnology implementation, that is, research centers, national agricultural programs, private companies, and organized farmers are available. Different international organizations, including the Food and Agriculture Organization of the United Nations (FAO), United Nations Educational, Scientific, and Cultural Organization (UNESCO), and United Nations Industrial Development Organization (UNIDO), participate in this important process, where the overall aim is to establish links between the technology available and the potential users who are mainly in developing countries.

THE ROLE OF FAO IN THE PROMOTION OF PLANT BIOTECHNOLOGY

FAO gives biotechnology high priority as a strategy to support member states, helping them improve their national programs for the genetic improvement of crops in order to attain nutritional self-sufficiency. In 1992 the Plant Biotechnology Program was created with the aim of supporting the most needy member states through the use of appropriate biotechnologies. The program has identified four main thrusts by which it hopes to offer greater assistance to those countries.

1.   Promoting Exchange of Biotechnical Information. FAO has promoted various mechanisms that facilitate access to scientific information, emphasizing the regional networks for plant biotechnology.

2.   Advisory Service to Member States in the Development of National Biotechnology Programs. The FAO Plant Biotechnology Program supports countries in the creation, evaluation, and priority-setting in the area of plant biotechnology. Currently, the program is assisting the following countries in the planning of goals, priorities, and medium- and long-term resources: Chile, Costa Rica, Cuba, India, Iran, Nigeria, Northern Brazil, Senegal, and Uruguay.

3.   Support to the Infrastructure of National Programs. FAO has helped member states to create a physical infrastructure and to acquire equipment and other facilities. Additionally, it has supported national programs in training high-level scientists in the areas of tissue culture and molecular biology. The program finances training courses in Latin America, Africa, and Asia and has supported international cooperation in collaboration with other U.N. organizations, including UNESCO, in African and Eastern European and Latin American countries.

4.   Promoting Research and Technology Transfer Adoption. The program promotes research on the identification of practical solutions to problems of improvements and preservation of plant genetic resources. This activity is carried out in conjunction with the international centers, mainly the International Plant Genetic Resources Institute, and with national programs.

BIOTECHNOLOGY AND PLANT GENETIC RESOURCES FOR TOMORROW

The constant need to increase food production has resulted in the neglect of the value of protective measures. The efficient use of plant genetic resources, which requires careful collection, conservation, evaluation, documentation, and exchange, has also suffered a lack of attention. Although germ plasm conservation is attracting more and more public concern, conservation and access to plant genetic resources are not simple affairs and involve cultural, ecological, technical, and political issues.

The possibility of developing complete plants from isolated cells, tissues, or organs, using plant tissue culture, has made the establishment of germ plasm banks feasible. During the last 20 years, *in vitro* culture techniques have been developed for more than 1,000 species, including annuals and perennials. The use of these techniques is more important for the conservation and multiplication of plants that produce recalcitrant (unable to withstand desiccation) seeds and also for vegetatively propagated species that are either sterile or do not have stable sexual reproduction.

In vitro storage has thus been proposed as a means to overcome some of the above mentioned plant conservation problems. *In vitro* technology has been a strong motivation for the planning, research, and development of alternative sources of conservation. In principle, tissue-culture techniques are appropriate for conservation, the development of a complete plant being the expected result in all cases. It is, therefore, logical to try to maintain a high level of tissue organization during storage. One of the major objectives of germ plasm conservation is to maintain the genetic diversity of a species in a stable condition; the storage techniques used thus should not endanger plant genetic stability.

Although tissue-culture techniques are already used for *in vitro* conservation, at present only 37,600 accessions are in such storage worldwide. *In vitro* collections are controversial since they must be maintained in a carefully controlled environment. Practical problems in their maintenance, associated with the risks of microbial contamination and genetic stability, have to be considered.

In vitro techniques imply the substitution of natural for artificial conditions, with the advantage that light and temperature are controlled in a reduced space. In many cases, for plants with short reproductive cycles, such as some roots, tubers, and other annuals, *in vitro* transfer intervals are less frequent than the harvest cycle in the field. Another important advantage is the possibility of producing virus-free plants with a high multiplication rate, independent of climactic conditions. In the modern context of conservation and with a rational use of genetic diversity, *in vitro* conservation should include the elimination of viruses from the stored material and the ability to micropropagate the germ plasm in large quantities when necessary. To guarantee future access to plant diversity for use in agriculture crop improvement, conservation of genetic resources is essential.

9

ADVANCES IN REPRODUCTIVE MEDICINE

DUANE ALEXANDER, M.D.
is Director of the U.S. National Institute of Child Health and Human
Development. The NICHHD is one of the major agencies of the National
Institutes of Health, which conducts research and awards grants and contracts
not only for research work in the area of child health and human development,
but in such areas as cancer and related diseases, heart and lung diseases,
neurological diseases, arthritis and metabolic diseases, environmental
health, and general medical sciences.

SCIENTIFIC ADVANCES in the twentieth century have produced unprecedented safety, success, and control in the area of reproductive medicine, along with the ability to extend healthy life spans. Because these changes affect fundamental aspects of human life and behavior, they have had a greater societal impact, particularly by way of facilitating equal participation of women in work, than scientific advances virtually in any other arena. Many of these scientific discoveries are just beginning to be exploited, so even greater changes can be expected as these developments continue. And continue they must, for as they affect our ability to control population growth, the ultimate environmental and public health issue, our very existence on this planet depends on progress in this field.

SAFETY

Imagine the fear of husbands and wives today if they faced a greater than 1 percent chance that the woman would die each time she became pregnant. We have come to accept pregnancy as almost a routine, nonrisk event, but in the first two decades of this century in the U.S. that was the risk, and it persists today in many developing countries. Through a combination of medical advances, representing one of the greatest of all health accomplishments, that risk in the U.S. has been lowered more than a hundred fold, to less than 0.01 percent, averaging 300 maternal deaths per year in more than 4 million births.

Numerous factors account for this dramatic change. The site of delivery has shifted, so that now more than 98% of births occur in hospitals, with their ability to minimize risk of infection and deal with any emergency and with care provided by specially trained physicians or nurse-midwives. Hemorrhage is averted, or readily treated, thanks to research that developed transfusion and blood banking. Antibiotics are available to treat infections when they do occur. Research has improved management of pregnant women with risky chronic medical conditions, such as diabetes or heart disease. The "grand multip"-a woman who has had many pregnancies-of Margaret Sanger's day has become a rarity. Pregnancies tend to be wider spaced, and fewer pregnancies are occurring in higher risk older women, as reliable family planning techniques have become available. Access to safe pregnancy termination has nearly eliminated maternal death from septic abortion, and safe cesarean delivery without risk of uterine rupture has markedly improved the ability to perform surgical delivery when necessary.

The most direct impact of these advances that have reduced maternal mortality is the ability of couples to contemplate pregnancy without fear of the mother dying. However there are two other social consequences as well. The most immediate has been the near elimination of a maternal death leaving no mother available to raise the children in the family, an all-too-frequent occurrence in earlier times. The longer term impact has been the steady increase of life expectancy for women, both in years and relative to men. At the turn of the century, women's survival advantage over men was three years; it has increased since to seven years, due in large part to reduction of the risk of childbearing. Women are thus even more likely to live well beyond their spouse, often alone, and to ages when numerous health problems occur.

SUCCESS

Success in reproductive medicine encompasses establishing a pregnancy, carrying it to term, and delivering a healthy infant who survives. Research has provided major improvements in success on all fronts.

Infertility is a frequent occurrence, with one in ten American couples unable to achieve a pregnancy during a year of unprotected intercourse. Approximately one-third of instances of infertility is ascribed to female factors and one-third to male problems. Despite research, the cause of the remaining one-third remains unknown. Until recently the only treatment available was for male infertility, by artificial insemination by donor (AID). Through research a variety of new treatment approaches have become available, allowing couples to have children who could never have had them before.

Underlying all this research were the studies of hormonal control of the male and female reproductive system, particularly the female menstrual cycle. Development of radioimmunoassay procedures replaced the crude animal bioassay methods for measuring reproductive hormones, initially permitting precise quantization of estrogen, progesterone, and testosterone, and then of the pituitary hormones (luteinizing hormone-LH and follicle stimulating hormone-FSH) that stimulate and control their release; of human chorionic gonadotropin (HCG) from the placenta that maintains pregnancy; and of the brain hypothalamic-releasing hormones that direct the pituitary's function. Analysis and chemical synthesis of the hormones followed, along with preparation of analogs of similar or greater potency for use as pharmaceutical agents. Ability to analyze HCG in small amounts provided the basis for development of home pregnancy detection kits, now widely used. The drugs in turn have provided for the first time a way to stimulate ovulation or sperm production for treatment of infertility. As experience has been gained, use of pulsed treatment with gonadotropins or of releasing factors has both increased the successful pregnancy rate and decreased the risks of multiple pregnancy (twins or greater) that have been a problem with this treatment approach, which created instant megafamilies and newspaper headlines but not an optimal outcome.

Most spectacular and attention-attracting among infertility treatments has been *in vitro* fertilization (IVF). First achieved by researchers in England in 1978, with the birth of Louise Brown after years of research, this procedure now accounts for more than 5,000 births a year in the U.S. It involves a long evaluation and workup; hormone administration to the woman to stimulate the ovary to ripen many eggs at once; retrieval of the eggs at just the right time (determined by ultrasound examination–another research advance), usually by an instrument inserted through the vagina; exposure of the eggs to sperm in a petri dish; culture of the fertilized eggs in media for one to three days; and then placing several fertilized eggs in the uterus that remains under hormonal stimulation, in expectation that implantation will occur. This complex process currently has a success rate (birth of an infant) of only about 15 percent and is too expensive for most couples to afford, so additional studies are needed to improve its success and reduce the cost, making this child-giving technology more widely available.

Success has also been enhanced by the development of prenatal diagnosis to avoid the birth of infants with severe birth defects or genetic disorders. A variety of procedures are employed. Amniocentesis was introduced in 1967. It involves inserting a needle through the abdomen into the uterus at 14-16 weeks of pregnancy and aspirating some amniotic fluid and examining the fetal cells it contains for chromosome abnormalities, such as Down's syndrome, or severe genetic disorders, such Tay-Sachs disease. Research demonstrated this technique to be quite safe, with a risk of below 0.5 percent of fetal loss. Chorionic villus sampling (CVS) was introduced in the 1970s as an improvement over amniocentesis because it can be done earlier (eighth week of pregnancy), provide faster results (one day instead of two weeks), and involves obtaining fetal cells from the developing placenta through the vagina, rather than inserting a needle into the uterus. Its safety was shown to be comparable to that of amniocentesis. Alpha fetoprotein screening of a maternal blood sample, followed by ultrasound exam of the fetus if elevated levels are detected, provides a way to detect severe physical abnormalities, such as neural tube defects (spina bifida and anencephaly).

Methods are now being tested for obtaining and analyzing fetal cells from a maternal blood sample at six to eight weeks of pregnancy. Unfortunately, when these diagnostic procedures detect abnormality, fetal treatment is generally not yet available, and the usual options are pregnancy termination or preparation for the birth of an affected child.

The newest development in prenatal diagnosis combines *in vitro* fertilization and new advances in genetics to make a diagnosis from a single cell. This technique avoids the need to consider pregnancy termination for fetal abnormality by making it possible to select only a normal fertilized egg for implantation. Called blastomere analysis before implantation (BABI) or preimplantation genetic diagnosis, it begins with IVF in couples known to be at risk for having an infant with a severe genetic disease (Tay-Sachs or cystic fibrosis, for example). The fertilized eggs are cultured to the eight-cell stage, at which time one of those cells is removed from each. Removal makes no difference; the remaining seven cells will continue to develop normally. The removed cell's genetic material is multiplied many times in a few hours by a new technique called polymerase chain reaction (PCR), the gene for the disease in question is identified, and it is analyzed in comparison with that gene in the parents. This procedure permits identification of fertilized eggs that have the defective genes and selection for implantation of fertilized eggs that are free of the disease gene. This technique, available in just the last few years, has so far been used to help fewer than 100 couples, who otherwise would not have risked pregnancy, have healthy children. Its use promises to significantly increase as more scientists develop the capability for this high-technology assisted reproduction procedure.

The final component of success is delivery of a surviving infant. Infant mortality has been steadily declining in most of the world and in the U.S. has reached an all-time low level of 0.8 percent. The major obstacle to even better survival is premature labor and low birth weight. Our ability to save smaller and smaller babies has steadily improved, to the point that half of the babies born weighing two pounds now survive through neonatal intensive care and new treatments, such as surfactant for respiratory distress syndrome. However there are still too many premature babies, and a major need from future research in reproductive medicine is to learn how to prevent premature labor and low birth weight.

CONTROL

The other side of the infertility coin is the ability to control fertility, both preventing unintended pregnancy and timing a wanted pregnancy's occurrence. While some methods of fertility regulation go far back in human history, the introduction of the oral contraceptive pill in 1958 represented a whole new approach to fertility control, producing the social equivalent of a revolution. Based on the same research described above, related to infertility that delineated the hormonal mechanisms controlling the menstrual cycle and synthesized estrogens and progestins, the oral contraceptive provided for the first time a female-controlled, safe, reversible, in apparent, and nearly infallible method of contraception. Women could now pursue education, career, or any life choice without concern that an unexpected or unwanted pregnancy would interfere and with the ability to plan pregnancy at a time of their own choosing. Much, though certainly not all, of the rapid entry of women into the work force at all levels can be attributed to the control over the reproductive aspects of their lives provided by the oral contraceptive pill.

With further research, the safety and freedom from side effects of oral contraceptives have been improved by modifying the chemical structure of the estrogens and progestins used, lowering the dose, and varying the composition during the cycle. Nonetheless, the basic approach and concept have remained unchanged, a tribute to the original developers.

Variations on the oral contraceptive theme also have been introduced. Injectables such as Depo-Provera® that provide midterm (three-month) protection have been developed to eliminate the need for taking a pill daily and solve the compliance issue, and improved products of this type are in testing. Implants such as Norplant® that provide long-term (five-year) contraception recently became available, and other implant variations (two-year protection, complete resorption) are undergoing trials. Vaginal rings that release a progestin or progestin/estrogen combination are also in use. A minor problem with all these is irregular vaginal bleeding in some women. Studies attempting to alleviate this complication are under way.

Other contraceptive approaches also have been introduced or improved. Male sterilization by vasectomy has been simplified and made safer, as has female tubal ligation by laparoscope rather than by open abdominal surgery; consequently, sterilization is the contraceptive method most used by older American couples. Barriers (cervical cap, diaphragm, male and female condoms) have been developed or improved, and effective spermicides help provide additional protection not only against pregnancy but against sexually transmitted diseases. With these diseases at epidemic proportions and with the advent of AIDS, major research efforts are now being directed toward developing improved barrier methods and spermicides that have better microbicidal properties.

New approaches to fertility regulation also are being explored, some based on research that demonstrated that hormones act by triggering specific receptors based on their physicochemical structure. Antiprogestins, drugs such as RU-486 that prevent the action of progesterone by blocking its ability to act on its receptor, were originally developed as abortifacients. Their long-term role for this application remains to be seen, but they have other possible uses as well. Results of early studies suggest that a very small dose of an antiprogestin throughout the menstrual cycle may be an effective contraceptive. The advantage here would be that it would not modify the normal hormonal levels. Another potential use is as a postcoital contraceptive (morning-after pill). Initial results indicate that a single dose of an antiprogestin given within 72 hours of unprotected intercourse provides virtually complete protection against pregnancy, without side effects. Testing to develop antiprogestins for this use is under way. Its importance is shown by the fact that there is no agent marketed for this purpose at present and by indications that half of all unintended pregnancies could be prevented if such an agent were available.

Some of the long-standing reproductive disorders of women that have been recalcitrant to other treatment approaches may also yield to antiprogestins. Endometriosis, for example, seems to improve with antiprogestin treatment. Clinical trials to test this therapy are now being planned.

Another new approach to fertility regulation is immunocontraception for both men and women. Studies of the process of fertilization have identified specific protein molecules involved in the process of recognition and binding of sperm to egg. These proteins are potential targets for development of "vaccines" that would bind to them to prevent sperm-egg union and provide contraception.

Farther on the horizon as a contraceptive technique is interference with meiosis, the process of cell division that reduces the cell's chromosomes from a paired set to a single set to form sperm and egg cells. No other cells in the body undergo meiosis. Scientists are attempting to elucidate the cellular control mechanisms involved in meiosis and find ways to alter them. Targeting meiosis would have the potential advantage of not affecting any other cells in the body and being a side effect–free form of contraception.

PROLONGATION OF HEALTHY LIFE

A unique contribution from reproductive medicine, and an outgrowth of the same research that provided hormonal contraception and infertility treatment, is perimenopausal hormone replacement therapy (HRT). Initially, this was developed as administration of estrogen beginning around the time of menopause to relieve the symptoms induced by cessation of estrogen production by the ovary. Most women obtained relief from hot flashes, mood and behavioral fluctuations, and vaginal dryness with this treatment. However, in addition to relief of these symptoms, it became apparent that the treatment was also associated with reducing the increased risk of heart disease that appeared after menopause, along with protection against osteoporosis. Initial concerns about increase in risk of endometrial cancer by estrogen-only treatment regimens have been alleviated by adding cyclic progestin to the treatment. The annoyance of continued mild menstrual periods is more than compensated for by the elimination of the endometrial cancer risk. Although ongoing studies have yet to determine whether a prolonged HRT regimen might slightly increase the risk of breast cancer, most physicians today highly recommend at least an initial HRT treatment and probably prolonged, multiyear treatment as well. In addition to the short-term benefits of symptom relief and the preservation of physical ability, there is no question about the extremely valuable long-term benefits of reduced risk of heart disease and osteoporosis. With the increased life expectancy of women today, ability to avoid the devastating impact of osteoporosis in their 1970s, 1980s, and even 1990s makes HRT one of the major contributions of reproductive medicine.

Males should not be overlooked in HRT consideration. While controversy exists over whether there is a counterpart to menopause in the male, and studies of hormone levels in males are not clear-cut, there are several studies that demonstrate that testosterone administration to post-middle-age males preserves muscle mass and improves the sense of well-being. These studies have been hampered by the need for administration of testosterone by frequent injection. A long-acting (two-month) form of testosterone now completing premarket testing should resolve that problem and permit the larger scale, long-term studies needed to assess whether aging males may also benefit from analogous HRT.

CONCLUSION

Despite the advances in making pregnancy possible, safer, and intended, and in prolonging healthy life, reproductive medicine and science face huge challenges. To this field falls the responsibility for containment of the AIDS epidemic for the near future. Through a combination of providing improved barrier contraceptives and microbicidal spermicides; efforts to influence sexual behavior to maximize their effective use; and employing treatment regimens in HIV-positive pregnant women that reduce the likelihood of transmission of HIV to their infant, reproductive medicine must hold the dike until effective treatment and a preventive vaccine eventually become available. To this field also falls the responsibility for developing and encouraging use of maximally effective contraceptive methods to avoid unwanted pregnancy and its triple undesired consequences: abortion, unwanted and poorly cared for children, and uncontrolled, unsustainable population growth. May we have the wisdom to provide the scientists and research support necessary for this task.

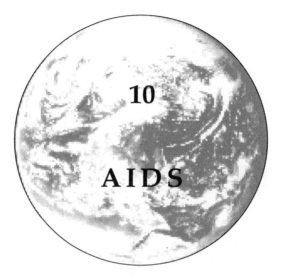

10

AIDS

JONATHAN MANN
is the Francois-Xavier Bagnoud Professor of Health and Human Rights at the
Harvard University School of Public Health. Dr. Mann is also Professor of
Epidemiology and International Health, Director of the International AIDS
Center, Director of the Francois-Xavier Bagnoud Center for Health and
Human Rights, and Founding Director of the World Health
Organization's Global Program on AIDS.

THE CHINESE SYMBOL for crisis is composed of two distinct words–"danger" and "opportunity." The global epidemic of infection with human immunodeficiency virus (HIV) and AIDS surely qualifies as a global crisis. The danger is clear, yet there is also opportunity to learn and apply vital lessons for the future of world health.

While the origin and past history of HIV are unknown, it is clear that the current worldwide epidemic started in the mid to late 1970s. By 1980, an estimated 100,000 people worldwide were HIV-infected; this number increased to approximately 10 million by 1990.

Worldwide, by 1 January 1995, an estimated 26 million people had been infected with HIV. Of these, about 23 million were adults, including 13 million men and 10 million women, and 3 million were children. The largest number of HIV-infected adults were in sub-Saharan Africa (17 million; about two-thirds of the global total). Overall, more than 90 percent of HIV infections have occurred in the developing world; only about 5 percent of HIV-infected people worldwide have been from North America.

The time between becoming infected with HIV and the onset of clinical AIDS averages 10 years. Therefore, as the pandemic is relatively new, there are many more people infected with HIV than the number who have AIDS. Worldwide, 8.5 million people have developed AIDS, of whom 7 million were in sub-Saharan Africa, about 700,000 were in Latin America and the Caribbean, and more than 550,000 were in North America, Western Europe, and Oceania combined. The 8.5 million people with AIDS includes nearly 2 million children, most of whom are also from sub-Saharan Africa.

While treatments exist that prolong life and enhance the quality of life for people with AIDS, it remains a fatal disease in most cases; a global total of 7.5 million people have thus far died of AIDS.

To understand the pandemic, it is essential to recall that it is a relatively new phenomenon. As such, it remains dynamic, volatile, and unstable, and its major impact is yet to come.

The dynamic quality of the pandemic is evident in three ways. First, HIV continues to spread in all already affected areas of the world. For example, it is estimated that in recent years, from 40,000 to 80,000 new HIV infections have occurred each year in the United States. Second, HIV has reached countries and communities that were thus far unaffected or little affected by the pandemic. For example, while very few people in Asia were HIV-infected prior to the late 1980s, countries such as India, Thailand, and Burma are now experiencing major HIV epidemics. The number of HIV-infected people in Southeast Asia (4.5 million) is now more than twice the total number of HIV-infected people in the entire industrialized world. Third, the pandemic has become increasingly complex. While the routes of HIV spread remain constant and limited (sexual intercourse, blood contact, mother-to-fetus/newborn), the pandemic reaches and spreads within different communities at different rates and times. For example, while the epidemic in Brazil started among gay men from the social elite, the epidemic is now centered among heterosexual men and women living in the large slums around Rio de Janeiro and São Paolo and among injecting drug users. Within large urban areas, such as Dade County, Florida, multiple simultaneous epidemics of HIV infection may be under way.

The second major characteristic of the pandemic is that its major impact is delayed, due to the long average period between initial infection with HIV and development of clinical AIDS. The situation in Thailand illustrates well the magnitude of this delayed feature of the HIV/AIDS pandemic. Given that at least 500,000 Thais are now HIV-infected, it can be predicted that the number of AIDS cases in Thailand will increase from several hundred over the past five years to at least 100,000 during the next five years! Therefore, even if the HIV spread stopped immediately, the effects of the pandemic would not.

During 1994, an estimated 4 million new HIV infections occurred worldwide, or an average of about 11,000 new HIV infections each day. How has the world responded to this expanding, accelerating worldwide epidemic?

The history of the global response to HIV/AIDS can be divided into four periods. During the first period, from the mid-1970s until 1981, there was no response, yet a major worldwide epidemic was under way. No response occurred until the disease AIDS was first recognized in the United States in 1981. The delay in discovery resulted from a combination of factors, including the time from infection to illness and the difficulty in recognizing a new disease. Then, during the period of discovery and initial response, from 1981 to 1985, an enormous amount of scientific knowledge was accumulated. More is now known about HIV than about any other virus that infects humans. However, the public health response was slow: most of the important work in protecting people during this period was carried out by nongovernmental organizations. Finally, AIDS was recognized to be a global threat, and the World Health Organization (WHO) launched a major effort, leading to the third period, of global mobilization, from 1986 to 1990. During this time: a global AIDS strategy was developed; national AIDS programs were launched in most countries; and community-based efforts were expanded and intensified. This mobilization was dramatic and unprecedented in world history.

During this time, it was recognized that an AIDS vaccine or an effective AIDS drug would not be available soon, and the emphasis was on preventing new HIV infections and on caring, as well as possible, for those who were infected and affected. From a large number of creative, innovative, and courageous projects (many launched and carried out by nongovernmental and community-based organizations), the key elements for effective prevention programs were identified.

There are three vital elements for HIV prevention. First, people must be provided with accurate and useful information and education. Most importantly, this information must be developed with the participation of the target audience. However, knowledge about HIV/AIDS is not enough. Therefore, the second key element involves health and social services closely linked with the prevention messages. For example, messages about condom use must be accompanied by programs to ensure that condoms are available, affordable, and of good quality. Also, recommendations about HIV testing can only be useful where confidential counseling and high-quality testing services are readily available. Similarly, drug users who are advised to stop injecting need rapid admission to effective drug treatment programs.

While these two elements (information/education and supportive services) are traditional public health measures, the third key element of successful HIV prevention–preventing discrimination against HIV-infected people and people with AIDS–was new. The rationale for this approach emerged from field experiences, in which it became clear that when and if those most likely to be infected were threatened with dire social consequences (e.g., loss of work, inability to marry, expulsion from school), they would "go underground" and avoid contact with the very public health services designed to help them. In short, support to those infected and ill was recognized as vital to efforts to protect public health.

When this "prevention triad" was adapted to local cultural and other circumstances, it was highly effective. Whether among homosexual men, commercial sex users, injecting drug users, adolescents, or heterosexual men and women, the "prevention triad" was as successful (or more) than any other public health programs based on changing individual behavior.

However, despite the global mobilization and successful prevention programs at the pilot project and community level, the fourth and most recent period in the history of HIV/AIDS (1990 to the present) has been deeply disappointing, for, paradoxically, as the global epidemic intensifies, the global response has plateaued or even declined. Successful pilot projects are not replicated; the gap between the rich and poor widens (currently about 90 percent of resources for prevention and care are spent in the industrialized world while the developing world bears about 90 percent of the HIV/AIDS burden); and the political and social commitment to HIV/AIDS has not kept pace with the pandemic. In short, the current period has been characterized by stagnation and fragmentation

Therefore, the dangers of the HIV/AIDS pandemic are clear. What about the opportunities?

The major opportunity has arisen from a recent discovery about the pandemic. Study of the evolution of the epidemic in countries around the world revealed a "societal risk factor" for HIV infection. It was discovered that those people within each society who prior to the arrival of HIV/AIDS were marginalized, discriminated against, and stigmatized had a higher risk of becoming HIV-infected. For example, in the United States the epidemic is increasingly focusing on inner-city and poor African-American and Latino populations. As another example, for women in East Africa, being married and monogamous is now considered a risk factor for HIV infection. Even if a woman knows that her husband is HIV-infected, she cannot refuse unwanted or unprotected sexual intercourse for fear of being beaten, without civil recourse or for fear of divorce, which translates into civil and economic death for the woman. Therefore, even though knowing about HIV/AIDS and despite condoms being available in the marketplace, these women cannot protect themselves. They lack the equal rights that alone would enable translation of knowledge into protection. Efforts to change the laws governing divorce, marriage, and inheritance are now under way, as part of a broad strategy to slow the spread of HIV.

Thus, the understanding of vulnerability to HIV/AIDS has expended to include not only personal and program-related but also societal dimensions. The failure to realize human rights and respect human dignity has now been recognized as a major cause–actually, the root cause–of societal vulnerability to HIV/AIDS. This understanding resulted from concrete and practical experience, not from simply theoretical considerations; it was discovered in communities, not in governmental bureaucracies or universities. It is now clear that HIV/AIDS is as much about society as about a virus.

This insight regarding the inextricable connection between promotion and protection of health and promotion and protection of human rights offers a new understanding of the pandemic and how it should be controlled.

A two-pronged strategy is now needed. The first part involves efforts to strengthen the existing, "prevention-triad"–based programs around the world. These efforts require support at community, national, and global levels.

The second, truly innovative part of the new global AIDS strategy requires that the societal roots of the pandemic be addressed directly. This will require a commitment to promoting and protecting basic human rights of people currently marginalized and discriminated against. This effort may initially seem unusual for public health until it is recalled that public health has been defined as "ensuring the conditions in which people can be healthy"–and the major determinants of health status are societal. Ensuring respect for human rights and dignity is a clear pathway to ensuring the presence of those "essential conditions" for HIV prevention and for health more generally.

Hope arises also from recognition by the United Nations that a truly coordinated global effort is required to confront the diverse challenges of HIV/AIDS prevention and care. Starting in January 1996, a new Joint and Co-Sponsored United Nations AIDS program will be in operation. This program will link together the six major U.N. agencies involved with HIV/AIDS: WHO, UNICEF, the U.N. Development Program (UNDP), UNESCO, the U.N. Fund for Population (UNFPA), and the World Bank.

Projections for the HIV/AIDS pandemic are grim. While estimates for the number of people HIV-infected by the year 2000 vary widely (from 40 to 110 million people), it is clear that the years to come will be much more difficult than the nearly 15 years since AIDS was first recognized.

Yet even as new insights, strategies, and programs are developed against HIV/AIDS, the experience of this pandemic serves as a warning for the future, for today's world is more vulnerable than ever before to the global spread of new and emerging diseases. The extraordinary and dramatic increases in movements of people, goods, and ideas worldwide have truly made this world a "global village." Whether involving old diseases or previously unrecognized pathogens, it is a matter of time (not a matter of "if") before the next global epidemic occurs. Therefore, along with the new understanding of the health and human rights connection (which applies to all major health problems of the modern world, including cancer, heart diseases, injuries, violence, and infectious diseases), perhaps the most important lesson from the "age of AIDS" is the message of global interdependence, for we can no longer believe that our borders will protect us; the health of the world is bound together. The photograph of Earth from space, that image of our entire world, blue, green, and brown against a black immensity, must guide and usher in a new era of understanding about the true meaning of global health.

11

THE FUTURE OF AIDS RESEARCH: WHAT TO DO?

LUC MONTAGNIER
is the discoverer of the AIDS virus and Head of the AIDS andRetroviruses
Department at the Pasteur Institute. Professor Montagnier is also Cofounder of
the Foundation for AIDS Research and Prevention, Directeur de Recherche au
CNRS, and recipient of the Legion of Honor and the Albert Lasker Clinical
Medical Research Award.

THERE IS CLEAR EVIDENCE that the AIDS epidemic is evolving according to two patterns: one in the North, with a slow progression; one in the South, with a very fast progression.

In the North, most of the AIDS cases, and a significant portion of the new infections, are still restricted to the initial so-called "high-risk groups": homosexuals with multiple partners and intravenous (IV) drug abusers, with a trend toward an increase of heterosexual transmission to female partners (from bisexual men particularly).

In the South, in tropico-equatorial areas, although the virus infection might also have started in the same high-risk groups, it has spread very rapidly through some parts of the heterosexual population: female prostitutes and single men, particularly migrants.

Clearly, the transmission of the virus from men to women and from women to men is more efficient in these southern areas. I believe that several factors, both biological and socio-behavioral, can explain these differences and also shed some light on the origin of the epidemic.

BIOLOGICAL FACTORS

The Virus

HIV is a retrovirus that first was isolated in 1983 from a French homosexual man with persistent lymphadenopathy, a sign precursor of AIDS. Since then, it has been extensively confirmed that lymph nodes are the main site of continuous virus replication. The virus cannot fully replicate in its main target cells, T4 lymphocytes and monocytes, unless they are at least partly activated. Moreover, the number of activated cells the virus can infect in the first weeks of infection, before the immune defense of the host put it under incomplete control, determines the length of the incubation period: the greater the virus replication at this stage, the sooner the onset of the immune depression leading to clinical AIDS.

In a healthy individual living in northern countries, most of the cells of the immune system are at rest, and therefore the virus has some difficulties in finding its way to the few activated cells. The passage of intestinal bacteria through the gut mucosa probably continuously stimulates the lymphoid cells in the vicinity (Peyer patches). Airborne bacteria, not great in number in these countries, are easily controlled in lung broncho-alveolar mucosa by macrophages and neutrophils.

In human beings living in the tropico-equatorial areas, the situation is quite different. Here the concentration of airborne microorganisms is much higher. The immune system is continually stimulated by bacterial, parasitic, viral, or fungal infections, especially at the level of mucosas, which are the *"porte d'entrée"* of many germs.

A recent study on Ethiopian African immigrants indicates a large degree of immune activation due mostly to parasitic infections. Similarly, ongoing studies of West Africans indicate an elevated level of inflammatory cytokines (growth factors regulating activation of cells of the immune system).

The nature of infectious factors could, of course, vary from one individual to another and vary also among the various parts of the tropico-equatorial belt, but they all stimulate a systemic activation of the immune system, which makes such individuals more susceptible to HIV infection. This is, in my opinion, the main cofactor explaining the ease of heterosexual transmission in Africa and the Caribbean Islands, in parts of South America and in Southeast Asia.

In the North, some practices can also obviously activate the immune system: multiple IV injections, under doubtful sterile conditions, could produce silent bacterial infections, if not septicemia, in IV drug users. Moreover, high psychological stress can release some neural growth factors that can activate lymphocytes of the immune system *(R. levimontalcini)* through personal communication. Such high stress is common in IV drug users and in some homosexual men.

In the latter population, anal penetration has been shown by epidemiological studies to be a very high-risk practice for HIV infection: the ano-rectal mucosa is particularly permeable to the virus, and activated lymphoid cells of the intestinal gut are in proximity. Moreover, bacterial, fungal, and parasitic infections are more frequent in homosexuals with multiple partners. Perturbations of the immune system in homosexual men had been described before the spread of HIV in European and North American gay men. Hemophiliacs also were exposed in the 1980s to abnormal immune activation, through frequent injections of highly impure preparations of antihemophilic factors (VIII and IX). These preparations contained a lot of more or less denatured plasma proteins accompanied by filterable bacteria or viruses, which can stimulate the immune system. The use of highly pure preparations of factor VIII since 1988 has almost completely suppressed this activation and sometimes was sufficient to restore to normal the T4 lymphocyte counts in HIV-infected hemophiliacs.

Local Genital Infections

Before the virus gets to lymph nodes, it has to intrude into a weak point of the organism–not the intact skin, which is protected by multiple layers of keratinized cells. This occurs, rather, in mucosas exposed to fluids containing the virus: sperm, vaginal secretions, and blood.

The oral mucosa is particularly fragile and exposed to HIV in newborns. This explains why newborns are so easily infected by the virus of their mothers during birth or after birth (by breast-feeding).

We have already mentioned the ano-rectal mucosa as highly permeable to the virus. The vaginal or urethral mucosas are more protective and make difficult the heterosexual transmission of HIV unless there are associated disruptive infections. Genital ulcers (caused by syphilis or herpes) increase the risk of HIV transmission to women and from women. Vaginal candidosis, a very common and often undetected and untreated fungal infection, is also a risk factor. Some silent infections of the cervical mucosa by papilloma virus, as well as mycoplasma infections, also are likely to increase the risk of transmission. It should be added that vaginal mucosa is more fragile in very young girls and in women after the menopause.

BEHAVIORAL FACTORS

As with other sexually transmitted diseases, increasing the number of sexual partners will favor the spread of AIDS in a given population. In tropico-equatorial areas young female prostitutes are good candidates for the virus. Prostitutes of the North, who are educated to avoid sexually transmitted diseases, are less at risk, except for those who also are IV drug users. A high percentage of the latter have been infected with HIV.

Another high-risk group in the South are single men, especially those who have migrated to large cities in quest of work and become clients of infected prostitutes.

In Thailand, it is a common practice in poor families to send young girls to serve as prostitutes in brothels in big cities, such as Bangkok. Many of these girls, when it is found that they are infected with HIV, are sent back to their villages, where they infect their husband and children.

Thus the spread of AIDS is promoted by the presence of four main factors:

> HIV – Human Immunodeficiency Virus
> HIS – Hyper Immunostimulation
> STD – Sexually Transmitted Disease
> MPS – Multiple-Partner Sex

The equation then reads:

> AIDS epidemic = HIV + HIS + STD + MPS

The last two factors, STD and MPS, are, of course, somewhat correlated. Sexually promiscuous individuals naturally are more at risk to contact a sexually transmitted disease. In some countries all four factors are present: Thailand, India (large cities), Ivory Coast (Abidjan), Zaire (Kinshasa), and Eastern Africa (Ethiopia to the north of South Africa).

The economic and sociocultural dependence of young girls and women also favors their infection in some of these countries.

Conversely, all four factors are not present in northern countries nor in many rural areas of the tropico-equatorial area. Therefore, it is inaccurate to consider AIDS a pandemic. Its progress is almost neutralized in developed countries due to the difficulty of HIV spreading to the general population by heterosexual transmission and thanks also to prevention campaigns in these countries. Even in the South, only a few countries meet the conditions for an explosion in targeted populations (female low-standard prostitutes, migrant single men, women depending on promiscuous men).

THE COFACTORS OF AIDS PROGRESSION

Once HIV is established in an organism (for example, it is easily transmitted to the brain through infected macrophages), a period of complex interaction between the virus and the immune system begins. Initially, symptoms usually do not manifest, and only sophisticated laboratory blood studies or biopsy specimens can tell the specialist that something is wrong. There is a progressive decline of the T4 lymphocytes, a key population that controls many immune functions, particularly those of the lymphocytes, whose function is to kill the infected cells. Current views insist on a fast turnover of the T4: The infected lymphocytes die of the infection or are killed by specific cytotoxic lymphocytes, and the released virus infects freshly activated lymphocytes. Since in each virus replication cycle the first step (reverse transcription of the viral RNA into DNA) is achieved by an enzyme prone to make many copying errors, the mutation rate is enormous (1 in 104 nucleotides). This allows the virus to escape the neutralizing antibodies produced by the immune system and also to become rapidly resistant to any viral inhibitor. This is the chief reason for the lack of success of chemotherapy in curing the disease and of vaccines in preventing the infection.

The destruction of the immune cells is amplified by some indirect mechanisms: more cells die than cells actually infected by the virus. An oxidative stress occurs, generated by the chronic virus infection itself and amplified by susceptibility to other infections caused by the immune depression (so-called opportunistic infections). Highly reactive oxygen molecules (free radicals) will, in turn, activate the virus in cells latently infected and cause damage to the main cellular components

(DNA, protein, lipids). The cytokine network is also highly disturbed.

Thus a vicious cycle is established, that can only be broken by a global therapeutic approach (see below). It appears that a hyperactivation of the immune system by infection cofactors will also accelerate the evolution toward full-blown AIDS by creating more targets in the virus, and by increasing the oxidative stress.

Thus the very same factors that favor HIV transmission could also accelerate progression to the disease after HIV infection.

The median time between HIV primary infection and AIDS is a little more than 10 years for a cohort of North American homosexual men. It is probably less in Africans and Southeast Asians. In these regions, tuberculosis, an airborne infection, is highly prevalent.

Tuberculosis progression increases due to immune depression induced by HIV, and in turn it accelerates the progress of the HIV infection (oxidative stress, activation of lymphocytes and macrophages by bacterial antigens).

The risks of a renewed tuberculosis epidemic, therefore, are high: a secondary event that could follow the HIV epidemic, making the situation even more critical.

What To Do?

Without intervention, the AIDS epidemic will badly hit some developing countries at the economical level, leading to political destabilization. It is estimated that 1 million seropositive persons exist in Thailand and along the Ivory Coast and 4 million in India. Similar numbers may be seen in the next decade in Burma, Malaysia, South China, and part of South Africa. According to WHO, 40 million persons will be infected by the year 2000, in addition to the millions already affected by AIDS. This will amount to an almost uncontrolled reservoir of HIV, giving rise to an unlimited number of variants, and a still more enormous reservoir for many infectious agents, already difficult to deal with at present. Clearly, our reaction must be commensurate with the score of this threat.

How?

1. To prevent HIV transmission we must simultaneously address the four factors:

> **a)** HIV: Vaccines are likely to be partly effective. We are not far from developing vaccines that will be protective for a short period of time (one year) against some of the main viral strains now prevalent. However, this protection will probably not be effective for all of the vaccinated population and will allow for the emergence of new variants.

We should therefore expect only a partial and long-term effect of such vaccinations.

b) HIS: The possibility of direct and massive intervention against this factor does exist, but this requires from governments vigorous health policies that so far have not been implemented. We have the medical means to decrease many infections affecting the immune system in tropico-equatorial areas: vaccines and antibiotics. Also, education campaigns and efforts to hygienically improve living conditions are highly advisable.

Will governments (*or* policymakers) understand the imperative need for such policies?

c) STD and MPS: Prevention campaigns against STD (promotion of the use of condoms) already have been successful in Thailand, decreasing the number of cases of classical STD by a factor of ten in ten years. However, more education efforts targeted to high-risk groups (prostitutes, very young girls and boys) are still needed. Information on silent genital infections should be given to medical doctors and young men and girls. Changes in behavior (to decrease sexual promiscuity) should be promoted at the secondary school level.

All of these efforts would require educational structures that are often lacking in poor developing countries.

2. To treat HIV disease: 90 to 95 percent of HIV-infected persons will eventually die of AIDS if they are not treated. The task is thus enormous, and classical medical structures will not be able to cope with millions of patients suffering from opportunistic infections.

Thus, I am proposing an early and global therapeutic intervention in asymptomatic HIV-infected individuals. This could best be carried out in clinical consultation centers equipped with special laboratories, prepared to regularly and comprehensively analyze blood samples for markers of the infection. Treatment should include association of several antiviral inhibitors (to reduce the risk of viral resistance), the use of broad-spectrum antibiotics, and the use of antioxidants and cytokines to restore the capacities of the immune system.

The aim of such centers would be first to stabilize the HIV infection in bringing it down to a level tolerable by the immune system. Eventual eradication of the HIV infection after a certain period of continuous treatment could be achieved.

The Foundation for AIDS Research and Prevention, created by Federico Mayor and myself, intends to create four pilot centers that will function according to these concepts, in regions of the world particularly affected by HIV infection. If successful, these centers could be the models for a world network of such centers, designed to efficiently combat the disease.

More than a century ago, Louis Pasteur and his disciples set up Pasteur Institutes in the Far East and in Africa to fight the diseases of their time. Our projects are following the line of this general approach, in responding to the challenges of new infectious diseases.

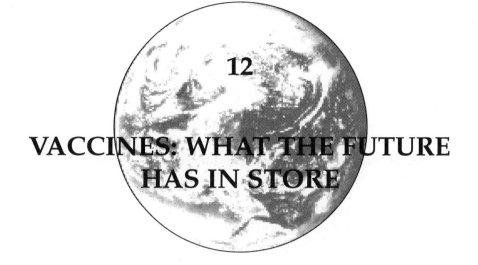

VACCINES: WHAT THE FUTURE HAS IN STORE

12

JONAS SALK
is the Founder of the Salk Institute for Biological Studies. Today, the Institute,
with a support staff and research facility of more than 500, is at the forefront
in the advancement of knowledge of the complex biological systems, including
the genetic system, the immune system and the brain. Dr. Salk developed the first
effective vaccine against polio. In 1986, he initiated the development of a strategy
for studying the prospects for the immunologic control of HIV infection and
AIDS. With the collaboration of several research groups internationally, he is now
coordinating studies to develop a method of immunization using a killed virus
preparation in investigating the prospects for the control of HIV infection before
disease develops and to prevent infection and/or disease in those not yet
infected. He has recently received FDA approval to launch the largest trial
yet of an AIDS vaccine for people infected with HIV.

UNTIL RELATIVELY RECENTLY, we thought the use of vaccines was for the purpose of preventing infectious diseases by stimulating the immune system to form appropriate antibodies or cells to counter the infectious agents. Vaccines have been developed against approximately 28 infectious diseases caused by viruses, bacteria, and their toxins.

Now, at scientific meetings dealing with vaccines, we learn not only about challenges for the development of combinations of preventative vaccines, but also about vaccines to be administered after infection to prevent the development of diseases, such as those that slow or arrest the progress of herpes and HIV infections. Vaccines also are being developed for the treatment of cancer, as well as the prevention of parasitic diseases, such as malaria and other tropical diseases, using sophisticated means for their design and delivery. All of this points to major evolutionary changes in the prospect for control of various pathogens, using the immune system either for the prevention, the arresting, or the reversing of the progression to disease. We hear also about anticholesterol vaccines for the prevention of arteriosclerosis and about the use of vaccines against autoimmune diseases, such as multiple sclerosis.

Thus, we have come a long way in recent years from the days when we were powerless against microbes or other causes of malfunctioning of the human organism. With the new science and advancement of technology, there will be available a more rapid expansion of the armamentarium for physicians and public health officials, influencing not only the prevention of the diseases of early childhood and of later life but prospects for the treatment of diseases amenable to immune-based therapies and for improved health and greater longevity as well.

This broadened perspective about vaccines reflects what the future may have in store as we become more aware of the further potential of advances in science and technology to change the human future in many different ways. The degree of success that will be achieved will be determined not only as a result of advances in these scientific pursuits but by the development of ways and means to apply them

Editor's Note: Dr. Salk died as *One World* was going to press. This was one of the last pieces he wrote. The editor would like to record here his indebtedness to Dr. Salk, not only for his many contributions to humankind but for the kindness Dr. Salk showed the editor as a young medical student working in his laboratory.

more widely for human use and to bring such benefits to all and not only to the more affluent. The development of appropriate socioeconomic and political systems will be needed to make this possible.

Hence, as we look into the future and consider what now can be accomplished, we realize the great potential of the knowledge we possess and the need for the wisdom with which to put that knowledge to use. It is important to emphasize the need for wisdom, in view of the fact that we have long had at our disposal vaccines that have not yet been used to their full potential. Therefore, it is necessary, in order to take advantage of the possibilities that exist, to turn our attention to how this might be achieved.

HOW VACCINES WORK

It has been shown that infectious agents of which humans are the exclusive reservoir can be eliminated by vaccination. This has been demonstrated for smallpox and will soon be achieved for poliomyelitis. Still, for such diseases as tetanus and diphtheria, and for the infectious agents that reside in nonhuman reservoirs, the continuing use of vaccines will be required. It will become increasingly possible to simplify immunization procedures by the inclusion in a single vaccine of many more antigens than has yet been administered together. This is now technically feasible and is scientifically sound. The efficiency and effectiveness of immunization procedures will improve as the number of antigens per vaccine are increased. We are entering a new era in the wider use of available vaccines, and new ones are in development for the future.

Until fifty years ago, it was presumed necessary for infection to be present for induction of immunity to virus diseases because noninfectious viral vaccines had, until then, been effective. When it was possible to provide sufficient quantities of antigen by propagation of virus in a developing chick embryo, or in tissue culture, it became possible to develop effective noninfectious viral vaccines. Still, attenuated infectious virus vaccines continue to be developed and used since it is still presumed that immunity induced by infection is more lasting than that induced with a noninfectious form of the virus. At last, the principles have been discovered by which lasting immunity can be induced with noninfectious vaccines as well, providing the basis for immunization without inducing infection.

In addition, in recent years advances have been made in using bimolecular approaches to developing protective antigens for use in such vaccines. These include recombinant DNA technology and synthetic antigens, as well as improvements in large-scale cultivation of viruses in continuously propagating cells for making noninfectious vaccines. The use of these approaches is based upon the knowledge that the infectious core of the virus is not needed in order to achieve effective and durable protection and that such protection can be induced by presenting to the immune system a sufficient quantity of the protective antigen in the appropriate form.

Whether the requirement is for antibody-mediated or for cell-mediated immunity, the induction of immunologic memory will be required for long-term persistence of protective effects. Vaccines will contain combinations of antigens for inducing simultaneous protection against a widening spectrum of infectious and parasitic diseases, of humans and of animals, for which either antibody-mediated or cell-mediated immunologic memory is needed.

The inclusion of multiple antigens in a single inoculum is also made possible by the use of more potent immunopotentiators. These have the advantage of reducing the amount of antigen required to immunize; permitting the inclusion of many more antigens in a single vaccine; enhancing the degree and duration of the immune response; and reducing the number of doses required for immunization.

Hence, it is likely that, in the course of the next century, many more diseases will be controlled by vaccination. The future has in store great promise. The challenge to take advantage of the opportunity that lies ahead will be met by the generations to come.

13

PROBLEMS INTRODUCING A
NEW MEDICAL FIELD

LINUS PAULING
first won international acclaim for his research into the physical configuration of
amino acids. This was material in earning him the Nobel Prize in Chemistry in
1954. Dr. Pauling also won the 1962 Nobel Peace Prize for his efforts on behalf
of a nuclear test ban treaty. More recently, he became known for his theory
that massive dosages of vitamin C can prevent and cure the common cold.

DURING THE LAST FIFTY YEARS I have devoted an increasing amount of effort to medical research and to the study of the health-care system in the United States. The main conclusion that I have reached is that the people of the United States remain in poor health because of two defects in the system. These two defects are the high cost of the process of approval from the U.S. Food and Drug Administration (FDA) of a new drug or treatment and the existence of bias against some kinds of treatment.

The cost of developing a new drug and gathering the information required for a successful application for FDA approval may be more than $100 million. I believe that great care should be taken in the effort to ensure that a new drug or therapy does not have dangerous side effects, and I support the FDA in most of its actions. The FDA should, however, recognize that some innovative treatments require special consideration.

One common situation is that of a treatment that cannot be patented or that for some other reason cannot be profitable to any company that might make an application to the FDA. A well-known example is lithium carbonate, which now constitutes the usual treatment of patients with manic-depression. There was a 20-year delay in the use of this substance in the United States because no pharmaceutical company could afford to spend the large amount of money required to win FDA approval when the substance could be obtained at a low price from any one of many sources.

Another example is intravenous EDTA chelation therapy for prophylaxis or treatment of cardiovascular disease or other problems. About 2 million individual infusions have been given to about 150,000 patients for these purposes, sometimes as an alternative to bypass surgery, mainly by physicians who have a special interest in innovative methods of improving health. Some years ago I asked a number of physicians about EDTA chelation and usually received the answer that the procedure was not approved by the FDA. In fact, the method of administering EDTA was approved by the FDA, but only for heavy-metal poisoning (lead, mercury, and cadmium) detoxification. It was not approved for other purposes because no one

Editor's Note: Dr. Pauling died in August of 1994. The Editor would like to thank Dorothy Munro, Secretary and Assistant to Linus Pauling, for her assistance with the final manuscript.

had made application to the FDA. The pharmaceutical firm that owned the U.S. patent rights to EDTA decided that the patent would expire so soon (seven years) that the income from sales would be less than the cost of winning FDA approval, and, of course, no other company could profit from applying for FDA approval.

For years, physicians and medical authorities showed a bias against EDTA chelation that was based on ignorance and misunderstanding of the sort just mentioned. If EDTA had been an ordinary drug marketed in the ordinary way, this bias would have been dispelled by the information in advertisements published by the company in medical journals.

Bias, based upon misinformation and misunderstanding, was especially significant in hampering the acceptance of vitamin supplements in the amounts required for optimum health. The idea that vitamins taken in small amounts as their only valid use to prevent those diseases incurred by their corresponding deficiencies lingered on for years despite the great amount of evidence to the contrary. Several years ago I shared an hour on a radio program devoted to vitamins and health with a retired university professor of biochemistry and nutrition. Our statements differed. Near the end of the hour, he said, "For 50 years I and other distinguished authorities have said that 60 mg of vitamin C is all that anyone needs." I then said, "That is the problem–you are 50 years behind the times; you don't know what has been discovered in recent years."

This bias against vitamins was shown also by the editors of the leading medical journals. In my book *Vitamin C and the Common Cold* I mentioned a physician from Johns Hopkins University who discovered that very large doses of vitamin C were effective in suppressing the signs and symptoms of the common cold and preventing the secondary bacterial complications in 95 percent of his patients. He wrote an article about his observations and submitted it, in succession, to 11 professional journals, every one of which rejected it.

One result of the failure of the major medical journals to accept papers dealing with new medical areas is that the papers must be published in journals that are not abstracted and indexed in the usual way. The usual processes of retrieval are then unsuccessful, and future investigators remain ignorant of the existence of the work.

My own experience has been mainly with vitamins and other orthomolecular substances. I shall emphasize this field in the remainder of this chapter. Orthomolecular medicine–a term I invented in 1968 to describe the new field of medicine–is the achievement and preservation of the best of health, and the prevention and treatment of disease by varying the concentrations in the human body of substances normally present in the body that are required for health. The vitamins are good examples of substances of this sort, but there are a great many other orthomolecular substances also required for life that for one reason or another are not classified as vitamins (one reason being that the substances are synthesized in the body).

As a result of reading a paper on the treatment of acute schizophrenics with large doses of nicotinic acid or nicotinamide, I was impressed by the fact that vitamins differ greatly from ordinary drugs in respect to the range of concentrations over which they have important physiological activity. Drugs are usually administered in doses to the seriously toxic or lethal levels. Conversely, a few milligrams per day of niacin is enough to prevent death from pellagra in most people, and a few milligrams a day of ascorbic acid is enough to prevent death from scurvy. Yet these vitamins are so lacking in toxicity that 10,000 times as much can be taken in one day without serious side effects, and the danger of death from an overdose of vitamins is almost nonexistent. The fact that vitamins are physiologically active over a tolerated range of hundreds or thousands of times their usual bodily concentrations caused me to raise the question as to the optimum daily intake of vitamins, the intake that leads to the best of health. The conclusion I have reached is that for people in what is called ordinary good health, the optimum intake of vitamin C may well be 100 or 200 times the RDA (the recommended dietary allowance set by the Food and Nutrition Board of the National Academy of Sciences–National Research Council, United States); that for each of the various B vitamins, except folic acid, it may be 25 or 50 times the RDA; that for vitamin E it may be 50 or 100 times the RDA; and that for vitamin A it may be ten times the RDA. People who are seriously ill may benefit from considerably larger amounts taken over long periods or by much larger amounts taken for a brief period of time.

My introduction into this field in the late 1960s was by way of the orthomolecular and megavitamin treatment (the use of vitamins in larger intakes than usual to treat disease) of mental disease, and it came at the end of a ten-year period during which my associates at the California Institute of Technology and I had studied the molecular basis of mental illness, especially mental retardation and schizophrenia. Several years later I assisted a psychiatrist, Dr. David Hawkins, in editing a book on various aspects of the subject.

Orthomolecular and megavitamin treatment of schizophrenia was then vigorously attacked in a report by the task force of the American Psychiatric Association. This report seemed to a number of psychiatrists to be not only biased but also thoroughly unreliable, and several criticisms of it have been published.

In 1970, my book *Vitamin C and the Common Cold* was published. The biochemist Irwin Stone had sent me copies of his papers about the optimum intake of vitamin C, published in 1966 and 1967, and, after checking his arguments and reading some pertinent parts of the medical literature, I had increased my own daily intake of vitamin C from the RDA, then 50 mg per day, to a value 60 times as great– 3000 mg per day. I observed an immediate striking decrease in the amount of illness due to respiratory infections I previously had suffered, and also what seemed to be apparent improvement in my general health. My wife and other people in communication with me reported similar results. My public statement of these observations aroused the ire of a physician who challenged me to find in the medical literature any report of controlled studies showing that vitamin C has any more value than a placebo in controlling respiratory infections. I checked the medical literature and sent him copies of papers in which as much as a 63 percent decrease in the amount of illness from the common cold was reported to have been achieved by an intake of 1000 mg per day, as compared with a placebo.

When I discovered the physician was unwilling to discuss the evidence in a rational way, and also discovered that the medical and nutritional textbooks and reference books misrepresented the published studies, I decided to present the evidence about vitamin C and the common cold in a short book. Within one month of the book's publication, a thoroughly unfavorable review of it appeared in a publication on drugs and therapeutics for physicians. I wrote the editors a letter discussing the false and misleading statements in their review and asked them to publish it, but this was not done. In the meantime, other unfavorable reviews of the book had appeared, and reports reached me that most physicians were telling their patients that vitamin C had no value against the common cold or other diseases, except for scurvy.

For many years, the stand of the American Medical Association (AMA) was that vitamin C had no value in preventing or treating the common cold or any other disease. In 1975, the AMA issued a statement to the press with the heading "Vitamin C will not prevent or cure the common cold." The basis for this quite negative statement was said to be two papers just published in the *Journal of the American Medical Association (JAMA)*, which did not provide any sound basis for the statement that vitamin C will not prevent or cure the common cold. I at once prepared a thorough but brief analysis of 13 controlled trials and submitted it to *JAMA's* editor, who returned it to me twice with suggestions for minor revisions, which I made. Six months later, however, the editor decided to reject it.

I think it is quite improper for major medical journals, or any others, to follow the policy of publishing only those papers that support one side of a scientific or medical question or to interfere with the proper discussion of questions by holding papers that are submitted, during which period, according to accepted custom, the papers cannot be submitted elsewhere.

Another example of this sort of action also relates to vitamin C. A paper about the destruction by vitamin C of the vitamin B_{12} in foods was published in *JAMA* in 1974. The authors stated that after the addition of 1000 mg of vitamin C and subsequent laboratory treatment similar to the process involved in digestion in the stomach, as much as 95 percent of the meal was destroyed. Some readers of the article noticed that the reported amount of vitamin B_{12} in the food was only about one-eighth that given by the accepted food tables, and that the method of extracting vitamin B_{12} from the food used by these investigators was not the approved one. Upon repetition of the experiment using the approved method of analysis, it was found that very little vitamin B_{12} was, in fact, destroyed. When the investigators submitted their paper correcting the work to *JAMA*, it was held for six months and then rejected, thus delaying its publication in another journal and preventing many of the readers of the original article from learning that the results first reported were incorrect.

In my check of the literature about vitamin C I had read a number of papers, mainly written in the period around 1940, about the apparent value of vitamins C and A in the control of cancer. An account of an address I had made at the dedication of the new Ben May Laboratory for Cancer Research of Pritzker Medical School, University of Chicago, appeared in the *New York Times* and was read by Ewan Cameron, Chief Surgeon of Vale of Leven Hospital, Scotland. Dr. Cameron had for 20 years been trying to find some way of alleviating the suffering of cancer patients but had not found any new treatment that seemed to have value. He wrote me to ask how much vitamin C should be administered to terminal cancer patients. I replied, with mention of the supporting evidence, that 10 grams per day or more should be given. Dr. Cameron began cautiously with one patient, administering this amount of sodium ascorbate intravenously each day for ten days and then orally thereafter. The patients responded well, as did several other patients, and Dr. Cameron and his associates continued to administer vitamin C to patients in Vale of Leven Hospital and the adjacent hospitals near Glasgow.

Dr. Cameron reported that it initially had seemed to him quite ludicrous to suggest that vitamin C would have value against cancer. He has said, "Here was I, a conservative Scottish surgeon, surrounded by conservative Scottish people; we could not believe that this simple, cheap, harmless powder, which could be bought in any drugstore, could possibly have any value against such a bafflingly complex and resistant disease as cancer. But the solid logic of the arguments persisted, the idea continued to make sense, together with the general idea that a high intake of vitamin C might make all of the body's natural protective mechanisms more effective, and, since vitamin C would not do harm to the patient, it seemed worth a try."

By 1973, Dr. Cameron and his associates had treated 50 "untreatable" cancer patients with vitamin C. The possible value of ascorbic acid in controlling cancer by protecting and strengthening the intracellular cement in normal tissues had been recognized by this time, and Dr. Cameron and I prepared a paper on the topic. As a member of the National Academy of Sciences, USA, I sent this paper to the *Proceedings of the National Academy of Sciences (PNAS)* for publication. The paper was rejected, though, despite the fact that members of the academy in general had the right to publish their papers in *PNAS* without editorial review; in the 60 years of existence of this journal no other paper submitted by a member had been refused publication. Enough progress in the attitude toward vitamins had been made by 1976, though, for a later paper by Dr. Cameron and me on supplementary vitamin C in the supportive treatment of cancer to be published in *PNAS,* and a second paper on survival time was also published in that journal two years later.

There is now clear evidence that far larger intakes of orthomolecular substances than usual may have great value in the control of cancer and other diseases. Over a period of ten years, R. F. Cathcart had treated about 10,000 patients with vitamin C, sometimes, but not always, together with conventional therapy. He has pointed out, supporting an earlier observation by Dr. Cameron, that the amount of this vitamin taken by mouth and tolerated by the gastrointestinal tract is far larger for a seriously ill person than for a well person. An intake of 10 to 20 grams per day by a person in ordinary health may have some laxative effect, with a larger amount having a still stronger laxative effect. Some seriously ill persons with viral infections, such as mononucleosis, viral pneumonia, and hepatitis, may have to take as much as 200 grams per day to achieve the laxative effect. The dose then needs to be decreased as the patient recovers from the disease. Cathcart has said that "you can't treat a 100-g-per-day cold by taking one gram of the vitamin." The common cold and other infections can be controlled by vitamin C, but the amount needed varies from person to person and from infection to infection.

The official attitude not only of editors of medical and scientific journals but also of agencies such as the National Cancer Institute (NCI) has changed over the years. In 1973, the NCI rejected out of hand the suggestion that I made, on the basis of Dr. Cameron's experience with the first 40 terminal cancer patients to be treated with large daily amounts of vitamin C, that the institute set up a randomized, double-blind, controlled trial of the value of vitamin C in relation to cancer. In the early 1980s, a decade later, the NCI began to support studies of vitamin C and other vitamins, especially vitamin A, in relation to cancer.

One of the problems in introducing orthomolecular medicine to the medical profession and to the public was that there was a great amount of misrepresentation about the toxicity of vitamins. This emphasis on toxicity and possible harmful side effects from intakes of the vitamins larger than the recommended dietary amounts was found both in articles in the popular press and in some scientific and medical journals, and it probably represented a bias based upon a lack of knowledge, especially about recent investigations. An example is provided by an episode occurring some years ago when a small boy swallowed all of the contents of a bottle of vitamin A and began to suffer nausea and headache. He was taken to the hospital, treated, and was then released. The physicians prepared an account of the episode for a medical journal, and news stories about this poisoning by vitamin A were published in the *New York Times* and hundreds of other newspapers. Every day someone dies of aspirin poisoning, but no newspaper stories about the deaths are printed. When a small boy becomes sick enough from eating a large number of vitamin A tablets to require treatment in a hospital, however, the physicians themselves and the newspapers consider the fact worthy of publication.

A great amount of work still remains to be done on the general problem of getting information basic to orthomolecular medicine. What are the optimum concentrations of orthomolecular substances in the body fluids? What are the optimum intakes of the various vitamins?

Evidence about the optimum intakes of various vitamins is provided from several sources. One indication that the optimum intake of vitamin C is about 200 times the RDA comes from a unique characteristic of this vitamin. Whereas the other vitamins are required from an outside source by all species of animals, vitamin C is required exogenously only by humans and the other primates and a few other species. The overwhelming number of animal species manufacture ascorbic acid in their own organs, the liver for mammals and the kidneys for birds. They all manufacture rather large amounts of the substance. An animal the size of a human manufactures about 10,000 mg ascorbic acid per day, with other animals manufacturing similar amounts, proportional to their body weights. It has been argued that the biochemistry of human beings is closely similar to that of other animals, that other animals manufacture this large amount of vitamin C every day because it puts them in better condition than a smaller amount would, and that, accordingly, the optimum intake for a human being is in the neighborhood of 10,000 mg per day. A related argument is that investigators who use monkeys in their work have carefully studied the question of how much vitamin C needs to be given to the monkeys in order to keep them in the best of health and have concluded that they should be given about 70 times the RDA for humans. Epidemiological studies have provided some support for the assumption that a high intake of vitamin C decreases mortality. Very large amounts of vitamin C, up to 200 grams per day, have been reported to cure viral diseases, such as mononucleosis, hepatitis, and viral pneumonia. The value of vitamin C in amounts of 10 grams per day or more, as an adjunct to appropriate, conventional therapy in the treatment of patients with cancer, has been reported by several investigators.

There is evidence that a high intake of beta-carotene, a precursor of vitamin A, has value in decreasing the mortality from coronary heart disease and also that vitamin C has some value in this respect. Statistical studies have shown that the mortality from heart disease increases with the increase in the total cholesterol in the blood and decreases with the level of high-density lipoprotein cholesterol. An increased intake of vitamin C has been shown to decrease the total cholesterol level and to increase the level of high-density lipoprotein cholesterol, each of these changes being favorable when correlated with heart disease.

Several troublesome conditions have been found to be controlled by an intake of about 25 times the RDA of vitamin B₆ per day. One of these conditions is carpal tunnel syndrome, for which previously there had been no treatment other than surgery to relieve the pressure on the nerve in the wrist. Another condition controlled by a high intake of vitamin B₆ is gestational diabetes, which troubles some pregnant women. The abnormality in tryptophan metabolism resulting from the use of the pill to prevent conception is also rectified by this amount of vitamin B₆.

Because of their remarkable low toxicity, vitamins should be considered as a class of substances different from drugs, which in general have high toxicity and often are prescribed in doses close to the lethal level. The water-soluble vitamins are especially innocuous. A number of years ago it was reported that persons who has taken between 1,000 and 3,000 times the RDA for months or years had developed some peripheral neurological damage, with diminished sensation in the feet and some interference with walking. There was no central nervous system damage, however, and when the intake of pyridoxine was stopped, the peripheral neurological damage disappeared. It is evident that the upper limit of regular intake of vitamin B₆ is 1,000 times the RDA, that is, 2000 mg per day. Other investigators have reported that the long-term intake of somewhat smaller amounts, 200 to 800 mg per day, has not revealed any toxic effects.

As people age, their physiological activity decreases–their enzyme activity in particular–perhaps in part because of a decreased intake of vitamins, associated with a deterioration in the appetite. The possibility of improving the health of the aging population through an increased intake of vitamins may be especially great, but it is also likely that younger people, too, can benefit by improved nutrition through the use of vitamin supplements. Highly reputable scientists and conventional physicians have begun to join alternative health practitioners to expand and legitimize the field of nutritional medicine. Recent epidemiological studies now indicate that vitamin C intake does have an overall positive effect in reducing mortality from degenerative diseases, such as cancer and atherosclerosis, and extending life span. Abram Hoffer's reported success in using megavitamin therapy in patients with advanced cancer demonstrates experimental validity for prescribing nutritional regimens in the life-threatening diseases, including multiple sclerosis, amyotrophic lateral sclerosis, and HIV/AIDS. It may turn out that the greatest contribution to public health made during the past few decades has been the recognition of the value of vitamins ingested at the optimum intake levels.

14

MEDICINE NEGATED

CHRISTIAAN BARNARD,
Emeritus Professor of Surgical Science at the University of Cape Town, was the
first surgeon to perform a successful human heart transplant. Dr. Barnard's pio-
neering heart transplant operation took place at the Groote Schuur Hospital in
South Africa in 1967. Medical applications of transplantation have increased
significantly since that time. To date, almost half a million patients
worldwide have received life-sustaining organ transplants.

WORLD POPULATION MAY REACH 6 billion by the turn of the century, and may double again in the twenty-first century, when 60 to 80 percent of the population will live in Third World countries.

At present, more than 400 million people in the world are suffering from malnutrition. If population trends continue as expected, this figure will increase dramatically. In general, U.N. projections paint a frightening picture: a world situation of economic, political, and social disorder in which the figures for hunger, disease, and death from starvation continue to rise. So disastrous is the prospect that many authorities have evoked the lifeboat image and seriously suggested that an overloaded planet can no longer afford the luxury of untrammelled humanitarianism.

In the meantime, health budgets worldwide continue to climb as the cost of medical training, hospitals, and high-technology medicine rises beyond the pocket of the ordinary man. World health projects on the scale envisaged to cope with even basic Third World problems are stalled for lack of funds.

In Pakistan, peasant corn is used to produce a corn sweetener for soft drinks. In Mexico, asparagus is grown by the acre for export to American restaurants. Throughout the Third World, mothers are encouraged by advertising campaigns that urge supplementary feeding to doubt their ability to breast-feed their children. Promotion of commercial baby foods continues in the face of evidence that such practices can lead to loss of breast milk and complete dependence on supplementary feeding. Thus, peasant mothers, who are either unable or unwilling to sterilize bottles or even to calculate the correct amount of formula to use, are buying the full amount of baby food required. The result is an increase in disease, malnutrition, and, inevitably, the infant mortality rate.

Once, after a visit to what is politely referred to as a developing country, I had occasion to pass through the country's major airport–a concrete, chrome and glass extravaganza. I noticed that most of the air-conditioning units had already stopped functioning and about half of the still-gleaming luggage trolleys had lost their wheels. My briefcase was packed with copies of research papers that had been delivered at a conference held in that country. They detailed, among other things, the differences in illnesses suffered by the affluent and the poor, industrial workers and peasants, the white Westerner and the black tribesman. They spelled out quite clearly that health is largely a matter of life-style, and that the life-style of an individual is largely determined by the ruling ideology. Choice did operate, but only within certain limits.

Among other outcomes of an inequitable society, disease, injuries, and malnutrition among infants and children bring crippling costs. These are not reflected directly in the budget, though we could point to the incredibly expensive intensive care required to nurse a single child back to a healthy condition. Possibly of more importance in the long term is the cultural deprivation and latent brain damage suffered as a direct result of disease processes. Once they have been psychologically and physically maimed, the cost of maintaining individuals so damaged throughout adulthood is an ongoing national expense. In contrast, the cost of attacking malnutrition and childhood diseases at their source is minimal. Medicine is negated each time we fail to drive that point home to the administrators and the budget makers.

Where does the medical profession fit into this global misdirection of effort? Medicine, too, has followed the pattern of "bigger is better," its real function being obscured under its fixation on the space-age technology of the twentieth century. The antibiotics, products of high technology and massive capital input and once hailed as a universal panacea, have not made possible a brave new world but rather a more disease-resistant old one in which it costs a lot more to be ill. The infant mortality rate of some Third World countries is on the increase, and even that of many so-called developed countries have shown no real positive change for some time.

Apart from our pat solution to clinical problems, a form of automated medicine, we have also lost our medical souls in terms of specialization. For that we have to thank the modern industrial model, where each individual has specialized to the point of lunacy: one mechanic fixes your car, another fixes your ulcers, a third your heart, a fourth your head, and so on. Your mind is the province of yet another expert who will de-coke you and restore you to mental health so that you can be sent back to the production line. And while the experts are doing all this, the figures for stress diseases, divorce, suicide, crime, and all the other indicators of a very sick society are climbing. So-called neutral technology continues to add more and more complications, more and more divisions of labor, more and more calls for growth and consumption, and more and more soulless ways of earning a living.

Medicine's place in all this is a bit like cleaning the Augean stables. We keep on wiping the floor without turning off the tap. Ideologies, social systems, and economic theories-all of which we consider to be beyond our legitimate ken–produce the disease processes we are fighting.

In my own country, it is only very recently that doctors took note of their responsibility for the diseases of the body politic and joined in an affirmation of the need to guide social forces in positive directions.

The acknowledged trend in medicine in South Africa over the past decade is toward preventive rather than curative work. Doctors hope to move away from the era of gigantic disease palaces, staffed by thousands and stuffed with millions of dollars of expensive diagnostic equipment, to a society that follows the basic health rules. It is not a new idea. The Old Testament prophets harangued the Israelites on the dangers of living in low-lying hollows and of eating suspect forms of food.

Nearer our own time, a man called Thomas Crapper made what was probably the largest stride in terms of preventive health measures in London in the last century when he developed the flush toilet. Possibly one of the few persons who really appreciated his gift to mankind was Queen Victoria, who knighted him. Sir Thomas Crapper, whose name still lives on evocatively in the English language, was not a doctor—he was a plumber. Before that, it was an English ironmonger who noticed the power in steam and used it to work a pump. His crude steam engines, used to drain seepage from the coal pits, made life more bearable for nineteenth-century miners. The pump also operated the piped water systems of the great cities of Europe, which did much to wipe out the mass diseases so common in medieval times.

Much later, it was a builder who first used plastic sheeting to damp-proof the foundations of modern mass housing. If all three gentlemen were assembled in one spot there would be a trio of worthy Nobel Prize winners, except that these prizes are seldom handed out for simple and straightforward effort.

It is a fanciful idea but worth pondering: a plumber, an ironmonger, and a bricklayer together did more for the human race than all the surgeons put together. It cuts down our loftier ideas about the practice of medicine to their proper proportions.

Apart from medicine's failure to concern itself with the steering of the boat, we negate our efforts in other ways. I have mentioned specialization and a preoccupation with technology. Related to this is the tendency toward heroic intervention—an officious striving to keep alive patients who have hope of little more than mere existence.

A televised report recently showed a home of congenitally disabled and retarded children. Many had been "stabilized" surgically. That is, through surgical intervention they had survived infancy and were now a charge on the nation. They had no hope of attaining anything beyond a meaningless existence chained to a hopelessly physically and mentally deficient body.

A generation ago, such children died at birth as a matter of course. Today's doctors, blinded to reality by technological gimmicks, sew, stitch, repair, intubate, pump, drip-feed, and intensively nurse these mindless cabbages in a travesty of medicine aimed as much at assuaging parental guilt and massaging professional pride as it is at humane considerations. Machines cannot give love. Life is more than air, and iron lungs can only give air. No sentient being can relate to intravenous feeding. Heart-lung apparatuses are hell on earth in the strict theological sense. Hell does not have to be a place of fire and brimstone; it is any place without love. And there can be no real love in a machine-supported life, despite the care and sense of duty of the nursing staff in institutions providing these treatments.

Anyone doing such work must be highly motivated, but motivation is not love. Love is warmth and touch and two-way communication. Anything else is sympathy. The television report showed children lying in babbling rows, mindlessly moving arms and legs, some incapable even of normal continence. They were awakened, cleaned, fed, dressed, exercised, lulled to sleep, and wakened again to begin another day of frustration and boredom. Even the mentally retarded can be bored, and boredom taken to infinity is torture indeed.

Perhaps there is a case for caging adults in life-support systems that keep them lingering between life and death, but medical practitioners should think hard before being a party to such situations. For example, there was strong political necessity for the teams of doctors who worked day and night shifts to keep Spain's General Franco "alive" until his successor was assured. In doing so they linked him to a respirator and kidney machine, dripped blood and sustenance into his veins, carried out three major abdominal operations, and successfully foiled several heart attacks. It is to be hoped that the old man, already in mental limbo, knew nothing of the assaults on his body.

President Tito was another who suffered medicine's final insult, and for the same reasons: the need to keep the national calm until another hand could be placed on the helm. In his late eighties, he was agonizingly held fast at death's door for weeks while daily bulletins were issued on his condition. If that be mercy, give me apathy.

Possibly the most horrifying example of the living-death syndrome is that of Karen Quinlan, a beautiful U.S. teenager who suffered brain damage from an overdose of drugs and alcohol. Skilled medical attention and prompt use of a respirator in the first few hours saved her from death by asphyxiation, but as time went on it became clear that Karen would never regain consciousness. Her parents–hope dwindling after daily visits to an unconscious form that was turned at intervals, pumped, tube-fed, and kept at constant temperature–at last requested the hospital to turn off the respirator. Unbelievably, the request was contested in court. Good sense won out, but the situation took on a tinge of the macabre when Karen continued to breathe without the respirator. A decade later, she continued to breathe. The difference was that the once beautiful teenager had become a shrunken skeleton, limbs fixed in the fetal position. A skilled nursing team worked around the clock, turning her body to prevent bedsores, tube-feeding her to stave off starvation, and, no doubt, treating her for infection as it occurred.

Sophisticated modern medicine has lost touch with the real needs of humanity.

Where once we sought to improve the quality of living for all, much effort is now spent on increasing the quantity of life for a few. The profit motive is not far away in these efforts. Hillary P. Ojiambo, a Kenyan professor of medicine, has told the *Kenyan Standard* that drug-dumping in the Third World is a major problem. A sizable proportion of the drug budget is spent on expensive drugs for use mainly in large, prestigious hospitals, at the expense of health care in poor rural areas. Because there are few, if any, pharmaceutical companies owned by developing countries, most of the drug budget is spent on buying the manufactured articles elsewhere.

In the Third World, most drug companies have a monopoly of information, as medical journals are few and far between. This means that doctors must rely on drug companies in order to keep up with the latest drug advances: in itself an undesirable situation. At the 1976 World Health Organization conference in Stockholm, the influence of medical technology was referred to as "psychic and cultural pollution." One delegate complained that our medical systems were not very well adapted to the healthy, let alone to the needs of the ill.

The Western habit of shrouding doctors with mystique has affected Third World medical practice. Patients accept medical advice as law, placing all responsibility of their own well-being on the shoulders of the doctors and ignoring the traditional concept of self-care.

In general, the technology of medicine has not been effective in coping with the major killers of mankind, such as malnutrition, heart disease and cancer. For example, the reduction of the incidence of tuberculosis in the developed world took place long before the drug advances of the 1940s. Medical intervention was not the decisive factor. More likely it was improved nutrition, housing, sewerage, and piped water that did the job. The efficacy of medical treatment has been doubted in many quarters: a commission of enquiry in the United States found that only 10 to 20 percent of treatment had been validated by the acid test of controlled trials.

For some countries, however, the problem with medicine is not technological but economic. Health costs are accelerating faster than income. For others, the crisis is the maldistribution of health resources, with the bulk of these being devoted to curative rather than preventive treatment. About half of health-care expenditure is devoted to people who will die within the next year. In addition, medical resources are concentrated in areas where health needs are lowest and, conversely, most sparse where death and disease are greatest.

Health is far too serious a matter to be left solely in the hands of the health professionals. The curative approach to health involves heavy expenditure on prestige hospitals. These massive institutions filled with sophisticated equipment are staffed by highly trained personnel whose expensive postgraduate training fits them to carry out costly research, but they are looking for trees while up to their eyes in wood. They provide a disease service rather than a health service; instead of promoting health, they try to displace the disease. Yet, in spite of the training and treasure poured out in the pursuit of this very laudable object, results have largely negated the practice of medicine as we in the West know it.

It wasn't the doctor who wiped out typhoid, it was the plumber. It wasn't the drug researcher who halted the advance of tuberculosis, it was the social planner who attacked poverty and overcrowding. Nor was it the pediatrician who cut the infant mortality rate, but more likely the school teacher and the district nurse. Few medical schools emphasize public health or social science subjects in their curricula. Most are heavily drug-oriented. What they do is to produce competent technicians who can recognize and treat a disease in isolation from its social context. I am not necessarily pointing a finger at any one country. We are all aware of examples in our own countries where the system produces the disease and the doctor makes it better, all at tremendous cost and with little alteration to the annual health figures.

The medical practitioner is on a merry-go-round. Today—more than four decades since the end of World War II—we continue our cycle of international interference, reading research papers, occasional breakthroughs in odd, obscure specialties, much trumpeting of scientific know-how and mutual backslapping. Yet we have not noticeably altered the world picture. More than 400 million people are dying right now of hunger and malnutrition. Millions more are suffering from a range of horrifying ills. In the crisis areas, one child in five will never see a second birthday.

We do not need more medical research to tell us what to do. It is staring us in the face.

It is time for a rethink, a spiritual and moral regeneration, and a realization that in the practice of advancing twentieth-century medicine we have negated its primary aim: a sociologically and physically healthy family of nations in which quality, rather than quantity, of life is the prime concern.

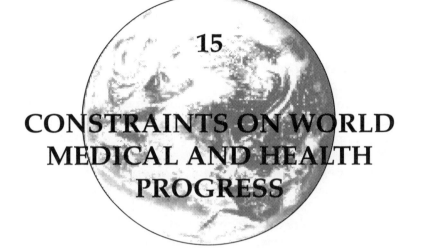

15

CONSTRAINTS ON WORLD MEDICAL AND HEALTH PROGRESS

T. ADEOYE LAMBO

has been Deputy Director-General of the World Health Organization since 1973. He was formerly Dean of the Medical Facility, Professor and Head of the Department of Psychiatry and Neurology, and Vice-Chancellor of the University of Ibadan, Nigeria. Dr. Lambo is the first President of the Scientific Council for Africa and in 1974 was appointed the first African Member of the Pontifical Academy of Science by His Holiness Pope Paul VI. He received the Nigerian Order of Merit and is a Commander of the Order of the Niger.

IN 1967, at the North American MENSA Meeting in Montreal, Canada, Buckminster Fuller, one of the great American scholars and philosophers, said:

> "Only one decade ago . . . it came so clearly into scientific view that leading world politicians could acknowledge it to be true, that for the first time in the history of man . . . there could be enough of the fundamental metabolic and mechanical energy sustenance for everybody to survive at high standards of living, . . . enough to take care of increasing population while also improving the comprehensive standards of living."

Since then, greater exponential growth and development of scientific knowledge has taken place, resulting in great advances in the medical and biological sciences. These have ranged from basic research at the molecular level to determine fundamental mechanisms of biological action through applied research and technological development with special reference to specific diseases and their control. It also includes the organization and management of health services whose ultimate goal is to provide adequate health care for individuals and the community.

In spite of these great advances, we have failed to improve man's position in the world and to place in the mosaic of our knowledge new ideas, concepts and intellectual achievements that could have made man's well-being the center of development in our time. The present world health situation is not only grave but it also has grossly deteriorated. More people today are hungry, sick, without shelter, unemployed, and illiterate than when revolutionary advances to erase all inequalities and the dearth of opportunities from the face of the earth were made.

Science and technology, directed, as they increasingly are, to enhancing military, economic, and political power, cannot by themselves upgrade the conditions of human life or solve the immediate problems of our society. The recent advances in medical science can be regarded with pride as one of the highest achievements of our century. However, improvements in health and the quality of life leave much to be desired. We face formidable challenges as the twenty-first century approaches. Good health continues to elude many, and this poses a challenge for humanity as crucial as that presented by slavery in the last century.

Why, then, do the goals of a good life, security, and equity seem ever more out of reach. It would seem that major constraints would have to be dealt with in order to guarantee better health, social equity, human freedom, and a quality of life characterized by full employment, housing, water and sanitation, education, access to good and low-cost medical care, and elimination of social and sexual discrimination. The twentieth century, which can be seen to be a century of major change and challenge, has brought in its wake many man-made problems–cultural, religious, psychosocial and economic–that continue to stand in the way to the attainment of these objectives.

The new philosophy and aim of the World Health Organization (WHO) emphasizes the need to generate new technology and new discoveries in medicine and to eradicate, or at least control, disease. In addition, it strongly stresses the need for society to expand its concept of health, for fostering potentialities, for growth and development, and for cultural innovation, irrespective of sex, while fostering a high quality of life. Recognition also is given to the needed technology and to desirable habitats. By these means, life can be materially and spiritually richer, more productive and rewarding. Let us recall the words of Sir Winston Churchill: "[Everyone is entitled to] a fair chance to make a home, to reap the fruits of their toil, to cherish their wives, to bring up their children in a decent manner and to dwell in peace and safety, without fear of bullying or monstrous burdens and exploitations. This is their heart's desire." This exemplifies the quality of life one would like to see achieved as a direct benefit of these advances. At the least, we should aim to reduce unnecessary human suffering and to promote human happiness as far as possible.

> "It is now clear that more than a decade of rapid growth in under-developed countries has been of little or no benefit to perhaps a third of their population. Although the average per capita income of the Third World has increased by 50 percent since 1960, this growth has been very unequally distributed among countries, regions within countries, and socio-economic groups. There are more poor and deprived people, especially in the developing countries, as well as groups of people who are more affluent and privileged than ever before. The gap is ever growing wider.
>
> "The crisis of development lies in the poverty of the masses of the Third World, as well as that of others, whose needs, even the most basic–food, habitat, health, education–are not met; it lies, in a large part of the world, in the alienation, whether in misery or in affluence, of the masses, deprived of the means to understand and master their social and political environment."

There are countries where rapid changes are wiping out the old and traditional ways while providing no valid or acceptable substitute; countries that now are confronted with a rising incidence and prevalence of psychosomatic diseases, mental disorders, anxiety and neurosis, prostitution, crimes, political corruption, and a variety of sexual diseases, including AIDS. The Social Breakdown Syndrome is characterized by the alienation of large segments of society and the depersonalization of individuals, with large groups of people living precariously on the periphery of society.

In 1957, at the Royal Society of Canada's Seventy-Fifth Anniversary Meeting, Professor Woodhouse of Toronto made a memorable statement: "Civilization requires to be defined in terms of the good life." According to him, education must extend its influence "from intellectual training, which is its center, to a refinement of sensibility–to the cultivation of understanding, imagination, sympathy and tolerance, and to the fostering of talent and of the kind of individuality that operates harmlessly and beneficially within the framework of a free society."

This is a new concept of total health and, to my mind, defines the true meaning of development manifested in the quality of life. We must continue to ask ourselves agonizing questions–questions concerning, for example, the lack of transfer of appropriate technology and the deterioration of the basic human values of dignity, equity, liberty, security, and social justice–questions concerning man's future, and his deeper needs. It no longer should be considered utopian to assess, plan, and be prepared for the problems of the future.

Sir James Goldsmith also asked the puzzling question. "How is it that humanity's great leap forward in material prosperity has resulted in extreme social breakdown, and that our greatest period of technological and scientific achievement has come to endanger conditions which allow life on earth? That is the extraordinary enigma which we must seek to understand."

In the perspective of these medical advances and achievements through scientific research and practice, our business in the world should be seen to be the provision of the best and most enduring of our human standards upon ourselves and our planet.

The enjoyment of the beauty and interest, freedom from want, freedom from extreme poverty, ignorance, and disease, the achievement of goodness and efficiency, the enhancement of life and its variety–these are the harvest that, as a result of this gigantic progress and medical scientific "quantum jump," our human uniqueness should be called upon to yield.

Man, today, is a victim of his own political, cultural, social, economic, ideological, and psychosocial constraints and his extreme prejudice, although he has at the same time become the sole representative of life in that progressive aspect and its sole trustee of any progress in science, the technology in the future. But he must release himself from this bondage, as Jean Jacques Rousseau has so aptly described in his writings.

What I am going to express in this chapter, I am sure, is not entirely new, but it has become more urgent; therefore, the best I hope to achieve is to restate the problem with a different emphasis and to highlight some of the contemporary critical issues associated with the need to overcome major constraints in our efforts to solve today's world ills, bitter and shattering social and health problems, through the application of new knowledge.

However, my approach will be unorthodox. I will be looking at the final product, man, instead of the classical approach of going into atomistic analysis of our modern medical and health system. It is health, resources, and development that must be focused upon.

Economic, cultural, psychological, and political constraints constitute major factors that impede our hopes for a better life, undermining our preventive and curative efforts to achieve it. There also are major social obstacles, such as the low status of women, coupled with a lack of education, in many developing countries.

The main question I would like to pose is: Can a modern medical and health system assist in or contribute to our total effort toward pushing humanity to retain its unique central position as the means and the end of development, as a living reality and aesthetic, ethical, and human persons, in the infinite variety of individual needs, potentialities, and manifold aspirations?

I would like to examine the problems of humans from the eyes of health politics, social reform, economy, and culture. Health, in its full context, is embedded in a matrix that is at once historical, social, political, economic, and cultural, especially in an epoch when medical progress, including molecular biology, has made some resounding breakthroughs, almost unparalleled in the history of medicine.

The solution of the complex problems of ill health that are associated with poverty and social deprivation does not depend on the collection of research findings and discoveries alone but also on the *acceptance* and the use of technologies that result from them. It should be pointed out that many developed countries have invested their resources in medical and scientific advances that have benefited not only the health of the people in those countries but also those in other countries. The development of new drugs; the near breakthroughs of vaccines against malaria and leprosy; better diagnostic tools; and in successful vaccines to combat hepatitis B and C and other diseases have been due to the dedication of many scientists in the developed countries. Their efforts have been supported by such institutions as the Centers for Disease Control in Atlanta, Rockefeller University in New York, Walter Reed Hospital, and many other research centers worldwide. National donor agencies and bilateral resources also have provided significant financial aid.

An example of international collaboration and cooperation is the WHO's Special Program for Research and Training in Tropical Diseases, which was initiated by the author and which mobilized brain power, know-how, and facilities across national boundaries in a concerted and coordinated attack on six major diseases of the tropics. It is jointly sponsored by the U.N. Development Program, the World Bank, and many European and American donor agencies operating under the umbrella of the WHO. The goal of TDR (Tropical Disease Research program) was to find solutions to these health problems by using new and improved methods and tools. The benefits and medical research achievements resulting from this effort have been most impressive.

Unfortunately, such international concern is decreasing, principally due to economic problems, although the AIDS program continues to enjoy the same kind of cooperation internationally. However, in spite of giant strides in molecular biology, immunology, and genetics, to name only a few, the lag between discovery and application continues to persist. Ignorance, likewise, persists and constitutes a barrier to more intelligent implementation of control measures.

In 1960, Henry Sigerist, one of the most outstanding medical historians of our time, made a profound and strikingly original contribution to health service organization. Not only did he expand our concepts of the functions of medicine but he redefined them in a manner that was later to be paraphrased by the WHO as follows: "Health is a state of complete physical, mental and social well-being, and not merely the absence of disease or infirmity." In current considerations of the relationship between medical science and health, it will generally be found that stress is laid upon sociocultural, political, and economic conditions. The advances of science and the every-increasing knowledge of nature and humankind have inexorably brought us closer to other disciplines, such as social science, pure and applied, geography, and political science. Thus, the medical sciences are increasingly becoming involved with social values, culture, and education.

In 1960, Sigerist also wrote the following: "The promotion of health, moreover, requires the provision of a decent standard of living, with the best possible living and labor conditions. The promotion of the people's health is undoubtedly an eminently social task that calls for the coordinated efforts of large groups: of statesmen, labor, industry, medical research scientists, of educationalists, and of physicians who, as experts in matters of health, must define norms and set standards." In this approach, the elements to be considered are the quantity and quality of resources; the size and dispersion of the population; its educational level and technical infrastructure; the global economic situation and its repercussions; political instability and insecurity in relation to world affairs; and, at last, those problems requiring solution, with an indication of priority.

The triumphs of natural science, both in discovering radically new knowledge and spectacular advances and in applying them practically to satisfy human needs, have been so important and fruitful that it would seem natural and obvious to extend the same methods to the field of social phenomena.

International concern for the health of the world is comparatively recent in origin. It began when the whole world realized the need to expand and to explore the natural resources of the Third World and to protect itself from the scourges of the East and the unknown part of Africa. The Sanitary Conventions, begun in 1851, were drawn up mainly for this purpose. These were followed by the establishment of the Paris Office, the League of Nations, and, finally, in 1948, the WHO. Even then, the Third World was an indeterminate entity, largely the responsibility of colonial governments. Thus, individual research centers were set up by a variety of countries–for example, the British Medical Research Council, the Pasteur Institute, and research centers of the Belgian government–remnants of which still exist in Africa and Asia today.

As long as much disease was contained within the boundaries of Africa and Asia, the concern of the well-to-do imperialistic powers was minimal. But the disappearance of most of the colonial empires within the last three to four decades has resulted in the emergence of new nations, new sets of social and political goals, and new ideologies, clamoring for deliverance from ill health and for the right to have the same standards of living as the rest of the world.

We have been told repeatedly that, on balance, the world is a healthier place to live in today than it was 50 years ago, and this, of course, is true in Europe and America. According to T. McKeown:

> "The transformation of health between the eighteenth and twentieth centuries was due essentially to the decline of infectious diseases, brought about mainly–until 1900, wholly–by better nutrition, provision of clean water, improvements in sewage disposal and a reduction in birth rates, the last being the indispensable complement, without which the other advances would have been offset rapidly by rising numbers. In the twentieth century, infectious deaths were reduced further by immunization and therapy."

However, one must question this view as it relates to the increasing millions in tropical and subtropical areas of the world. The common lot of those living in African jungles, the savannas, the semideserts of the world is birth, life, and death, without help from the medical advances that continue to benefit the sophisticated peoples of the world. In spite of noble statements about what more could be done to help the developing countries, many of the Third World countries are still so incapacitated by social and economic exploitation that it is impossible for them to realize the dream of development cherished by economists. People of the Third World should not have to wait for long-term development (especially for a moderate-to-high gross national product [GNP]) when intelligent use of resources and the goals of health for all and primary health care by the year 2000 could benefit them today.

In developing countries, the profound and phenomenal shift from old to new ways is occurring steadily and rapidly; and change has, in most cases, been dictated from outside. These nations confront exceedingly difficult problems. Across many parts of the continents of Africa, Asia, and South and Central America, drastic population growth and abject poverty have contributed to extremely severe health problems that put enormous constraints on progressive development. As Abdus Salam stated in 1975, "The developing world–some nine-tenths of humanity–is bankrupt. We, the poor, owe the rich–one-tenth of mankind–some 50 billion dollars. The poorest amongst us cannot even pay the interests on our borrowings–far less find 10 billion dollars we collectively need to import 10 million tons of cereal every year to feed ourselves."

Good and relevant research and good medicine, even application of research alone, will not give the underprivileged social justice, self-reliance, and a fair deal in this contemporary world of ours. The fierce verbal battles that were fought in recent times on the floor of the World Health Assembly concerning such topics as essential and rational use of drugs and infant feeding bear witness to this. As physicians, health managers, and administrators, we also should make contributions to concrete social progress. This call is not new; as far back as 1858, the greatest pathologist of that century declared that physicians were the natural attorneys of the poor and social problems fell within their jurisdiction.

By the year 1848, Europe was in turmoil and the *Communist Manifesto* of Karl Marx and Friedrich Engels, similar to Thomas Paine's eighteenth-century *Declaration of the Rights of Man*, had been published. A Pomeranian shopkeeper's son, Rudolf Virchow, a graduate of the Army Medical Academy in Berlin, serving a year as assistant prosector on an outbreak of a typhus in Upper Silesia, sent the government no mere pathological report. Virchow covered the whole history and economic background of this unhappy area, calling for social as well as health reforms. (The people of Berlin elected Virchow to the National Assembly, but he was ruled too young to take his seat. Despite this early reverse, he sat in the Reichstag for most of his life and was the greatest annoyance that ever confronted Bismarck.)

Health is a fundamental human right, as the constitution of the WHO recognized more than 30 years ago. Health has long been defined by the 164 member states of this body as "a state of complete physical, mental and social well-being and not merely the absence of disease and infirmity."

The ultimate goal of development is to enhance the quality of life and promote total human well-being. This goal can be said to encompass health in its *broadest sense*, for all the people of the world. In view of this, it would seem increasingly important that, for all peoples of the world to benefit from scientific and technological advances, one would need the participation of other disciplines (social psychology, sociology, law, political science, economic, culture, and behavioral science). Human attitudes have always played a role in the achievement or failure of many well-formulated and costly medical and health projects.

In the famous North-South dialogue, a cornerstone of Willy Brandt's report is to identify the complex, multidimensional, and multifactorial process involved in global poverty and to make suggestions. Nobody would quarrel with most of the courageous recommendations of the eminent political and influential public figures who participated in this dialogue, especially the detailed analysis of the world's economic and social predicament as it affects the developing countries. It offers a viable solution to modern man's malaise–abject poverty. The members of the commission showed a deep awareness of the importance of change, from a perspective that was predominantly socioeconomic. But their report significantly stated that "since even quite common men have souls, no increase in material wealth will compensate for arrangements which insult their self-respect and impair their freedom."

In *Past and Present*, Thomas Carlyle said that "we have profoundly forgotten everywhere that cash-payment is not the sole relation to human beings . . . . How far from it!" Deep, far deeper than supply and demand, are laws of fair play–obligations as sacred as life itself.

It is not unreasonable to postulate that economic development must be more widely distributed if international relations are to improve. To what extent is it true that in recent years "rich" nations of the North have been growing richer while the "poor" nations of the South have been getting poorer? If this has been the trend, what factors explain its direction and magnitude? Will the gap increase or decrease if present national and international policies are continued?

Many of us, moderately well-adjusted, comfortably circumstanced, are not keenly aware of the frustrations and deprivations of others or of the contradictions of the human condition. In recent times, a number of authors have divided people into "the laughing multitude and the screaming few." Without doing injustice to their profound literary insight and creative minds, I am sure, they would not mind turning this around to reflect the present circumstances or "the laughing few and the screaming multitude."

The people of conscience who participated in the North-South dialogue stressed the urgent need to redefine the social and economic relationships between the North and the South.

Pope John Paul II put it more strongly and succinctly when he wrote in his 1984 "World Day of Peace Message":

"Although the tension between East and West, with its ideological background, monopolizes the attention and fuels the apprehension of a great number of countries, especially in the northern hemisphere, it should not overshadow another more fundamental tension between North and South, which affects the very life of a great part of humanity. Here it is the question of the growing contracts between the countries that have had an opportunity to accelerate their development and increase their wealth, and the countries locked in a condition of underdevelopment. This is another gigantic source of opposition, bitterness, revolt or fear, especially as it is fed by many kinds of injustice."

Unfortunately, much of the Third World has not yet recovered from the historical consequences of almost five centuries of colonial control, which concentrated economic power overwhelmingly in the hands of a small group of nations. To this day, at least three-quarters of the world's income, investment, and services, and almost all of the world's research, are in the hands of one-quarter of its people. The developing nations are still struggling with the problem of how to bring about socioeconomic equity and a palpable improvement of their lot.

Nearly 500,000 scientists and technologists, almost half of the scientific and technological human resources, are devoting their efforts to military research and development, costing between \$20 and \$25 billion. This funding represents 40 percent of all public and private research and development expenditure mankind appropriates.

Biotechnology had been termed "new science for the Third World," for what could become the most revolutionary scientific establishment for the developing world. However, very few developing countries have the scientists or research resources to embark upon the most sophisticated research in biotechnology, in spite of its enormous potential benefits.

It would be foolish to think that the scientific and medical development that has revolutionized industry, agriculture, and weaponry will prove useless applied to the health of the family, of the nation, or of the human race, if not for the ideological, social, economic, psychological, and cultural differences that limit either or both its application and its acceptability.

Pervasive lack of resources and disease constitute an exceedingly heavy burden on the nations of the developing world. Their burden of early death and long-term disability is, likewise, exceedingly heavy. Malnutrition and infectious disease take the lives of a great many infants before they reach one year of age, and thousands are disabled for life. In most of these countries, disease is a way of life. Dave Rowe of the WHO Special Program for Research and Training in Tropical Diseases, writes that it is difficult for those living in temperate climates, with good standards of public health and medical care, to realize the impact of disease on rural communities in the tropics:

"For example, if you are born to live in the African bush, you are liable to harbor four or more different disease-producing organisms simultaneously. And yet, as a parent, you must be fit enough to work, or your family will starve. In your village, every child at times suffers the paroxysms of malaria fever, and you and your wife will mourn the death of one or two children from this disease. The snails in the village pond carry schistosomiasis, and you do not consider it unusual when children pass blood in their urine.

"You take for granted the disfigured faces and fingerless hands of the beggars in the village street, suffering from leprosy. If you live near a river where blackflies breed, one in ten of your friends and neighbors will be blind in the prime of life. You know that waves of killing diseases such as measles and meningitis and, perhaps, sleeping sickness are liable to strike your village. But, lacking effective remedies, you tend to respond with fatalism in the face of sickness. You make the effort to walk the ten miles to the nearest dispensary when you or your child is ill, but there may be no remedies, and it may be too late."

He goes on to say that malaria is one of the most widespread diseases in the world, affecting some 200 million people. In some regions, malaria transmission is so intense that present efforts at mosquito control and disease treatment are totally inadequate.

In Africa, about one-fourth of all adults suffer from malaria fever at one time or another; and others who are infected have developed a relative immunity and rarely have attacks. After the age of 12 months, almost every child in tropical Africa has malaria; at least one million children die of the disease every year. In other countries, such as India and Sri Lanka, where malaria had regressed, it is now resurgent.

Malaria, schistosomiasis, and filariasis are the three massive tropical infections, but there is a score of other tropical diseases, most of them caused by organisms that prey on man—his liver, blood, heart, brain, and gut.

The WHO, in a recent publication, reported "that in the 31 least developed countries, life expectancy at birth is 45 years and infant mortality 160 per 1000 liveborn children; only 31 percent of the population has a safe water supply, and the adult literacy rate is 28 percent. Infectious disease is still the predominant cause of death, and malnutrition, defective hygiene, and excessive growth of populations are the major influences."

The remedy lies in the utilization of scientific knowledge, coupled with the humanization of the whole pattern of social, economic, and cultural relations. F. A.

Von Hayek, a pillar of economic orthodoxy, wrote that "the individual, in participating in the social process, must be ready and willing to adjust himself to changes and to submit to conventions which are not the result of intelligent design, whose justification may not be recognizable, and which to him will often appear unintelligible and irrational." More than that, he must be "willing to bow before moral rules whose utility cannot be rationally demonstrated." These kinds of things appear to men like John Ruskin and Thomas Carlyle, to be submitting the individual to the ruthless operation of an impersonal economic machine.

The human race today, engaged in a mighty outward and inward struggle for a new and universally binding order of life, stands at a point where two worlds meet, amid an almost inconceivable devastation of traditional values. No clear orientation is possible, nothing can yet show us the way ahead, all bearings have been lost in this whirlwind of forces striving for form. Human existence itself, in all its dubiousness and uncertainty, must submit to a thorough re-examination. The colossal material investment in war technology alone should direct our gaze more imperatively than ever to the realm of social and spiritual reality.

A U.N. report prepared in 1981 states:

"Poverty in the world is widespread and increasing. More than two billion people in the world are forced to exist on less than thirteen percent of the global income. This disparity between rich and poor is profound: in 1950, the per capita Gross National Product of the poor countries was 7.9 percent of the per capita GNP of the rich countries; in 1975 it was only 7.6 percent. To the extent that poverty generates ineffective or inappropriate resources usage, the resource costs of global poverty could be extraordinarily high . . . . [This] gives a very rough idea of the distribution of resources between the developed and the developing world, and it is clear that the developing world commands a significant share of the world's resources. It is in everyone's interest to see them used as efficiently as possible."

According to Lester R. Brown in the *Human Interest* (1974), he depicted the situation of extreme affluence and unimaginable poverty with such realism. He writes, "In reality, our world today is two worlds, one rich, one poor; one literate, one largely illiterate; one overfed and overweight, one hungry and malnourished; one affluent and consumption-oriented, one poverty-stricken and subsistence-oriented."

The world has produced many facts and figures in its efforts to stir the conscience of the leaders and the public in the affluent North, and in 1981 it produced another report. The report is the parting shot from Robert McNamara, who retired as president of the World Bank after 13 years of trying to galvanize the international community into action and who indicated that the outlook for many countries had darkened during the previous year. The economic situation was most serious in the three dozen of the poorest countries with a combined population of more than 1000 million, or more than a quarter of the world population. Without more help, these countries would achieve little or no growth in per capita income during the 1980s, and he said, Africa would actually see income per capita decline. A further 100 million people would be plunged into absolute poverty, a condition already experienced by nearly a fifth of the world. Whether the next decade would be better or worse than the 1970s would depend on how well rich and poor countries adapted their economics to higher energy costs, as well as on the willingness of the industrialized North to resist trade protectionism and help the most vulnerable nations in the South.

Nothing more clearly illustrates the need to reform the present socioeconomic imbalance, as well as promote total human well-being, than the recurrent crises that have overtaken the world the last decade.

It is now half a century since the U.N. charter was signed and inaugurated, in an international effort to establish a new international order. This constituted one of the most striking and hopeful features of the United Nations. Among many obscure pronouncements on humanitarian ideals were some concrete instruments whose goal was to guarantee security and needs in a new human context and to formulate a policy by the great "civilized" governments to extirpate social and economic slavery from the world.

Today, those hopes for creating a better life for the whole human family, and of transforming society, have turned out to be illusory. It has proved impossible to meet the world's minimum health and social needs. In fact, more people today are hungry, sick, without shelter, and illiterate than when the United Nations was inaugurated to, among other purposes, eradicate these inequities. To these preoccupations must also be added the realization that the next few decades may bring a doubling of world population, another world on top of this one, equal in numbers, demands, and hopes.

But we need not despair of the human enterprise, provided we undertake efforts to make the necessary changes. It should be emphasized that the failure to provide a safe and happy life for all is not caused by any present lack of physical resources. The problem today is not primarily one of shortages but of economic and social maldistribution and misuse. Mankind's predicament is rooted primarily in economic, social, and political structures and in behavior within and between countries.

Despite the apparent paralyzation that is occurring, the disenchantment with the prevailing international socioeconomic order, and the allergic reactions to exploitation and alienation, there is still–at the level of the search for health and at the level of the collective search for solutions to many major disease problems–hope. And hope for the growing unity of mankind can never be misplaced hope. Earlier in this chapter, I pointed out that scientists from all corners of the world are working together on problems vital to the improvement of humankind, supported by national resources in the United States, the Scandinavian countries, many of the European countries, and others.

Only through the interdependency of nations will the eradication of ignorance and other cultural factors that impede the practice of good health and health education–and, most especially, through the education of women and their full participation in all human affairs–can we achieve real progress.

Our faith in the omnipotence of technology has been eroded. Paradoxically, the technology that has brought many medical advances also has the power to demoralize and estrange us from one another: We no longer know how to look, to listen, or to feel. Too much emphasis is being laid today on obtaining hard data through technology, and too little on human values. We see technologies grow in importance and sophistication while people seem to deteriorate. Medical science and technology are powerless to achieve the quality of life we all desire, unless their development is accompanied by education and social reforms.

The eminent poet, Pierre Emmanuel, representing the French Academy, pursued this theme. "Medicine today," he said, "enjoys the prestige of the magician and electronic engineer, yet it loses sight of the indivisible individual; failing to correlate old wisdom and new knowledge, and does not recognize the existence of the potentially sick." The fact that people in the modern era do not have time to be ill adds to the inherent fear of suffering and death already aggravated by the tendency to segregate the sick in hospitals, which virtually are ghettos. People feel alone and dismembered before physicians who ask what to treat rather than who to treat.

"For thousands of years," according to Sigerist, "the treatment of the sick was considered the primary task of medicine, while today its scope is infinitely broader. Society has given the physician four major tasks which, although they can hardly be separated, since there are no sharp borderlines, yet may be discussed separately for simplicity's sake." The four functions of medicine, as conceived by Sigerist, include the promotion of health, the prevention of illness, the restoration of the sick, and rehabilitation. To this, I would add total human well-being. These are some of the new parameters of a changing orientation toward health. There has been growing disillusionment with many international development efforts to meet the world's basic health needs, partly because of the obvious disparities between the proclaimed social goals and the still-existing problems.

The goal of "Health for all by the year 2000," announced by the WHO, is an irrevocable commitment and a passionate protest against the doctrine of inequity and want.

It is necessary, if we are to achieve health for all (which includes social justice, equity, and security for all), to learn to understand and respect the feelings of human beings: their anguish and joy, their fears and insecurity, their search for selfhood. These, to me, are as important to our effort as microelectronics or biotechnology. Einstein was asked whether he thought that everything could ultimately be expressed in scientific terms. He replied, "Yes, this is conceivable, but it would make no sense. It would be as if one were to reproduce Beethoven's Ninth Symphony in the form of an air-pressure curve."

The world of the twenty-first century could be one in which most human beings would be better fed than at present and would have more hope for the future. The main thesis presented here is that a man should be the measure of all things. It presupposes that a revolution, by which I mean far-reaching changes in economic, social, and international relationships, in the management of resources, in political power, in culture, in value systems, and in the concept of individual freedom, in both the developed and developing countries, is needed and is possible. We are indeed in a race with time, and time is not on our side. Being under enormous pressure, our present situation presents the best chance of learning what might work.

We need to cross the barriers of social and economic deprivation, outmoded cultural beliefs, and lack of health education, drawing heavily on local and community organizations and health education strategies in order to make basic changes in the way we live. David Hamburg has written, "Behavior, we are coming to understand, profoundly influences our health, for better or for worse, and the society we live in can make it easier or harder for us to change behavior for better health."

The political, economic, and cultural factors that influence the profile of health and disease in different countries in many instances may constitute a formidable array of constraints. Social and economic changes are potent determinants of health and disease, as is the need for changes, from the harmful to the constructive, in human behavior.

Today, man's capacity to interfere with natural causation and dominate his environment, to create and invent, imbues him with the "arrogance of one who regards himself as master of the world and therefore wants to mould it to his own liking." Scientific and technological advances have created a paradox situation of both loss and gain in terms of human developments. This situation can be summarized in the following outline.

MAJOR OBSTACLES AND CONSTRAINTS CONSTITUTING BARRIERS TO THE APPLICATION OF EXISTING KNOWLEDGE

I. POLITICAL FACTORS

(i) Lack of political will and purpose; and lack of stability; lack of political direction.

(ii) Reduction or subjection of health, medical care, and social services to party politics. Health has nearly always been accorded low priority.

(iii) Lack of clear-cut policies.

(iv) Diversion of resources to areas of political prominence and power, rather than to agriculture, women's education, and the modernization of industries.

(v) National and local conflicts provoked by ethnic rivalry, hatred, religious bigotry, and political ideologies.

(vi) Inadequate allocation of resources to health services, research and training, and education.

(vii) Lack of cooperation and coordination between various departments of the government, e.g., health, social services, works, and finance. Department ministers tend to underrate this need.

II. ECONOMIC FACTORS

(i) Global recession and its impact on medical and health delivery systems. Breakdown of global morals and ethnic behavior and corruption among leaders, the privileged, and financial institutions. Fragile international trade relations, which continue adversely to affect global development, and scientific and technological support in particular.

(ii) Changes in donor policies, giving less emphasis to medical and health programs due to failures and mismanagement at national levels.

(iii) Donor-driven projects formulated and designed according to donors' priority and "sold" to the Third World countries.

(iv) Low priority given to social welfare, social services, social development, health, and health research.

(v) Unmanageable and uncontrollable rural migration to cities with little or no infrastructure.

III. CULTURAL FACTORS

(i) Great suspicion of–and resistance to–programs on women and development, women and health, i.e., the empowerment of women. Severe resistance to women's equality, rights, education, and participation in social and political affairs and in national policy formulation. This is true both of the developing and developed nations.

(ii) Failure of medical and health programs which do not consider or respect local sociocultural, historical, and traditional ways. Imposition of Western traditional ways on Eastern countries, affecting such programs as those concerning family planning and AIDS, especially community-based projects.

(iii) Medical ethics, legal, and legislative factors which are culture-bound, adopted without adaptation from foreign countries, and at variance with indigenous social, religious, and cultural traditions.

IV. MANPOWER

(i) Lack of appropriate manpower, especially with scientific and managerial skills and especially in the developing countries.

(ii) Overall shortage, mismanagement, and severe degree of maldistribution of health manpower, especially imbalanced between rural and urban areas.

(iii) Emigration of skilled manpower–doctors, research scientists, nurses, pharmacists, nutritionists, teachers, dentists, technologists–from the developing countries as a result of low wages, lack of facilities, and lack of incentives. Today, many African, Asian, Caribbean, and other well-trained, highly motivated medical and health workers and research scientists and technologists have emigrated from their countries to Europe, North America, Saudi Arabia, and Australia; others are preparing to follow.

(iv) Deficiency of health information for scientific and comprehensive planning.

V. DEMOGRAPHY AND LIFE-STYLES

Changes in age and social structure populations and the consequent emergence of new health and medical problems. Increase in pre-senile dementia, alcoholism, drug abuse, hypertension, cardiovascular diseases, cancer, stroke, mental disorders, and AIDS. Education plays an important role in altering life-styles.

VI. ILLITERACY

This factor constitutes a major impediment to the application of modern medical and health advances. The cost involved in wiping out illiteracy in most developing countries is staggering. Families vary in their attitude toward whom to educate (a daughter or a son?). The need for political and economic support for education, especially of women, is urgent.

Illiteracy plays a crucial role in nearly every factor–cultural, political, economic, and manpower–that impedes development, especially of health services. Man must be reeducated to know that he and the society will gain immeasurably when a woman is no longer regarded as a "beast of burden, a plaything, a child-bearing machine" in the words of M. A. Simet-Lutin, president of "Maternit consciente."

16

ADAPT, ADOPT OR QUO VADIS?
A DILEMMA IN THE
DEVELOPING WORLD

OLADIPO AKINKUGBE
is Professor and former Dean of Medicine at the University of Ibadan,
Nigeria. He was also Vice-Chancellor of the Universities of Ilorin and Ahmadu
Bello, Zaria, and Pro-Chancellor of the University of Port Harcourt. Professor
Akinkugbe is Commander of the Order of the Niger and Officier de l'Ordre
National de la Republique de Côte d'Ivoire.

A NOTABLE DEVELOPING COUNTRY, on shedding the yoke of political dependence nearly 50 years ago, embarked upon the Herculean task of removing the last vestiges of colonial influence from its national corpus. One such, in its assessment, was the imported and exotic language of science. It began to render the imperial system of measurement in its own neojargon: the test tube and microscope acquired local names. But it soon found all this effort misdirected and futile and has since turned its attention to more tangible ventures.

So great is the emotional reaction in many emergent nations to real or imagined threats to intellectual independence and self-confidence that many a national Third World medical scientist often unwittingly disperses his energies in such futile pursuits. The more pragmatic ones have come to realize that you do not have to rewrite Harvey's "De Mortu Cordis" or rediscover penicillin to make a scientific mark in today's world.

Knowledge in its varying dimensions and complexity has never been a permanent monopoly of any cultural, economic, sociological, or political group. Its advancement depends on a wide variety of factors, such as talent, resources, opportunity, and circumstances. A critical mix of these elements often results in a leapfrog advance, but lack of one or the other may drag a nation back many decades. Most medical scientists recognize that while the groundwork of the scientific basis of modern medicine was laid in the last century, the present one has advanced the cutting edge of scientific progress more extensively and decisively than all previous centuries put together.

In the developing world, the main burden of illness is attributable to conditions that are largely preventable: infection, malnutrition, and undernutrition. The low level of education, poor infrastructural services, generally unhealthy environment, and unbridled increases in population further aggravate the situation. Modern medicine has gone a long way toward providing the knowledge needed to contain these problems, but emerging nations are short on implementation.

We might pause to consider these questions:

- Can limitation of resources be a valid apologia for the minuscule contribution of the Third World to medical science over these centuries?

- Might it be that we make too much song and dance over inadequate resources and that, instead, we should aim to make maximal use of our ever-dwindling assets and, in the fashion of Schumacher, aspire to make small beautiful?

• How much budgetary outlay does a mass immunization program or an education program in family health require to make the desired impact on a remote community?

• How much use has been made of the immense research potential and consequent therapeutic properties of the rich flora of the developing world?

Gleaming new university teaching and tertiary care hospitals in the developing world are bustling with complex research activities in molecular biology, imaging techniques, and sophisticated drug trials, and enthusiastic national experts (products of the industrial world's research training) vie with one another in replicating what has been done elsewhere with bigger and better equipment. This robotics limping after the Western scientific tradition is altogether unnecessary. Developing countries would do better to identify those resource materials at hand that can be utilized or improved for their own practical application and ultimate benefit.

WHICH WAY FORWARD?

Missing Link Role

Frontiers of knowledge are often advanced by efforts in international collaboration. Developing countries can supply the missing links in the etiology and natural history of a great variety of diseases that afflict mankind. Genetic and environmental differences can be exploited to provide clues that would otherwise be hidden in the context of advanced-technology research in industrialized countries.

Scientific research in the field of cancer, in genetically determined conditions, and in cardiovascular diseases can all be advanced if there is a deliberate effort by both industrialized and Third World scientific communities to complement each other's efforts. The extreme rarity of a clinical condition in a regional setting could provide the long-awaited clue to its apparent prevalence in another region. Situations operating within an environment may point to the importance of certain risk factors and thus assist in focusing on specific preventive measures.

This concept of the missing link is well illustrated in the area of tropical medicine. The World Health Organization/United Nations Development Program/World Bank Special Program for Research and Training in Tropical Diseases has for nearly two decades devoted considerable attention to a group of diseases estimated to affect over 600 million people in the developing world: malaria, schistosomiasis, filariasis, leprosy, and trypanosomiasis. This important program is aimed at developing research on a global bias and integrating the wide variety of research facilities scattered throughout the world, with a long-term view of instituting effective control strategies. Previously, the European schools of tropical medicine in the colonial era served as orientation, training, and research centers, attracting indigenous doctors. Mosquitoes were imported from tropical Africa and myriads of parasites and worms were elegantly prepared for clinical demonstration. Scores of scientific papers, monographs, and dissertations flowed from research into these communicable diseases, and diplomas were awarded in tropical medicine, public health, and related fields.

Unfortunately, the newly independent status of most of the countries in the tropical world has not, to any great extent, changed this colonial approach to scientific pursuits. A few of the more innovative schools have developed "research outposts" in tropical diseases, which are at last beginning to make broad impact, but we are still some way from the ideal: the mutuality of respect that stems from a knowledge of the importance of functional interdependence, the partnership of opportunity that recognizes the strengths of independent input from differing backgrounds.

Communication

The mechanics for disseminating information and stimulating adequate responses is a subject eminently worthy of pursuit in the developing world. In epidemiology, for instance, the preparation and handling at the national level of data relating to health services research, health manpower development, economics of health care, and major causes of morbidity and mortality in defined populations have real implications in the context of coverage and the quality of service in health- care delivery.

The contribution of health to the total effort of national development, and the apportioning of resources commensurate with such a contribution, has always been an obscure area in the evolution of national development plans. Research can assist in bringing parameters for health evaluation into sharper focus and relating them to such social services as education and welfare, housing and environment, food and agriculture.

Primary Health Care and the Quality of Life

The grim realization that developing countries will continue for a long time to grapple with the dilemma of manpower and material resource shortage should constitute a challenge to find ways of minimizing this hardship. Until a few years ago, many Third World countries had, almost by default, given the most health care coverage to the privileged, urban segments of their populations, leaving the rural majority with a paucity of services. Their professed bias toward preventive (as opposed to curative) medicine was notable more for the breach of this practice than in its observance.

Within the past decade, however, attitudes seem at last to have been changing, and again the World Health Organization (WHO), through its member states, is beginning to regard health not so much as the absence of disease but as an area in which man could demonstrate this real concern for human development and social justice. This has led to regarding the community as the prime target of health-care concern, and this care has now been related to other important parameters of social development. But it has needed a strong political will to take this credo beyond mere rhetoric. Member states of the WHO also have been quick to recognize that primary health care is the major platform from which a pervasive and effective health strategy can be launched. To this end, most nations are now fully committed to providing optimal coverage in essential health-care services to their communities. The ultimate objective of this WHO mission of "Health for All" is the attainment by the year 2000 of a level of health that will permit all citizens of the world to lead a socially and economically productive life.

The degree of access to primary health care, the percentage of newborns with low birth weight, the infant and maternal mortality rates, the extent of immunization coverage, life expectancy, the doctor/population ratio–all have some bearing on development, as do the gross national product, per capita income, productivity in agriculture, safe water supply, extent of atmospheric and water pollution, adult literacy, rural-urban trends, absenteeism from work, and so on. All these are ways in which the scientific approach can be exploited in order to understand factors that support or undermine health in relation to human development and to monitor ways in which such development can be used to enhance the quality of life. This effort toward developing a national agenda of health issues does not necessarily carry far-reaching budgetary implications, through which its ethos and discipline can be steered toward a purposeful, science-oriented goal.

Constraints, Culture and Creativity

In the developing world, the best is often made the enemy of the good. It is self-evident that the lot of ordinary folk in these societies can be vastly improved, not through the quest for new ideas and discoveries but by the application of existing knowledge in an organized, meaningful way. Many examples readily come to mind: the expanded program onimmunization, oral rehydration therapy for childhood diarrhoeal diseases, and life-style changes that take into account such cardiovascular risk factors as smoking, alcohol, fatty foods, excess consumption of salt, obesity, and lack of exercise.

In recent decades, however, abuse of the democratic process and militarization of the polity have in many parts of the developing world given rise to new concerns. The unrelenting wave of assaults on the gains so painstakingly achieved (in health, education, and infrastructural development) has threatened not only the social fabric but also the intellectual output. In many of these countries it has left the citizenry, including committed scientists, deeply frustrated and bewildered and has forced many to flee their countries to seek solace in the industrialized environment.

The capacity of endogenous culture to enhance or retard intellectual creativity is illustrated in the evolution of scientific activity in China, India, and Japan. The Chinese invented printing and the magnet and discovered gunpowder, but this creativity had little impact on the social and intellectual lives of the ordinary folk until these products were transmitted to Europe. Chinese science, including medicine, for many centuries lacked the stimulation of mobile intellectual currents and appropriate economic incentives and so was destined to remain empirical rather than rational. The fusion of the theoretical genius of the Chinese intellectual class with the native capabilities of the practical world of artisans, technicians, and farmers has thus taken a long time to be implemented.

Indian medical scientific genius has for a long time remained dormant for a number of reasons. There were few intellectuals with the will, time, and energy to devote themselves to the exercise of curiosity for its own sake; and those few who did so found little or no support from endowments and organizations solely devoted to medical scientific research. The vast population, the traditional system of villages, the low status of the productive classes, and the generally accepted credo that "action is inferior to thought" made it difficult to test speculation through experiments.

Similarly in Japan, the notion of science for its own sake was anathema. While retaining its uniqueness, it borrowed what it needed from the West and did not make heavy weather of basic or original research–hence, its remarkable versatility in adapting.

What lessons are there for the developing world in these cultures that vary widely in their political forms basically and are traditional and agricultural societies trying desperately to become industrial ones? The competing claims of social justice demand an egalitarian approach to education and health and, indeed, to the provision of a basic infrastructure to enhance the quality of life. Much of this infrastructure derives from the application of knowledge acquired in the industrialized milieu. Thus, we find that in Asian and African countries, the rationalistic, empirical approach is often in conflict with traditional indigenous values. This situation has given rise to two intellectual classes, with no real synthesis evolving, to the detriment of creativity in art, science, and scholarship by international standards.

The work of medical scientists in the developing world will have little relevance if all their energies are spent in acquainting themselves with the work in developed countries and then imitating it. What is needed is the extension and enrichment of one's own tradition through a creative assimilation and adaptation of modern intellectual traditions. Scientists in developing countries should concern themselves with work that is relevant to their environment and situations in which local cultural values and traditional characteristics can be made to relate their scientific efforts to the predominant modern world of rationalistic empiricism. This is their only durable passport to creativity and intellectual respectability.

17

REFUGEE EMERGENCIES: NEW CHALLENGES FOR HUMANITARIAN ACTION

SADAKO OGATA
is the United Nations High Commissioner for Refugees and former
Chairman of the Executive Board of UNICEF. The UNHCR's main functions
are to provide refugees with international protection and to seek permanent
solutions for their problems. In discharging the first function, the Commission
seeks to promote the adoption on an international level of minimum standards
for the treatment of refugees in such fields as education, employment, residence,
and freedom of movement. The UNHCR also tries to safeguard
refugees against being returned to countries where they
have reason to fear persecution.

In 1994, more than 23 million persons benefited from the international protection and assistance of the United Nations High Commissioner for Refugees (UNHCR). This number includes 16.4 million refugees, 3.7 million internally displaced persons, and 3 million others, including returnees and affected civilians. This number has steadily increased from 1.7 million in 1951, the year UNHCR was established, to 8.2 million in 1980 and to 17.2 million in 1990. Since 1986, the global total has risen at an average rate of 1.5 million people per year. The five largest countries of origin of refugees are Afghanistan (2.9 million), Rwanda (2.2 million), Liberia (848,000), Somalia (516,000), and Eritrea (425,000). The five largest concentrations of internally displaced persons are in Bosnia-Herzegovina (2.7 million), Mozambique (791,000), Azerbaijan (778,000), Croatia (520,000), and Tajikistan (520,000).

UNHCR has been mandated by the international community to provide international protection and assistance to refugees and to seek solutions to their problems through either local integration or repatriation. The 1951 Convention and the 1967 Protocol relating to Status of Refugees bind the 128 states party to them to internationally agreed standards for the admission, protection, and treatment of refugees. The principle of *non-refoulement* prohibits states from returning a refugee to a territory where his life or liberty could be threatened. The underlying principle is that refugees should have crossed an international recognized border before they can benefit from international protection.

War, violence, and basic human rights violations are the direct causes of refugee movements. These, combined with social inequalities, economic disparities, political exclusion, ethnic and religious intolerance, and environmental degradation, make a powerful mix for massive population movements. In recent years, interstate conflicts have been replaced by intrastate violence. The abundance of modern weaponry has allowed conflicts to be pursued with unspeakable savagery and total disrespect for the most basic principles of international humanitarian law, without distinctions between combatants and civilians. Massive population displacement is a direct consequence, and sometimes the very objective, of these conflicts.

Since the wars of decolonization and independence in Africa and Asia during the 1950s and 1960s, UNHCR has been providing emergency relief to millions of refugees. However, the nature and characteristics of refugee emergencies have changed significantly in the 1990s. Whereas before, the large majority of refugees crossed into neighboring countries, where they were granted asylum and were provided assistance in refugee camps for extended periods of time, present-day emergencies are more complex:

1. Frequency: In recent years, the number of refugee-producing emergencies has increased significantly. The breakup of the former Soviet Union has emanated conflicts within and between its former republics. By late 1992, the conflict between Azerbaijan and Armenia had created more than 800,000 refugees and displaced persons, while the civil war in Tajikistan uprooted another half million. Fighting in Chenhya has caused more than 230,000 people to flee to Dagestan and Ingushetia. More than 260,000 people in Georgia were displaced following the fighting in Abkhazia. In 1992, a quarter of a million Rohingas fled Myanmar to poverty-stricken Bangladesh. Some 300,000 Sierra Leonans fled to neighboring Guinea and Liberia. The continuing fighting in Angola and Liberia cause refugee emergencies at regular intervals.

2. Scale: The largest refugee emergencies in recent years are the result of intrastate conflicts. Since 1991, four refugee emergencies affected more than a million people each. In April 1991, 1.7 million Iraqi Kurds fled to Iran or Turkey. More than a million Somalis in Kenya, Yemen, Djibouti, and Ethiopia have been assisted by UNHCR. In the former Yugoslavia, 3.7 million refugees, displaced persons, and affected populations are being assisted, in addition to the estimated 700,000 who have departed for other countries. In addition to an estimated 750,000 internally displaced persons, more than 2 million Rwandans sought refuge in Tanzania, Rwanda, and Burundi in the summer of 1994.

3. Diversity: Refugee movements are often fluid, as fleeing to a neighboring country does not necessarily provide the needed safety. Governments are increasingly reluctant to keep their borders open in situations of mass movement of people and exert pressures upon the refugees to quickly return to their countries of origin. Increasingly, governments call upon the international community to create "safety zones" inside the country of origin to cope with the population displacement.

Although UNHCR has no specific mandate toward internally displaced persons, UNHCR is increasingly requested by the U.N. Secretary-General and governments to operate inside countries involved in conflict or internal instability, such as the former Yugoslavia, northern Iraq, Sri Lanka, Rwanda, and the Caucasus. By providing protection and assistance to displaced persons inside the country of origin, UNHCR seeks to prevent them from crossing an international border in search for protection and aid. A successful cross-border operation was undertaken from Kenya into Somalia. This has facilitated the return and reintegration of the Somali internally displaced and somewhat lessened the huge burden on neighboring countries of asylum, in this situation Somalia.

The fluidity in refugee emergencies requires great operational flexibility. Since the repatriation in 1989 to Afghanistan from neighboring Iran and Pakistan began more than 3 million refugees have returned. The continuing fighting, however, has displaced more than 330,000 persons, among them many returnees, inside the country, and has led to repeated outflows. In many situations, refugees, returnees, and internally displaced and affected civilians are intermingled, making distinctions between those who need protection and assistance difficult. This is true of the former Yugoslavia and Afghanistan. Furthermore, continuing fighting threatens the delivery of assistance to and the protection of refugees and displaced persons and hampers relief efforts.

4. Solutions: Local integration in the country of asylum of large numbers of refugees is not feasible in most instances, given the high burden the refugee population poses on the local communities. Voluntary repatriation in safety and dignity is the most desirable solution but is difficult to achieve in war-torn societies. Despite the problems, in the past five years nearly 9 million refugees have repatriated to northern Iraq, Afghanistan, Cambodia, Somalia, Mozambique, and a number of other countries. The communities to which refugees and internally displaced persons are returning have often been devastated: villages razed; roads and fields mined; schools, clinics, and other basic infrastructure in ruins. In war-torn societies, such as Angola, Afghanistan, Liberia, and Rwanda, the already weak economic, social, health, and judicial infrastructures have been nearly completely destroyed. Continuing violence, insecurity, and human rights abuses inhibit rehabilitation efforts. The re-integration of returnees, therefore, often poses formidable challenges; and a failure to do so sometimes leads to a renewal of the emergency state, as in Afghanistan, Liberia, and Angola.

The diversity and complexity of today's refugee crises require a multidimensional and simultaneous approach to address the entire spectrum of problems, from emergency response to eventual solution. This chapter focuses on the steps taken by UNHCR to enhance its emergency preparedness and response capacity, and seeks to identify measures to further strengthen these.

UNHCR REFUGEE EMERGENCY PREPAREDNESS AND RESPONSE

Response to any refugee emergency is dependent upon preparedness, which in turn has to be linked to standby capacities that guarantee the rapid mobilization of personnel and equipment. Timely and early presence in the area affected by the emergency is critical to ensure the delivery of humanitarian relief, to provide protection to the victims, and to identify early opportunities for a solution. Close cooperation and coordination among all the international and national agencies involved are essential to avoid duplication of efforts, to identify and address shortcomings, and to make the best use of scarce resources.

Following the outbreak of the Gulf War in December 1990, U.N. agencies drew up contingency plans for an anticipated flow of refugees from Iraq into Turkey. In April and early May 1991, as government troops closed in, 500,000 Kurds fled to the Turkish border and 1.2 million to the Iranian border. A major human disaster could not have been averted without the crucial assistance of the 13-nation Coalition Force, around 30 bilateral donors, and more than 50 non-governmental agencies (NGOs) employing more than 20,000 staff and 200 aircraft. Following Security Council Resolution 688, the Coalition Forces established in northern Iraq a "safety zone" designed to encourage refugees back into more accessible areas where they could be more easily fed and sheltered. The speed with which the refugees fled Iraq was matched by that of their return. Health, food, logistics, shelter, and sanitation systems set up to respond to the exodus had to be dismantled and transferred inside northern Iraq to provide assistance to the returnees. In April 1991, the United Nations and Iraq signed an agreement allowing U.N. humanitarian centers to be established inside Iraq. By mid-July 1991, when the Coalition Forces withdrew, the responsibility for humanitarian assistance in the "safety zone" was transferred to UNHCR. By December of that year, only 70,000 Iraqi refugees were left in Iran and some 10,000 in Turkey.

The crisis revealed the serious shortcomings in emergency preparedness. It revealed the limits of humanitaritan assistance and raised the issue of humanitarian intervention, particularly the relationship of humanitarian military approaches.

One of the major consequences was that UNHCR revamped its emergency preparedness and response system. These reforms included the following measures:

> **1. Emergency Response Teams:** A special unit exists consisting of five Emergency Preparedness and Response Officers who are on standby for any emergency. A roster of qualified staff with special expertise in protection, programming, logistics, and communications and supported by health, water, sanitation and shelter specialists has been drawn up. Within 72 hours, a completely operational and self-sufficient emergency team could be deployed.
>
> In emergencies, staff should be multidisciplinary to cope with the com-

plexity of issues involved. Accordingly, special training programs have been developed for UNHCR staff, government officials, and NGOs. The development of contingency plans, identifying the constraints, needs, and capabilities in potential areas of operation, is essential for emergency preparedness.

2. Standby Arrangements: Agreements have been signed with a variety of NGOs, governments and other international organizations to provide personnel, especially technicians, and equipment within a short period of time for a limited duration. This ensures that extensive staffing resources can be called up at short notice and withdrawn once the crisis is over.

3. Emergency Stockpiles: Procurement of equipment and relief supplies can take considerable time. Therefore, emergency stockpiles have been set up in cooperation with governments, NGOs and other international agencies upon which UNHCR can draw. The equipment includes vehicles, communication equipment, food, shelter, blankets, prefabricated warehouses, and tents. In addition, agreements have been signed for the lease of aircraft and trucks.

4. Emergency Fund: Donors' response to the launch of a financial appeal, based on a needs assessment, can often take several months. Therefore, UNHCR established an emergency fund of $25 million U.S. dollars, which can meet immediate financial needs up to a maximum of $6 million U.S. dollars per emergency until an appeal is launched.

The first priority in any emergency is to save lives. Thus, it is important that refugees are granted protection from danger. It is equally important to meet their immediate physical needs, including health care, shelter, food, water, and sanitation, and to provide social services.

During flight, refugees might have little or no food or clean water, may have long distances to walk, and are sometimes exposed to harsh weather conditions, as well as harassment, physical violence, and trauma.

As a result of the lack of clean water and adequate sanitation facilities, from 60,000 to 80,000 refugees suffered from cholera in Goma during the summer of 1994. Increased availability of potable water immediately brought the cholera epidemic under control. Irregular distribution of food can lead to malnutrition, lowering natural resistance to infectious diseases. Lack of shelter can cause respiratory infections and pneumonia, particularly among the very young and the elderly.

Not surprisingly, excessive mortality rates are a defining characteristic of an emergency. The crude mortality rate (CMR) is the principle yardstick in measuring the effectiveness of the relief effort. It represents the number of persons dying each day per 10,000 population. Relief programs should aim at achieving a CMR of one death per 10,000 population per day shortly after the onset of the emergency. This rate still represents approximately twice the normal CMR for nondisplaced populations in most developing countries. A higher rate, or significant fluctuations in it, represents gaps in the emergency response that need to be rectified immediately.

The first days and weeks of an emergency represent the greatest risk, in particular among children under 5 years old. Preventable diseases, such as malnutrition, measles, cholera, diarrhea, acute respiratory infections, and malaria, are the main causes of death.

The CMR for Goma represented the highest rate in recent history. On average 1,500 persons, or an estimated total of 50,000 persons, died per day during the first weeks of the emergency. The majority of the victims were children, women, and the elderly. Although UNHCR had emergency teams in place in the

Table 1: Monthly Crude Mortality Rate (CMR) in Selected Refugee Populations, with Baseline CMRs in Countries of Origin, 1978–1994

Month/Year	Host Country	Country of Origin	Refugee CMR	Baseline CMR
Jan./Dec 1978	Bangladesh	Burma	6.3	1.0
Oct. 1979	Thailand	Cambodia	31.9	2.5
Aug. 1980	Somalia	Ethiopia	30.4	2.0
Jan./Mar. 1985	Sudan	Ethiopia	16.2	2.0
Sept. 1985	Sudan	Chad	24.0	1.6
Jan./June 1987	Malawi	Mozambique	1.0	1.5
Sept. 1988/ Aug. 1989	Ethiopia	Somalia	3.8	1.8
July 1990	Ethiopia	Sudan	6.9	1.7
June 1991	Ethiopia	Somalia	14.0	1.8
Apr. 1991	Turkey	Iraq	12.6	0.7
July 1994	Zaire (Goma)	Rwanda	60–105	0.6

(Source: UNHRC)

region since April 1994, the size and suddenness of the movement overwhelmed the capacity of the emergency response. In addition, the inhospitable environment in which the refugee camps were set up provided little natural water resources and shelter.

In situations of flight, when the social fabric is torn apart and family members often are separated, women and children are especially at risk. Extrapolated demographic information indicates that women constitute some 48 percent and children some 40 percent of the global refugee population. A significant proportion of refugee households are headed by single women, who in addition to traditional female family tasks may have to cope with new responsibilities previously undertaken by men. They have special protection and assistance needs. Women and children may need to be protected from sexual violence, abduction, military recruitment, or irregular adoption.

Although women are especially vulnerable in refugee emergency situations, they should not be viewed solely as victims. In times of social breakdown, women often become the stabilizing force in the community, maintaining traditional structures and a semblance of normality. The particular role and responsibilities of refugee women in family and community support must be recognized and reinforced through the provision of humanitarian assistance.

Social services are important to meet the basic needs of the refugee community even in the earliest stage of the emergency. These services aim at identifying persons with special physical, mental, or health needs; setting up care for unaccompanied minors; seeking the involvement of the refugee community in camp management, maintenance, and relief distribution; and setting up education programs. These measures help refugees to attain self-sufficiency and avoid the dependency syndrome.

The delivery of assistance in refugee emergencies is a complex challenge, often hampered by logistical problems, such as inaccessibility of the refugee camps, lack of transportation and communication, bad road conditions, and insecurity. To meet the immediate basic needs of the 800,000 Rwandans who fled to Goma, the daily requirements were: 40 medium trucks or 10 planes to transport 400 tons of food and 300 to 400 water trucks to provide 4 million liters of water.

Such requirements go beyond the capacity of any single humanitarian agency. Only governments, in particular the military, have the manpower and logistical capacity to deliver the necessary equipment, material, personnel, and systems to meet the needs within a matter of days. Following UNHCR's cooperation with the Coalition Forces in northern Iraq, ways to improve UNHCR's emergency preparedness and response through the use of military assets have been tried and assessed.

Working under UNHCR's supervision and control, military teams provided by donor governments have helped to sustain airlift operations to Sarajevo and eastern Zaire. Following the influx into Goma, UNHCR appealed to governments to provide eight self-contained and independent service packages in areas in which UNHCR's capacity was overwhelmed or had no immediate expertise: airport services, logistics base services, road servicing and road security, site preparation, provision of fuel, sanitation facilities, water management, and airhead management.

Another area of cooperation with the military has opened up with the increasing support of U.N. peace-keeping or enforcement forces to humanitarian activities. UNPROFOR in Bosnia-Herzegovina ensures security at the Sarajevo airport, provides protection to land convoys and for "safe areas," as well as undertaking tasks, such as road and bridge repair and demining. The relationship between military and humanitarian actors in a refugee emergency, however, is complex and has raised issues of principle, particularly relating to neutrality and impartiality. Military contributions to humanitarian action should be under civilian control to ensure that common objectives are shared.

STRENGTHENING PARTNERSHIPS

The increasing complexity of today's refugee crises requires the adoption of further measures aimed at strengthening the emergency preparedness and response mechanisms through improved partnerships among all the actors involved in refugee emergencies:

1. A wide diversity of actors participate in a refugee emergency: international governmental agencies, national and foreign governments, national and international NGOs, donor, media, and individuals. Ensuring coordination and cooperation among all these actors is a difficult task. The objective should be to fill the gaps but avoid overlaps, taking into account the differing competencies and expertise required for emergency response and rehabilitation, humanitarian action, and development.

2. To meet all the needs in a refugee emergency goes beyond the capacity of any single agency. Partnerships must be reinforced with nongovernmental agencies, governments, and other international organizations to enhance the effectiveness of the emergency response.

UNHCR has a long-standing partnership with NGOs and has agreements with some 250 agencies. The commitment, speed, and community-based approach, which is a particular strength of NGOs, make them ideal partners in meeting the varying needs of refugee emergencies.

Memoranda of understanding among the international agencies, outlining mutual agreements regarding emergency responses, terms of reference, and respective responsibilities will facilitate cooperation and coordination. A general agreement facilitates the immediate mobilization of resources, obviating the need to negotiate on a case-by-case basis. UNHCR has signed such an agreement with the World Food Program regarding the delivery of food supplies to refugees.

The unique capacity of the military to deliver humanitarian assistance, and of peacekeeping operations to provide security to humanitarian aid workers and a stable environment in which humanitarian action can take place, must be further explored. In doing so, the comparative costs, capacities and appropriateness of military and civilian actors must be assessed and balanced. To be effective, a better understanding of the respective roles, mandates, and limitations between military and humanitarian actors is required.

Although humanitarian action is neutral in principle, impartial, and non-political, it clearly does not take place in a political vacuum. Conflict resolution and peace negotiations should take into account the refugee question, so as to enable the refugee population to return as soon as possible to their country and participate in its reconstruction. To avoid any gaps in the transition from emergency relief to development and to ensure the sustainability of projects, development programs need to take into account the reintegration needs of the returnees. The planning process should also take into account the totality of a country's needs and establish a coherent list of priorities. In the absence of such a blueprint, the impact of the individual parts of the system is likely to remain limited or even futile.

CONCLUSION

The emergency preparedness and response of humanitarian agencies have improved significantly in recent years, although ways to further strengthen these remain essential in the face of growing demands. The response should not be limited simply to meeting the immediate basic needs of refugees and the internally displaced but should be accompanied by measures that contain the causes of the emergency, and consequently of human suffering, and a search for solutions. The international community has neither the resources nor the willingness to protect and assist refugees in protracted emergencies. Compassion fatigue sets in quickly when the public and donors see no quick fix to the problem.

Prevention of refugee emergencies–if it can be accomplished–is the most effective form of protection for people in danger of becoming refugees. Despite the richness in early-warning data of impending crises, the international community repeatedly fails to take appropriate action to prevent or contain crisis situations prior to their developing in large-scale population movements. Prevention, at the general level, addresses the root causes of conflicts and involves the whole amalgam of measures directed at improving economic and social development, human rights and minority policies, political participation, and responsible governance. These measures go far beyond the role of humanitarian action. However, without the necessary political will, humanitarianism can only help to staunch the wounds and cannot avert disaster.

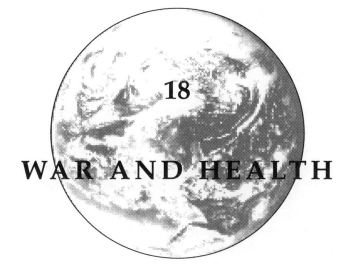

18

WAR AND HEALTH

JEAN-CLAUDE MULLI
is Deputy-Head and Spokesperson for the International Committee of the
Red Cross. In addition to recognition of new national Red Cross societies,
the International Committee of the Red Cross works for the development
and   observance of international humanitarian agreements (especially Geneva
conventions). It also acts as a neutral intermediary in time of war or internal
strife to, ensure the victims of such conflicts of protection and assistance;
and, in particular, it serves the welfare of prisoners of war, making
appropriat recommendations for ameliorating their condition.

WHY STUDY WAR'S EFFECTS ON HEALTH?

LONG BEFORE OUR TIME, people were of course aware of the disastrous effects of war: the word itself has always conjured up pictures of ruin and destruction, wounds and death, epidemics and famine. So at first sight it seems absurd to consider what effects war has on health: these cannot be anything but harmful. However, it makes sense to study the consequences of war on health if the aim is to identify them precisely in order to define the necessary remedial action. What such study does is to assess the needs of war victims, whether individuals or groups, and of war-damaged structures or systems; this is, in fact, the first step essential to any kind of humanitarian action. If we wish to acquire a deeper understanding of the complex relationships existing between conflicts and health, it is, above all, to be able to act more effectively. A close examination of the problem will show to what extent the action required is itself complex, going far beyond the mere provision of medical assistance to conflict victims.

War

One result of war is to diminish society's ability to solve its problems while at the same time increasing them. War destroys infrastructures, diverts human and material resources, and disrupts services. At the same time, it augments society's needs because of the many casualties it produces: the sick and wounded, the physically disabled and mentally traumatized, the shipwrecked, prisoners, widows, orphans, abandoned children, homeless and displaced persons, refugees, unemployed people–and the list is not complete. In addition to these immediate and direct effects of war, there are the indirect and long-term results. After a war, a country's economy takes time to recover, development may be halted for a long period, and the population's standard of living remains low for many years.

War is an extremely complex social phenomenon, which cannot be described and analyzed from a single point of view. It may be considered in relation to its scope (worldwide, regional, or local); its intensity (high or low); its duration; its motivation (war of extermination, war of religion, power struggle, territorial conflict, minority or separatist conflict); the methods of warfare and the weapons used (bombardment, mines, weapons of mass destruction, chemical weapons); the strategy employed (guerrilla warfare, opposing armies, blockade, total war); and its nature (civil war, war between states).

The context in which war is waged may aggravate its effects, for example, adverse climatic conditions (bad weather, drought) and underdevelopment. Fighting also has varying consequences depending on the surroundings in which it takes place (urban, industrial, or rural areas).

Health

Health, defined as a state of complete physical, mental, and social well-being in individuals and groups of people, is also the result of complex social phenomena. It is not measured solely in terms of access to medical care (curative and preventive), but also in relation to the availability of food and water, the existence of proper sanitation and environmental hygiene, of housing, education, and employment, and of security and protection against assaults on personal and collective dignity. It involves, especially in the modern communities of developed countries, the uninterrupted operation of complex systems: the production, transport, storage and distribution of food, water, and energy; the disposal of solid and liquid wastes; the construction, repair, and maintenance of housing and other infrastructures; social and health services; the police and the judiciary; and so on. These systems are vulnerable on many levels, any or all of which may be affected by war.

War, Health, Human Rights, and Humanitarian Activities

In a less materialistic context, health may be regarded as linked with respect for human rights. One of the chief characteristics of war is that it undermines this respect: in the midst of fighting there is, in the best of cases, only relative compliance with international humanitarian law, which constitutes, so to speak, the "hard core" of human rights. In the worst of cases, even humanitarian law is no longer observed, and it is then that the consequences of war are most grievous. This is true especially when war displays one or more of the following features:

- Disorganization of the parties to the conflict, absence of any authority controlling the combatants, several militant factions, and, in extreme cases, total anarchy. The result is maximum insecurity for civilians and humanitarian organizations.

- Marked cultural or religious antagonism between the belligerents, ideological, or religious fanaticism. The worst atrocities are then possible in the name of principles considered by the adversaries to transcend any humanitarian considerations.

- Absence of democratic control by the authorities in place (dictatorship, warlords), leaders' indifference to moral, diplomatic, political, or economic pressure from outside. The war may become total. Any sanctions imposed from abroad have no influence on those in power but exert all their harmful effects on the population.

• No distinction is made between combatants and civilians (civil war, guerrilla warfare waged by a movement within the civilian population). The need for effective "antiterrorist" action is used to justify the neglect of human rights by the forces of repression.

• Infrastructures vital to civilians are taken as military targets. The Gulf War gave striking examples of this situation: the "surgical" destruction of electrical power stations, justified in military terms in order to weaken the Iraqi army, had the "side effect" of cutting off supplies of drinking water to civilians and making it impossible to pump away wastewater, with disastrous epidemiological consequences.

When war occurs in the midst of underdevelopment and poverty, or when natural disasters coincide with war, human needs are redoubled, the constraints on humanitarian action become enormous, and humanitarian aid may even fall prey to aggression. In the worst cases, banditry may occur, increasing the insecurity.

Finally, when war is waged for the purpose of eliminating a population or ethnic group, denial of rights to such a group is absolute. Humanitarian action is then totally opposed to the very aim of the war. It is no longer only the health but the life of a whole community that is at stake. This is when genocide occurs.

Combatants and Civilians Killed

The prime victims of war, those most directly affected, are the combatants who are killed. The following figures have been cited:

Thirty Years' War (1618–1648)	6,000 soldiers killed per year
Napoleonic Wars (1805–1815)	51,000 soldiers killed per year
American Civil War (1861–1865)	125,000 soldiers killed per year
World War I (1914–1918)	2,520,000 soldiers killed per year
World War II (1939–1945)	5,561,000 soldiers killed per year
Korean War (1950–1953)	666,000 soldiers killed per year
Vietnam War (1965–1975)	106,000 soldiers killed per year

As clearly recognized since the beginning of the twentieth century, war tends more and more to affect the civilian population, directly or indirectly. It is generally agreed that the wars in the eighteenth and nineteenth centuries directly caused comparatively few civilian casualties, whereas the civil wars and wars of national liberation of the twentieth century have been characterized by the increased proportion of civilians among those killed: from 19 percent in the World War I, the figure rose to 50 percent in the Spanish Civil War and 48 percent in World War II and the Vietnam War. It has been estimated that the proportion of civilians among those killed during 1991–1992 in the war in Croatia was 64 percent.

If the indirect effects of war (food shortages or famine, water supplies impaired or completely cut off, disrupted sanitary or medical services, breakdown of social infrastructure in general) are taken into account, it must be admitted that the figure for civilian war victims is gravely underestimated, particularly since the "side effects" of war continue long after the end of hostilities. The figure has been given of 14 deaths due to indirect effects for each death caused directly by the fighting in the low-intensity conflicts in Angola and Mozambique during the 1980s.

The Wounded and Disabled, Amputees and Mine Victims

To the figures for the dead must be added those for the wounded, always many times more than those killed, and especially for those disabled for life. In particular, there are the countless war amputees. The majority of these people are victims of antipersonnel mines, which go on maiming and killing men, women, and children years after the fighting has ceased. The figures are not always accurate, but estimates of amputees are:

- 25,000 out of 8 million inhabitants in Cambodia, i.e., 312 per 100,000

- 20,000 to 30,000 out of 12 million inhabitants in Afghanistan, i.e., 166 to 250 per 100,000

- more than 20,000 out of 15 million inhabitants in Angola, i.e., more than 133 per 100,000

to give only these three examples.

According to U.N. estimates, more than 100 million land mines (some experts double this figure) have been scattered across the world. Every month, more than 800 persons are killed by these devices and thousands injured.

Mental Trauma, Stress, Sexual Violence

Among other direct victims of war are those mentally traumatized by their experiences. In Bosnia-Herzegovina and Croatia, for example, 700,000 people are estimated to have suffered grave posttraumatic psychological disturbances requiring urgent specialized help, and 700,000 others were considered to have less serious reactions that would nevertheless justify their receiving treatment in peacetime conditions.

One particularly odious form of violence inflicted directly on civilians has been the systematic rape of thousands of women, notably in Bosnia, Korea, Bangladesh, Liberia, Uganda, and among the boat people of Vietnam.

Displaced People

The consequences of war on the civilian population are especially grave when fighting leads to the massive displacement of a region's inhabitants, as in Somalia, Afghanistan, Rwanda, and Bosnia-Herzegovina, where refugees and displaced persons are counted in the millions. Such groups are extremely vulnerable and include subgroups that are even more vulnerable: children (especially those who are unaccompanied), women, the elderly, and the chronically sick. Their mortality rate, particularly in developing countries and during the initial phase of displacement, amounts to 12 to 25 times the normal mortality rate in their countries of origin. This increase in mortality is due to the greater incidence of communicable diseases related to poor hygiene and difficulties in obtaining water supplies but also to malnutrition, exhaustion, injuries, and exposure to the elements. Among the refugees arriving in Zaire from Rwanda, the daily crude mortality rates reached 41.3 per 10,000 people.

Three of the ways in which war affects public health on a large scale deserve special attention: food shortages (which may turn into famine), the breakdown of drinking water supplies, and epidemics.

Hunger and War

Scarcity of food is a permanent characteristic of conflicts due to the disruption of commercial activities, the reduction of food production, and other disturbances to the economy arising from the fighting. Famine, an exceptionally urgent lack of food characterized by a sudden increase in acute malnutrition and in mortality, is usually considered as the result of natural disasters (e.g., drought) occurring in the context of underdevelopment; but it is always aggravated by war, which is frequently its main cause. If the principal famines in Africa during the past thirty years are examined, it is evident that some were due to drought and underdevelopment, at times accompanied by culpable negligence on the part of the authorities in situations of internal political tension, such as: Sahel, 1972–75; Ethiopia, 1973–74; Sudan, 1984-85. Other famines were due to drought and conflict: Ethiopia, 1984–85; Mozambique, 1986; southern Sudan, 1988–90; Mozambique, southern Sudan, and Somalia, 1992–93. (It should be noted that while the drought in 1992–93 affected all the countries of southern and eastern Africa, real famine existed only in those three countries ravaged by war.) Famines have occurred in other countries at war, when there was no drought: Biafra, 1969; and Angola, Liberia, and southern Sudan, 1994.

Water and War

Certain recent conflicts have had considerable repercussions, deliberate or accidental, on water supplies to the civilian population, requiring humanitarian organizations to take action at increasingly sophisticated technical levels and on a wider and wider scale. Below are some examples, which are not exhaustive.

During the Gulf War in 1991, the destruction of electrical power stations in Iraq meant that the systems for pumping, treating, and supplying drinking water, and those for disposal of wastewater, whose operation depended on the power stations, were put out of action. Whole cities were left without drinking water, and the incidence of diseases, such as dysentery, hepatitis, and typhoid fever, greatly increased. During the fighting in Liberia, Lebanon, and Yemen, water supplies to cities such as Monrovia, Beirut, and Aden were also impaired by the destruction of pumping and treatment stations or of supply networks. In Bosnia, the intentional destruction of water-collecting stations and the deliberate cutting off of water supply systems were used by belligerents as means of warfare in dozens of places, in flagrant violation of international humanitarian law. In Rwanda, the flight of hundreds of thousands of refugees and their crowding together in places with poor water supplies resulted in epidemics of cholera and bacillary dysentery.

Epidemics and War

Conflicts throw health services into disarray, restrict their resources, deny the population access to these services, diminish the possibility of controlling and eradicating disease vectors, force people to leave their homes and to crowd together in unhygienic conditions, and aggravate malnutrition. By so doing, they generate and spread epidemics. In addition to the outbreaks of diseases linked to lack of clean water, as mentioned above, there are, for example, the epidemics of measles observed in many camps of refugees and displaced persons in Africa, the epidemic of relapsing fever that occurred among Ethiopian soldiers during their demobilization in 1991, and the epidemic of kala-azar that has raged since 1984 in the Upper Nile region of Sudan and that is thought to have already affected over 50,000 people. An unusual example of the indirect effects of war on health is the epidemic of heliotrope food poisoning that occurred in Tajikistan in 1992 following a late harvest and the relaxation of health regulations as a result of the conflict.

WAR AGAINST PUBLIC HEALTH / WAR AGAINST HUMANITY

While the consequences of war on public health are usually "accidental" or at least partly "involuntary," there are occasions when they appear beyond a doubt to be intentional. Such is the case in Bosnia-Herzegovina, where public health is clearly under direct attack. In Rwanda, a further stage of horror has been reached, amounting to genocide.

In fact, the most terrifying aspect of wars such as those in Bosnia-Herzegovina and, even more so, in Rwanda is that they are waged against the civilian population, not merely "by chance" or "by mischance" but deliberately targeted. The aim of the fighting is not to destroy the military power of the enemy but, above all, to eliminate a section of the population by killing or by harassment and intimidation to force mass flight. These wars are not solely struggles to gain power or land: Their purpose is to acquire control of a territory that has been "ethnically cleansed." The methods of this "ethnic cleansing" are the massacre and forced displacement of those considered undesirable.

In Rwanda, the extent of the killings and the speed with which they were committed are clear proof that they were not the result of loss of control but were planned and organized with the deliberate intention of eliminating political opponents, mainly (but not exclusively) identified with the members of the Tutsi ethnic group. In addition to the physical elimination of potential adversaries (men and youths), the massacres were intended to terrorize the whole population, not sparing women and children and the sick in hospitals.

In Bosnia-Herzegovina, the same reasoning led belligerents to terrorize the civilian population, forcing it to flee. I am a physician, not a tactician, but I fail to see the military value of shelling cities and hospitals, historic monuments and churches; blowing up mosque minarets and burning villages deserted by their inhabitants; deliberately destroying installations for collecting, treating, or supplying water; attacking aid convoys; and so on.

It should be repeated: The wars in Rwanda and Bosnia-Herzegovina are wars waged against entire civilian populations, not solely against armies. Their immediate (and intentional) consequences are thus the massive destruction of vital infrastructures, the reduction to extreme vulnerability of hundreds of thousands of people, and a profound upheaval of the social order. One day, perhaps, the economic effects may be estimated, but will it ever be possible to assess the long-term psychological consequences? When states fought in accordance with the ritual of military confrontation, in the name of relatively abstract political or geostrategic interests that were, after all, ephemeral, the return of peace gradually effaced the hostile attitudes engendered in the combatants by training and among civilians by wartime propaganda. Fifty years after World War II, the French and Germans no longer regard each other as mortal enemies simply because their states fought one another.

However, wherever human beings were massacred or tortured, robbed of their human dignity and their possessions because they were Tutsi or Bosnian Muslims (or Jews or Armenians or Kurds), the survivors' memory perpetuates the fear, the hatred, and the desire for vengeance: The seeds of future hostilities remain, ready to germinate, in their individual and collective consciousness. At the start of the war in the former Yugoslavia, the memory of the atrocities committed half a century earlier by the Ustashas and the Chetniks was a powerful instrument in the hands of the Serb and Croat leaders to stir up animosity among their followers.

If I have stressed the emotional and psychological aspect of the consequences of war, it is in order to emphasize the scale of the measures needed to restore lasting peace. It is not enough to repair the material damage, to restore the health structures and services, to revitalize the economy: Efforts must be made to change the attitudes and calm the emotions that continue long after violence has ceased to affect the victims. These efforts necessitate medical and psychological assistance to the victims, but that is not enough. Justice must be done to them, and their confidence must be restored by guarantees of respect for their rights.

War Against Health and Humanity Concerns Us All

When a conflict breaks out somewhere in the world, the international community's reaction can range from total indifference to massive intervention. Between these two extremes, it is possible to observe all the variations of involvement by states, by intergovernmental organizations, by humanitarian aid agencies and by those engaged in defending human rights, and by all levels of public interest, greatly influenced by the more or less constant media coverage of the events.

The reaction of states depends essentially on considerations of a geostrategic nature and on economic and security interests, even though human rights and democratic ideals may be ritually invoked to justify intervention. By that, I do not mean that the latter motives are completely divorced from the reasons for intervention by states but that they are subordinate to the former. The international reaction to Iraq's invasion of Kuwait would not have been on the same scale if the Middle East were not a region of major geopolitical importance and of oil production.

In Rwanda and in Bosnia-Herzegovina, the economic and geopolitical interests at stake are not as great. It is true that the regional consequences of these conflicts are far from negligible: In both cases, the influx of huge numbers of refugees threatens the stability of neighboring countries and places a heavy burden on their economies. Nevertheless, political analysis of these crises does not appear to have resulted in the identification of any threat to world peace and security that would justify anything other than measures of containment and diplomatic action accompanied by military intervention, confined essentially to protecting humanitarian activities; or else economic sanctions, which appear to have a dire effect on the population rather than favorably influencing the development of the political and military situation.

Must we really believe that the humanitarian, political, and economic consequences of these crises are merely local and regional and that they will have no marked repercussions at a global level? It all depends on our definition of the term "repercussions." If we consider only the material consequences of these conflicts, we may at least hope that massive international aid will make it possible to rebuild what has been destroyed and to reestablish decent living conditions for the people affected. But the dead cannot be brought back to life, and material help to survivors does not wipe out the memory of what they have suffered.

The consequences for the international community of the wars in Rwanda and in Bosnia-Herzegovina cannot be summed up in the material aid that will be required. In medicine, it is not sufficient to treat the body, it is also necessary to dress the wounds of the soul. In addition to the curative approach, there must be a preventive approach based on knowledge of the causes of the disease. War, when it occurs, may be regarded as a disease to be cured but also as the symptom of a profound disturbance, possibly threatening not only one organ but the whole organism. The crises in Rwanda and Bosnia-Herzegovina are perhaps the symptoms of a latent disease jeopardizing the whole planet in the medium or longer term. If that is the case, they concern all of us, beyond the scope of their immediate repercussions.

Bosnia-Herzegovina: Health, the Victim of "National Racism"

The racist nature of "ethnic cleansing" requires no proof. This racist attitude amplifies, exacerbates, and justifies total war, which cannot be explained solely by political and territorial ambition or nationalist sentiments. Without going so far as to exterminate "inferior" races systematically, as in Nazi Germany, the war aims to destroy the bases of health, well-being, and dignity of the people to the point where they no longer have any choice but to flee. The worrying question that we face is whether such racism is merely a local "Balkan" phenomenon or whether it exists everywhere, ready to burst forth in other conflicts and to make them uncontrollably violent and dangerous.

Rwanda: Malthusian Genocide?

The massacre of half a million people in Rwanda cannot be explained merely by unusual savagery on the part of extremists "possessed by the devil" and made fanatical by the infamous *Radio des Mille Collines*. Political antagonisms and tribal hatreds were perhaps only the sparks that set alight a fire, whose cause might perhaps be sought, according to Maurice King, in a particularly dramatic case of "demographic entrapment." If this theory is to be believed, the lesson to be learned by the international community is that other conflicts could well break out in all the places where a population with uncontrolled growth is entrapped in a territory without sufficient resources to sustain life and is unable to leave in order to find sufficient living space elsewhere. This is true not only for overcrowded countries with limited resources but also for the poverty-stricken outer areas of major cities. Rwanda, in that case, would be only the dress rehearsal for apocalyptic events in the most diverse places, from Bangladesh to Nigeria and from Lima to Kinshasa.

For the international community, this means that the Rwanda crisis must be interpreted as a grave warning and that it must consent to an immense effort to try to prevent the repetition and multiplication of such a situation rather than waiting for it to happen, hoping each time to be able to limit the damage by sending humanitarian aid or a few contingents of peacekeeping troops.

The effort to be made is no less than the struggle against underdevelopment, social injustice, and overpopulation or, rather, the concentration of people in regions with inadequate resources.

IN CONCLUSION

War, if not the chief threat to health in the world, is at least an aggravating factor among all the other threats. It is both a disease that we must try to prevent, and whose effects we must treat, and a symptom whose significance we must diagnose. Even a local war is of concern to the whole human race, which must recognize the effort necessary to counter its consequences and, if possible, its causes, the most deep-rooted of which are social and economic inequality, cultural and religious intolerance, and ethnic discrimination. If we are to succeed in this, humanitarian aid must not only be redoubled, it must also be protected and completed by comprehensive action at various levels.

The victims of war must be safeguarded by securing respect for international humanitarian law and human rights. We must not only restore to the victims the possessions they have lost and reestablish the services of which war has deprived them. We must give them back their dignity by promoting development and by ensuring the unimpassioned but inescapable punishment of war crimes.

19

THE END OF THE COLD WAR: A CULTURE OF PEACE

FEDERICO MAYOR
is the Director-General of the United Nations Educational, Scientific, and Cultural Organization. UNESCO was established in 1945 for the purpose of advancing, through the educational, scientific, and cultural relations of the world, the objectives of international peace and the common welfare of humanity. UNESCO promotes the international exchange of knowledge and ideas through conferences and other contacts among scientists, artists, writers, and educators around the world. In addition to establishing missions to assist governments in such projects as improving literacy, teacher training, and improving scientific and technical education, UNESCO also sponsors research in such fields as racial problems, disarmament, human rights, and peace studies.

SOME YEARS AGO, I wrote these lines:

> *In the dawn of your life*
> *don't come docile*
> *when I start my second half.*
> *But later on,*
> *please come and tell me*
> *that you and I did not remain docile*
> *. . . still very alive!*

No docility but no violence. Never accept the unacceptable. But never violence. We must forge and develop from the very beginning attitudes of openness, of inter-action, of otherness, of discussion, of persuasion. We must know the most power-ful thoughts of our common past, the progress achieved through research, discovery, and invention, in the infinite space of the mind, and not only the list of the battles to defend or enlarge our territory. We must "disarm history" and real-ize that welfare and dignity depend more, particularly in a global frame, on our tal-ent than on our wealth. At what a difficult, hopeful, turning point we are! We are in the crucial transition from the reason of force to the force of reason. From a con-text in which physical strength is utilized more than the intellectual capacities distinctive of humankind, from an impulse of domination and coercion, to a last-ing peaceful settlement of rivalries.

A transition, above all, from violence to nonviolence; from a culture of war to a culture of peace. What an immense price we have paid because only death is irre-versible, dying too young for causes that deserved to be defended and served throughout a lifetime.

Vision means to transcend the borders of our daily lives and look beyond our immediate concerns, beyond our families, our friends, our parties and beliefs. Vision means to feel and think beyond our personal interests and to take first into account the interests of all people.

That very vision led to the creation of the European Organization for Nuclear Research (CERN) and was perhaps a unique (and uniquely American) factor in the transition from the habits of war to the practices of peace. It was the great American theoretical physicist, Isidore Isaac Rabi, who argued in the midst of the burgeoning Cold War that world peace was safer if European physicists participated on equal terms with Americans in nuclear physics research for peaceful purposes.

I recently had a meeting with the director of CERN. He requested that UNESCO, the "mother" institution, enlarge the European scope of CERN to its present global reach. I remember thinking what vision those Americans had. Still horrified by the terrible conflagration of World War II, by genocide and unbelievable warfare practices, they were able nevertheless to see the essentials and to be concerned for others. It is to be hoped that we will not always need to be shaken by war to become lucid and wise.

Today we have advanced Professor Rabi's vision from his troubled time into our own era of unexpected prospects for peace and well-being. We have done it together, UNESCO and its partners in the public and private sector. By forging new partnerships, creating new synergies, we are creating new and stronger modalities for sharing scientific knowledge.

A few months ago, it was my honor and privilege to participate in the launching of the Report of the International Commission on Peace and Food at UNESCO Headquarters in Paris. Chaired by the renowned Indian architect of the Green Revolution, former Agriculture Minister M. S. Swaminathan, and including such distinguished members as Professor Abdus Salam of the ICTP in Trieste, Mrs. Rosalynn Carter, Mary King, Martin Lee, and a number of experts in agriculture and social development, the commission underlined *the basic role of farming and food production* in creating sustainable development and full employment. Entitled "Uncommon Opportunities: An Agenda for Peace and Equitable Development," this important and no doubt controversial report argues that conflict can be prevented by eliminating the frustration, marginalization, ignorance, and misery that so often give rise to the interreligious and interethnic violence that have marked the post-Cold War era.

The commission members urged important reforms on the U.N. system and the reduction of military expenditure throughout the world. The "peace dividend" thus created some $400 billion that would be used to redeploy manpower and promote education, scientific and technological knowledge, and productive enterprise to combat rural and urban poverty, as well as national and global environmental degradation. It would be used to address the new threats of overpopulation, poverty, and pollution, as well as natural hazard, which we are unprepared to face. We also are unprepared to face natural hazards such as flooding and drought. Even when these are recurrent, they are addressed with very poor or nonpreventive and post facto measures. We are prepared for threats that belong to the past. We are prepared for wartime. We are unprepared for peace. We have in our budgets the cost of war. We do not yet have the price of peace.

The commission also calls for the harnessing of the military's logistical and technical know-how, as well as private investment, to generate commercial agriculture, agro-industries, and agro-exports throughout the rural areas of the world's poorest countries. In fact, the enormous population shifts to the shantytowns surrounding Third World cities are the result of this dire rural poverty with its severely limited access to health care, education, and remunerative work.

Biotechnology can help increase harvests and reduce crop spoilage. Improving the quality of life of rural areas is essential to mitigate or to prevent emigration. Millions of people will flock to the already overcrowded urban centers if the opportunities mentioned above do not reach them and if there is not better sharing. This is not only a matter of global solidarity. It is a matter of global security.

We at UNESCO not only have supported the work of the commission but are mindful that many of its recommendations have important implications for the role of education, science, culture, and communication throughout the world. They are preventive roles and therefore not as dramatic as the peacekeeping forces and emergency humanitarian assistance that have unfortunately come to dominate the perception of the United Nations in our contemporary world. Prevention, if successful, is invisible. No conflict, no war, no pathetic scenes on TV. I like to repeat that the generals who won a battle are decorated. Those who prevented a war are not. The perception and awareness of the intangibles should become a crucial factor in the art of governance. Education is prevention from the grass roots up. Education is liberation, is awakening of human creative capacities, is empowerment for each person's choices.

We have been taking practical measures along these lines for some years now. UNESCO's alliance with the World Bank, the United Nations Development Program, UNICEF and the U.N. Fund for Population Activities (UNFPA) and for Education for All is perhaps the best example. No matter what the religious or cultural context, be it in North Africa, South Asia, sub-Saharan Africa, or Latin America, the education of women and girls is the best guarantee that uncontrolled population growth can come under control within the foreseeable future. Increasing the education opportunities for women and girls invariably means falling fertility rates. December 1993 was a watershed in this respect. In the frame of the U.N. alliance, I took the initiative with Jim Grant of UNICEF and Nafis Sadik of UNFPA, of convening a summit meeting of the nine most populous developing countries of the world. Their populations comprise 72 percent of the world's illiterate people between 15 and 60 years of age, and more than 50 percent of the planet's population. President Suharto of Indonesia, and Prime Minister of India P. V. Narasimha Rao, personally signed the commitment to increase substantially the resources invested in education, particularly of women and girls, before the year 2000. It was reported that India–this was an unforgettable moment of hope–had jumped from 3.6 percent of gross national product to 6 percent! Afterward, I witnessed the signature by President Mubarak of Egypt in Cairo; by Prime Minister Mrs. Benaezir Bhutto of Pakistan in Islamabad; by Prime Minister Li Peng of China in Beijing; and by President Carlos Salinas de Gortari of Mexico in Mexico City. If these nine countries shift their priorities in this way, population growth will be curbed, poverty will be reduced, and emigration will decrease. In addition, what really matters, the excluded will be included, and the unreachable will be reached.

Education empowers every man and woman to master his or her own life, to act according to personal models and values, and to avoid those imposed from outside, often as a condition for financial assistance. Education, in its broadest sense, is also the answer to creating that feeling of global awareness–of intercultural sensitivity–that beckons minds to transcend local circumstances and embrace the world. Up until now, too much education in our inherited culture of war has focused on narrow messages of nationalism and even chauvinism. Our history books celebrate battles and generals without paying due attention to those whose thoughts and actions created the economic, scientific, cultural, and, indeed, agricultural breakthroughs that can bring societies together and advance the human agenda for us all.

For several years now, these ideas and these concrete actions in the fields of education, science, culture, and communication have formed the basis not only for my priorities as director-general of UNESCO but for my efforts as an author. I have recently published a book entitled *The New Page*, (Dartmouth/UNESCO, 1995) that tries to express in practical, autobiographical terms the great opportunities made possible by the end of the Cold War to move from a culture of war to a culture of peace. It would be a poor outcome indeed if we moved only from a Cold War to a Cold Peace. In my book I said:

> "The 'new page' which we are turning . . . is one of a culture of peace, based on a culture of democracy. It is a transition fraught with all the dangers of moving into the unknown without much guidance from our personal or collective memories. If this transition can be successful, we will at long last have the possibility of changing radically our economic, social and political perceptions and entering a new renaissance of hope and creativity in our lifetimes. It would be foolish (and self-limiting) to try to predict precisely the outcome of such a process. As Alejo Carpentier wrote, 'El hombre nunca sabe para quien padece y espera' ('Man never knows for whom he labours and waits'). But it is clear that the beginning of this 'new page' can be written by all of us living right now."

Universities have a particular role here. How can we train teachers, even of the youngest children, without giving them the intellectual and scientific knowledge to confront the immense possibilities of our own time and to try to begin to solve the dramatic tragedies that often dominate the headlines. It's a moment of hope! Who, ten years ago, would have foreseen the collapse of the Soviet Union, the peace process in the Middle East, El Salvador, and Mozambique, and the creation of a democratic and multiracial South Africa? These were the impossible of a few years ago.

In science and the humanities, throughout any university program, researchers and students are busy trying to grasp the importance of the intangibles that shape our lives. From molecules to prejudices, from the AIDS virus to the communications "meme" that can vector good or bad behavior, our research and actions focus on things we can rarely see and perhaps never touch. At the same time, no accurate representation of the world, be it in science or political science, can avoid grappling with complexity. Our world is not simple and simple solutions almost always mislead.

What can be more intangible and more complex than theoretical physics? Yet for I. I. Rabi, Abdus Salam, Professor Lee, Professor Langenberg, and even for a biochemist like me, theoretical physics has a crucial contribution to make in building a culture of peace. Science is impossible in the absence of free enquiry, and free enquiry is relatively useless if its findings cannot be shared through "the free circulation of ideas by word and image," as UNESCO's Constitution states. *The Culture of Peace is impossible without the Culture of Democracy.* And democracy is not a value system and set of behaviors that can be exported prepackaged and ready for consumption like a Big Mac. All of us, scientists, engineers, philosophers, historians, and politicians, must speak out on the complexities of creating democracy and the need to begin with three essential elements: freedom of the press and media, free speech, and an independent judiciary. From these roots, tolerance and political fair play can eventually grow, but no transfer of the American or any other system should be expected to take root in cultures that have their own histories and specificities.

Thus, when UNESCO proposed to the General Assembly that in 1995 the Fiftieth anniversary of the United Nations be celebrated as the International Year for Tolerance, we were speaking to both the scientific and humanistic communities. All of us have a responsibility through our contributions to economic development, and therefore to social development, to advance the ethics of tolerance and mutual respect. We must make available in all languages to all schools, to all scholars, to all scientists, to all children the messages of Martin Luther King, Jr., and Mahatma Gandhi: "Rebellion, yes, but not violence. Dissent, yes, but not violence. Change, radical change, yes, but not violence." Perhaps we do not yet know the best way of teaching tolerance, but history shows us that totalitarian regimes–including some of their scientists–taught intolerance very effectively.

That is why UNESCO has established a new interdisciplinary program on the Culture of Peace that is not merely a program of study and research. In El Salvador, in Burundi, in the Philippines, in Mozambique, and in other areas of recent or potential conflict, UNESCO is working with all parties to create conditions of dialogue and mutual trust. I will never forget my visit to a Central American country in which the government requested me to visit the guerrillas up in the hills at the end of a long process of peace negotiations. There I met a young boy scarcely taller than his rifle who asked me, "*¿Hemos ganado o perdidi?*" "Did we win or lose?" And to be able to answer, "We all won," meant that I should immediately design a tailor-made, intensive, deformalized education and training in order to provide him–and all others in similar circumstances–with the possibility of reaching, without prerequisites, the level of those who were "on the other side" of the conflict. Otherwise, reconciliation and social rearticulation would not be feasible. Yes, our answer must always be that the train of education (up to and including higher education) will always come through again with programs adapted to those who have never had a chance to go to school. The United States, with its "GI Bill" of the 1940s and its system of high school equivalency diplomas, the junior college, and the great land-grant universities, has much to emulate in this regard.

Culture is expressed in how we behave every day. Too often, decision-makers have a plastic or even ornamental concept of culture. If today the cultural aspects have suddenly appeared as protagonists of the political agenda, it is because culture defines citizenship. Our behavior depends on our knowledge, memories, beliefs, experiences, conditions of life, expectations, thoughts, dreams, science and technology, prospects, hopes. It depends on all of those combined complex factors we call "culture."

Science is universal. It cuts across cultural differences while at the same time respecting religious practices and beliefs. It advances largely through teamwork, in which individual scientists from many backgrounds work together toward the common goals of solving problems that often are obstacles to human well-being. Because science, like the phenomena it studies, crosses national and cultural barriers, its common methods and shared language make it possible for former enemies to learn to share in the ways of peace, of tolerance, even of love.

The science laboratory is not only a place for the advanced study of arcane but important particles, quanta, and quarks. It is a laboratory in which researchers and students all go beyond their personal local concerns and learn to share knowledge on a global basis to solve common global problems hand in hand. For this to happen, governmental institutions and the private sector must cooperate. Development is possible not only through advances in science and technology but also through our ability to apply our findings in the social settings where poverty and ignorance thrive.

We must understand that our own security now requires a new and broader definition in which it is taken into account that environmental trends, uncontrolled population growth, and the ignorance and hatred they can breed can affect the stability of our global and local environments. The culture of peace is one attempt to build conceptual bridges so that the intimate links between our well-being and the suffering of so many on the planet can be seen as a whole, a whole in which solutions can be found, knowledge can be shared, and health and happiness can be passed down to new generations on this blue planet.

20

BETWEEN ENEMIES: RECONSTRUCTION OF CIVILIZATION AWAY FROM WEAPONS OF MASS DESTRUCTION

CARL SAGAN
is the David Duncan Professor of Astronomy and Space Sciences at Cornell University. Dr. Sagan is the Pulitzer Prize winning author of *Cosmos*, the best-selling science book in the English language in the twentieth century.

OUR LONG NUCLEAR NIGHTMARE has ended. At least, that's the prevailing view. Launchers are being destroyed, de-MIRVing has begun, nuclear testing is sharply down, the Soviet Union is no more, and leading former Soviet weapons scientists have been offered jobs by the United States. The Looking Glass command-and-control aircraft have been mothballed, and the Russians, they say, have taken U.S. cities off their targeting lists. Former U.S. President Bush proposed reducing the U.S. arsenal below 5,000 warheads and the Russian President Yeltsin saw him and raised him—or rather, lowered him, suggesting half that number. Presidents Bill Clinton and Yeltsin have agreed to speed up the Start II process. We are witnessing an arms race in reverse.

In light of all this, the dangers of global thermonuclear war are, in almost everyone's estimation, much reduced, but there are still many tens of thousands of nuclear warheads in the world. Under the new agreements, warheads are being destroyed at a rate of between 1,000 to 3,000 a year in each country. The agreements, however, do not dictate what is to become of the warheads taken out of service or of the uranium and plutonium they contain.

The U.S. defense budget, still well over $300 billion a year when hidden costs and the interest in past wars is included, is the most obvious source of funding for the urgent domestic problems that have been allowed to fester over four decades of the Cold War. (The U.S. tab for the Cold War is about $10 trillion—enough to buy everything in the United States except the land.) Almost all Americans would agree that some U.S. military force, still formidable by world standards, should be preserved for national security. But—in light of such problems as declining productivity, education, toxic waste, homelessness, inadequate health care, the collapsing infrastructure, AIDS, ozone layer depletion, and global warming, to say nothing of the national debt—unless we change our way of doing things, there may not be much that's worth defending.

All bureaucracies attempt to maintain themselves when their primary mission fades. They invent new tasks, preferably urgent ones, and the resulting inertia becomes especially high when jobs and profits are at risk. The U.S. Defense Department, with its laboratories and contractors, tends to inflate possible future perils. The statues of Lenin have not all yet been melted down and already we hear that there may be grave dangers from breakaway republics or from fundamentalist Muslims or China or North Korea or, under certain circumstances, Israel. The Japanese are increasingly depicted as a menace. How realistic are these fears, and how large a defense establishment is needed to offset them? How much of these alleged dangers is a frantic search for some replacement, even if short-term, for our former Cold War adversary?

A credible, sufficiently dangerous enemy is a great convenience for politicians unable to deal with proliferating domestic problems and potential discord. If such an enemy doesn't exist, it's usually easy enough to arrange for one.

Many methods are being proposed to maintain the weapons establishment: maybe weaponeers can teach school or make trains or interdict drugs while preserving their military aegis. One particularly instructive search for a new enemy can be found in the weapons laboratories and in the U.S. Defense Department's interest in asteroids and comets.

The inner solar system is filled with small worlds, some of which intercept the Earth's orbit. It is easy to show that sooner or later one of these objects will hit the Earth, as has happened–with catastrophic consequences–in the past. The longer the wait, the more devastating the impact. On average, once a millennium there will be an impact event equivalent to the largest nuclear weapons explosion; every 10,000 years, one that might have global climatic effects; and every million years, an impact event equivalent to a million megatons of TNT that would work a global catastrophe, killing a significant fraction of the human species. In 100 million years, you can bet on something that seems to have extinguished all the dinosaurs and most of the other species of life on Earth, perhaps by an "impact winter"–analogous to nuclear winter but still more severe.

However, in this grisly actuarial calculus the equivalent number of annual deaths worldwide is at most in the thousands. With the effects amortized, it might be argued that this is far from our most pressing problem. If a big impact happens, though, it would be an unprecedented human disaster.

Along parallel and only weakly interacting tracks, the planetary science community and the military, aware of the aforementioned scenarios, have been pursuing these questions: How to monitor all sizable near-Earth interplanetary objects; how to characterize their physical and chemical nature; how to predict which ones may be on a future collision trajectory with Earth; and, finally, how to prevent a collision from happening. In the early 1980s, some in the weapons establishment argued that the Soviets might use near-Earth asteroids as first-strike weapons; the alleged plan was called "Ivan's Hammer." Countermeasures were needed, but maybe it wasn't a bad idea for the U.S. to develop something similar.

There are two methods of prevention that have been discussed. First, a nuclear weapon of unprecedented yield might blast the asteroid or comet into fragments that would disintegrate and atomize on entering the Earth's atmosphere. This method might require nuclear weapons of much higher yield than the highest-yield nuclear weapon ever exploded (about 60 megatons).

Since there is no theoretical upper limit to the yield of a thermonuclear weapon, there are those in the weapons laboratories who consider such impact prevention as not only a stirring challenge but also as a way to give continuing nuclear weapons development a permanent seat on the save-the-Earth bandwagon.

Another approach under discussion is less dramatic but still useful as a way of maintaining the weapons establishment–a plan to place comparatively low-yield nuclear weapons on or near an errant object and explode them near perihelion to deflect the object's trajectory away from the Earth. This procedure also offers a way to deal with a suddenly detected long-period comet on imminent collision trajectory with the Earth. The comet would be intercepted with a small asteroid in a game of celestial billiards.

Russian and American nuclear weapons scientists–their interests perfectly consonant on this matter–have been meeting to discuss appropriate technologies. Armadas of launch-ready nuclear-tipped rockets are envisioned. Maybe this will one day be needed, but it's hard not to suspect motives in the weapons establishments. Is this world security or job security?

Another problem is that if you can deflect an object away from collision with the Earth, you can also deflect an object not on collision trajectory so it *does* collide with the Earth. There is no other way in which a comparative handful of nuclear weapons can do so much harm. Can we humans be trusted with civilization-destroying technologies? If we must wait a million years for a significant fraction of the human population to be killed by an impact, isn't it more likely that in much less time this technology will get into the hands of a Hitler or a Stalin, some misanthropic sociopath, someone in the grip of unusually severe testosterone poisoning, or technicians incompetent or insufficiently vigilant in handling the controls and safeguards? The risks seem far greater than the potential benefits.

Tracking asteroids and comets is prudent, it's good science, and it doesn't cost much. But, knowing our weaknesses, why would we even consider developing a technology today to disintegrate or deflect small worlds? Shall we imagine the technology in the hands of many nations, each providing checks and balances against misuse by the others?

Doubtless other dangers will be discovered or concocted that have the effect of preventing too steep a reduction in the military weapons establishment. In the ancient scientific tradition, such claims also ought to be looked at with the keenest skepticism.

The end of the Cold War permits the reconstruction of our global civilization away from weapons of mass destruction, away from massive conventional firepower, and toward solutions to such urgent problems as poverty, overpopulation, the deteriorating global environment, education, health, and social justice. We find ourselves unexpectedly between enemies. This is an opportunity that has not come often in this century. It arrives not a moment too soon.

21

CLIMATIC CHANGE: UNDERSTANDING GLOBAL WARMING

JAMES HANSEN
is Director of the NASA Goddard Institute for Space Studies in New York,
Adjunct Professor of Geological Sciences at Columbia University, and Principal
Investigator of the Pioneer Venus Orbiter and Galileo (Jupiter Orbiter)
Photopolarimeter Experiments. Dr. Hansen was trained in physics and
astronomy in the space science program of James Van Allen. In the last
fifteen years, he has worked on studies and computer simulations of
the Earth's climate for purposes of understanding man's
potential impact on global climate.

THE GREATEST THREAT to the long-term health of our planet, as the danger of nuclear war declines, is probably global climate change. Yet the media debate about climate change has served more to confuse than to enlighten the public. As we enter an era in which climate change is expected to become increasingly apparent, it will be crucial that the public understands better the nature of climate change and how science research really works.

I use here a series of personal experiences to provide a perception of the basis for anticipating global climate change. This will illustrate the difficulty in communicating this science issue to the public and to emphasize the central role that the public must play in determining the ultimate fate of the planet.

There is a scene fixed in my memory, when the mysteries of the greenhouse effect first took hold of me. It was late one Sunday afternoon in the summer of 1976, as my wife and I walked on Long Island's Jones Beach with our three-year-old son. Whitecaps crashed onto the shore, foam racing across the sand and bubbling against our feet. The wind picked up, blowing our hair sideways, and sea spray turned a hot afternoon to one that produced goosebumps. The sea appeared to extend without limit, merging with the sky in a distant gray line. The height of the waves reminded me that they were still but a tiny fraction of the ocean's average two-and-a-half mile depth. How incredible to think that puny man-made greenhouse heating could compete with such awesome natural forces.

Earlier that year Yuk Yung, a postdoctorate student of Mike McElroy at Harvard, had convinced several of my colleagues and me to estimate the heating effect of all man-made greenhouse gases that had accumulated in the Earth's atmosphere since the beginning of the Industrial Revolution. These gases absorb infrared (heat) radiation emitted by the Earth and radiate part of that energy back down, thus keeping the Earth's surface warm. This process is roughly analogous to the way the windows in a greenhouse trap heat. Scientists had speculated for a century about climate effects of excessive atmospheric carbon dioxide, which is increasing due to burning of coal, oil, and natural gas. Now the problem was becoming more fascinating as we realized that the emissions into the atmosphere of several other gases, such as methane and nitrous oxide, were also increasing, apparently as a result of human activities.

We calculated that the total heating by all man-made gases was nearly 2 watts per square meter. One watt is the power of a miniature Christmas light bulb, the tiny bulbs that are cool to the touch, being designed to use as little power as possible. Could two of these bulbs over each square meter of the Earth's surface significantly alter the temperature, winds, and precipitation? How could such a small force have a noticeable effect, given the size and apparent buffering capacity of the earth, its atmosphere, and especially its massive ocean? How long would it take for the ocean temperature to adjust to this small heating since, before the "bulbs" could do much warming, the winds would mix the surface water to great depths? If we waited long enough for the ocean to fully adjust to this small amount of heat, just how much warmer would it get?

My distraction that day on the beach was driven by the realization that the tools of science allow us to estimate how the Earth should respond to this man-made forcing, and that the results and tools could be tested against observations.

What made me confident, on the beach of Long Island, that the world must respond eventually to these man-made greenhouse gases was my knowledge of Mars, Earth, and Venus, which I had studied as a graduate student and in post-doctoral days. Mars, which has only a thin atmosphere of greenhouse gases, is only a few degrees warmer than it would be without any atmosphere, given the amount of energy it absorbs from the sun. Venus has a thick atmosphere of carbon dioxide and a greenhouse warming of several hundred degrees, making its surface hot enough to melt lead. Earth has an intermediate amount of greenhouse gases, keeping the surface about 35° C warmer than it would be without these gases.

Scientists have worked for years developing global climate models, which are computer programs that allow numerical simulation of the Earth's climate. Global-warming critics and the media give the impression that predictions of climate change are based mainly on such models, but that conclusion is naive and misleading. In reality, expectations of climate change are based on a understanding of the climate system, which derives mainly from analysis of observational data. Climate models are just one of our tools, albeit an essential one, as they help us sort out the importance of many processes that occur simultaneously in the world's complex climate system.

A climate model lets us experiment with a facsimile of the climate system, helping us to think about and analyze climate in ways that we could not, or would not want to, experiment with the real world. Climate modeling is complementary to global observations, laboratory experiments, and basic theory. Each of these tools has limitations, but together, especially in iterative combinations, they allow understanding to advance. Although models are very imperfect, they structure the discussions and help to define needed observations, experiments, and theoretical work.

New York City was a great place to find the physics, mathematics, meteorology, and computer programming talent needed to develop a climate model. A broad range of talents is needed as a climate model must simulate absorption of solar energy, radiation of heat energy, transfer of heat and moisture by winds, evaporation from the ground and vegetation, turbulent motions, ocean currents, and many other processes. I was fortunate in the latter 1970s to receive support from NASA (National Aeronautics and Space Administration) to assemble a team of people for this purpose. Our laboratory, the Goddard Institute for Space Studies, was located on Broadway of Manhattan's Upper West Side, on the floors above Tom's Restaurant, recently famous as the location of the "Seinfeld" sitcom.

We completed our first model, "model zero," in 1979 and tested it with an experiment in which we doubled the amount of carbon dioxide in the atmosphere. Similar experiments had been carried out earlier by Sykuro Manabe, the climate modeling pioneer at Princeton's Geophysical Fluid Dynamics Laboratory. After running many simulated years, our model produced a global average warming of almost 4° C, about twice the 2° C warming in Manabe's then most recent model.

To try to understand this difference, we analyzed the mechanisms causing the warming in our model. Only about 1.2° C of the warming was directly due to carbon dioxide, but the warming allowed the air to hold more water vapor, just as the air is moister in summer than in winter. Because water vapor is a greenhouse gas, it increased the warming to 2° C, similar to Manabe's result, and in our model the warming also reduced the cloud cover and the amount of sea ice, thus increasing the amount of sunlight absorbed by the Earth and making the total warming 3.9°C. Manabe's model did not have such strong positive feedbacks because he fixed the cloud cover and there was less sea ice in his control run.

Which model was closer to the truth? There was no way to tell. At the request of the White House, the National Academy of Sciences convened a panel in 1979 to report on the carbon dioxide greenhouse effect. Mainly on the basis of Manabe's and our simulations, the panel concluded that doubled atmospheric carbon dioxide would probably cause eventual global warming of 1.5° C to 4.5° C. A warming of 1.5° C would have significant effects on society, but it might not be too difficult to adapt to the changes. However, a warming of 4.5° C would dramatically shift climatic zones, altering the very face of the planet.

Climate models thus helped identify aspects of the climate system, such as clouds, sea ice and water vapor, which needed to be observed and modeled more accurately. However, the models were too imprecise to adequately illuminate policy issues. When the many uncertain components in the models were combined they multiplied to yield a huge range of possible results.

Current conditions did not seem to present a case for concern about global warming. Indeed, there was a widespread impression among climatologists that the Earth gradually had been growing cooler since about 1940. Some cooling tendency was expected as a result of the fine particles (aerosols) that humans were adding to the atmosphere, such as dust and sulfates from the burning of fossil fuels. There were probably as many scientists predicting global cooling due to aerosols as those predicting global warming due to greenhouse gases.

But in 1980, when my colleagues at the Goddard Institute and I studied global temperature records, we found that the perception of a cooling trend was a misconception based on Northern Hemisphere data up to 1970. Including data from the Southern Hemisphere, we showed that the world had cooled moderately between 1940 and 1965 but had since been warming, with a net warming of about 0.4° C over the period 1880 to 1978.

In addition, we made calculations with a climate model to estimate the expected global warming due to measured increases in atmospheric carbon dioxide. We tested the effect of several other climate-forcing mechanisms in our simulations, including variable stratospheric aerosols resulting from occasional large volcanic eruptions and hypothetical variations of the luminosity of the sun. The results suggested that increasing carbon dioxide was probably the predominant cause of global temperature change between 1880 and 1980.

We spent almost a year writing and revising the paper describing our study, which was published in the journal *Science* in 1981. We tried to find a balance between stressing the limitations of the study and the implications of continued warming if our projections were accurate. We pointed out the great uncertainty about climate sensitivity to a global forcing and the uncertainty about the rate at which heat perturbations mix into the ocean. But after considering broad ranges of these quantities, we found that, despite the uncertainties, the warming of the past century was consistent, with the greenhouse mechanism being the main cause of global temperature change.

Using our model to project climate change into the future, with a climate sensitivity matching the warming of the past century, we estimated that the continued increase of fossil fuel use would lead to about 2.5° C global warming by the end of the twenty-first century, making the Earth warmer than it has been in millions of years–in fact, approaching the warmth of the Mesozoic, the age of dinosaurs. We pointed out that such climate changes would likely have many effects, including a rising sea level and the possible opening of the fabled Northwest Passage.

Reactions to our conclusions by the press, the scientific community, and the funding agencies illustrate the difficulty of doing research in areas that have social and economic implications. When our paper came out in *Science*, it was reported by Walter Sullivan in a page one story in the *New York Times*. A few days later, a lead editorial in the *Times* discussing our conclusions noted the implications for energy policies, as the United States at that time was in the process of shifting to heavier use of coal and synthetic fuels, the most prolific producers of carbon dioxide. The editorial concluded: "The greenhouse effect is still too uncertain to warrant total alteration of energy policy. But this latest study offers fair warning; that such a change may yet be required is no longer unimaginable." Similar editorials appeared in the *Washington Post* and other newspapers.

Reactions from scientists were mixed. Criticisms, such as were published in letters to the editor of *Science,* are a normal part of the scientific process, and, together with rebuttals, tend to strengthen the ultimate conclusions. A letter in the journal *Climatic Change,* suggested that we "emphasized the worst case to get the attention of decision makers who control funding," thus questioning our scientific integrity. We responded simply that "as scientists we did our best to present an unbiased projection of likely climatic effects of carbon dioxide. We also fulfilled what we believe is a responsibility of scientists: to point out clearly the consequences of their findings."

Reaction by the agency that funded research on the climate effects of carbon dioxide, the U.S. Department of Energy (DOE), was unambiguous. A promise by DOE to provide continuing funding for our research was rescinded. The DOE position was further clarified when they told an independent researcher that his funding would be terminated if he used results from our climate model, which they described as an "outlier."

In the 1980s, the critical data emerged that was needed to define just how much the climate responds to a global forcing. This data was provided by holes drilled through the two-mile-thick ice sheets covering Greenland and Antarctica. These ice cores allowed sampling of bubbles of air that had been trapped as the ice sheets built up from snowfall year by year. The air bubbles provide a record of how the Earth's atmosphere has changed over the past 200,000 years.

With remarkable clarity these ice cores revealed that the composition of air had changed dramatically as climate changed. During the ice ages there were smaller amounts of the greenhouse gases, carbon dioxide, methane, and nitrous oxide, and there was more dust and other fine particles in the air than in the interglacial warm periods. This does not mean that these atmospheric changes "caused" the ice ages. Indeed, the greenhouse gas changes usually lagged behind the climate changes, suggesting that the ocean and land probably release more of these gases when they are warmer, thus providing a positive feedback.

Paleoclimatologists, those who study ancient climates, focus on trying to understand the sequences and the causes of climate changes. These are extremely complicated. A key factor seems to be changes of the Earth's orbit about the sun and the tilt of the Earth's spin axis. These orbital changes alter the seasonal distribution of sunlight on the planet and are observed to be synchronous with glacial to interglacial climate changes. The orbital changes occur over thousands of years, as the Earth is gravitationally perturbed by the major planets. The change of seasonal sunlight can make it easier or more difficult for ice sheets to grow, can alter vegetation distributions, and can change biochemistry and atmospheric composition in ways that are not well understood.

In looking at the Earth from a perspective of planetary science, it was clear that the new information from the ice cores allowed derivation of the most fundamental climate parameter, global climate sensitivity, without knowledge of the sequences and causes of glacial to interglacial changes. Data averaged over the thousands of years of an ice age or an interglacial period show that the Earth must be in radiation balance with space, emitting as much energy in heat as the solar energy it absorbs. As a result, the equilibrium climate sensitivity of the Earth is simply the ratio of the observed glacial to interglacial global temperature change divided by the net change of radiative forcings.

The change of global temperature between the last ace age, which peaked 20,000 years ago, and today is about 5° C. With the new information available on the change of atmospheric composition, the slowly changing factors influencing planetary radiation to space, that is, the climate "forcings," were all now also known. On the Earth's surface, the increased area of ice sheets and changes of vegetation altered the amount of absorbed solar energy, and in the atmosphere changes of gases and aerosols altered both the amount of absorbed solar energy and the heat radiated to space. The total change of these radiative forcings between the ice age and the current interglacial period was about 7 watts per square meter.

The implied climate sensitivity, 5° C for a 7-watt forcing, is equivalent to 3° C for doubled carbon dioxide because doubled carbon dioxide is about 4.3 watts of forcing. Thus, the empirical climate sensitivity based on a large observed climate change is right in the middle of the range that had been estimated from climate models. But the empirical sensitivity is more convincing and more precise, the 3° C for doubled carbon dioxide now being uncertain by no more than 1° C.

The high sensitivity of the climate system was no longer "only a model result": it was based on real-world data. And the ice age data provided a reminder of just how dramatic climate changes can be. During the last ice age, an ice sheet more than a mile thick covered North America as far south as Minneapolis, Seattle, and New York City.

The great thing about this empirical way of obtaining climate sensitivity, as opposed to models, is that it does not depend upon whether we know about every climate feedback process. All climate feedbacks in the real world are included automatically in the observed climate change. The derived sensitivity implies a net positive climate feedback factor of 2.5° C, because a 7-watt forcing with a simple blackbody planet, that is, without feedbacks, would yield a temperature change of only 2° C (just as the 4.3-watt forcing for doubled carbon dioxide would cause a 1.2° C warming without feedbacks). The positive feedback factor of 2.5° C as suggested by the models, presumably is caused by the fact that a warmer climate contains more water vapor, less sea ice, and probably some cloud changes.

We realized this net positive climate feedback had a rather staggering implication for the time constant of the climate system and thus also for potential policies to deal with the greenhouse effect. Researchers had usually assumed that the time required for the climate system to respond to a climate forcing was only a decade or two, but the climate system responds first only to the direct climate forcing. The feedbacks come into play only slowly, in response to the temperature change, not in response to the forcing. However as the feedbacks finally come into play, the initial heating of the ocean surface layer has already partly mixed into the deeper ocean. This is one of the problems I had puzzled about on Jones Beach.

It turned out to be easy to show that the time required for the ocean surface to respond is approximately proportional to the square of climate sensitivity. This extreme nonlinearity means that if climate sensitivity is about 3° C for doubled carbon dioxide, then the time required for the climate to reach two-thirds of its equilibrium response is about a hundred years!

One implication is that about half of the eventual warming that will result from man-made greenhouse gases added to the atmosphere in the past century is still "in the pipeline." The existence of this as yet "unrealized" warming obviously calls into question the wisdom of a "wait and see, and if necessary make midcourse corrections" policy. The strong positive feedback and long time constant of the climate system, together with the long time constant associated with carbon dioxide emissions, argue strongly for slowing down the inadvertent anthropogenic "experiment" being carried out on the climate system, so that the magnitude of the increasing climate change "in the pipeline" can be minimized.

In 1987 I was asked to testify about the greenhouse effect to the U.S. Senate Committee on Energy and Natural Resources. It was an opportunity to discuss the dangers of continued rapid increase of greenhouse gases, but I had testified at congressional hearings before to no effect. A global warming of half a degree, with the possibility of a few degrees in a hundred years, does not sound like much to politicians on two-six year election cycles.

Still a global warming of several degrees could alter the face of the planet. People are affected by climatic extremes, and the frequency of extremes would change greatly. I tried to illustrate this with a bar graph showing the average number of days per year that the temperature in Washington, D.C., exceeds 90° Fahrenheit, including an estimate of how this would change in a doubled carbon dioxide climate. With 4° C global warming, I found that the number of days exceeding 90° F. had increased from about 35 per year to 85 per year. This, at least, raised some eyebrows, and it even was reported in the *Washington Post*.

After that hearing, in discussions with congressional staff assistants, I said that I did not want to participate in the next hearing unless it were held in the summer, when people might take global warming more seriously. Although summer is not a popular time for hearings, Senator Tim Wirth of Colorado agreed or had a similar perspective, and he instructed the staff of his Committee on Energy and Natural Resources to schedule a hearing at a time they thought would be suitably warm. Apparently they were astute weather forecasters: On the date of that hearing, June 23, 1988, it was about 100° F. in Washington, D.C., with a drought in the Midwest so severe that the Mississippi River had practically dried up.

In my brief testimony that day I made three assertions: First, that global warming had reached a magnitude such that we could say with 99 percent confidence that it was a real change, not a chance fluctuation; Second, that the warming trend was probably due to the anthropogenic greenhouse effect; and third, that the greenhouse effect in our climate model simulations for the late 1980s and 1990s was already significant enough to affect the frequency of occurrence of extreme events, such as summer heat waves and droughts.

I emphasized that anthropogenic greenhouse warming would remain smaller than regional climate fluctuations for the next few decades, so we should look for greenhouse influence first in the frequency of warmer than normal seasons. In response to a question by one of the senators, I stated that no specific drought could be blamed on an increasing greenhouse effect, which only alters the probabilities.

A statement I made to reporters in the back of the room– "It's time to stop waffling so much and say that the greenhouse effect is here and is affecting our climate now"–accurately represented my opinion but by itself left a lot to the readers' imaginations. So did the one-sentence clips of my testimony on evening television, which were juxtaposed with images of the Midwest drought. Thus, it wasn't surprising that the television program "Jeopardy" incorrectly claimed I had testified that the Midwest drought was caused by the greenhouse effect.

After seeing the media interpretation, I realized that many people would misunderstand it the next time the temperature in a given season was colder than normal, in which case the attention drawn to the greenhouse effect may have done more harm than good. So I made up a set of large colored dice. The dice for the 1951 to 1980 period, which I used to define "normal" climate, had two red, two white, and two blue sides, representing unusually warm, average, and unusually cool seasons, respectively. The second dice represented our model calculations of how greenhouse warming should alter these probabilities in the 1990s. It had four red sides, one white, and one blue. The point I wanted to make was that even though climate fluctuates chaotically, greenhouse warming should load the climate dice enough for the informed layman to notice an increase in the frequency of warmer than normal seasons.

I used these dice on one or two television programs. I am not good at such things, and I don't enjoy them. Especially not that summer. Shortly after my testimony my wife told me she had been waiting until I was not so busy to tell me that she probably had breast cancer. She did. My father died that summer. Scientific reaction to my testimony was less than enthusiastic. I sent my colored dice to Carl Sagan, who I knew well from planetary research days, and suggested that he try to make the story clearer.

The next spring I was invited by then Senator and now Vice President Albert Gore to testify about the greenhouse effect before the Senate Committee on Commerce, Science, and Transportation. I thought this would be a good opportunity not only to correct misimpressions resulting from the media's exclusive focus on drought in 1988 but to discuss our recent studies at the Goddard Institute concerning regional climate extremes.

I told the Senate that extremes of climate have a great impact on people and on the rest of the biosphere. We need to understand how intense drought, 100-year floods, unusually strong storms, and record temperatures will change in frequency and severity if global warming increases. Unfortunately, current climate models cannot simulate realistically regional climate patterns, so we cannot have confidence in predicted changes for any particular place. Therefore, our procedure was to study the processes in a general sense without trying to predict change at a specific locality.

The bottom line of our study was evidence that an increasing greenhouse effect would cause a disproportionate increase in climatic extremes. The intensity of both extremes of the hydrologic cycle–droughts and forest fires, on the one hand, and heavy rainfall and the associated storms and floods, on the other hand– were found to increase with global warming. Qualitatively, this result seemed to make sense. Although the exact location and timing of droughts and floods move around in ways that are not generally predictable, it is clear that increased heating of the Earth's surface tends to increase evaporation, especially over oceans, where water is always available. The added evaporation leads to a corresponding increase of rainfall, and, moreover, there is a tendency for the rainfall to occur in more intense events in our model as the increased latent heat of vaporization powers deeper penetrating moist convective updrafts. The height of thunderstorms increases by several hundred meters in our simulations for doubled carbon dioxide. Yet in those places and times where the soil is dry, so that little evaporation is possible, the increased greenhouse heating intensifies the heat and drought conditions.

The increase of climate extremes is, I believe, a potentially useful indication for the layman and scientist to recognize greenhouse climate effects. I mentioned above the expected effects of global warming on the frequency of warmer than normal seasons, which I expect to be noticeable in the next several years. Another sensitive indicator is the number of daily record warm temperatures in a year as compared to the number of daily record cold temperatures.

The changes we calculated for the global hydrologic cycle imply that an increased greenhouse effect also will lead to an uncharacteristically large number of, say, 50-year or 100-year storms, floods, and droughts. With the present 0.5° C global warming, it may be difficult to clearly detect changes in the frequency of such hydrologic extremes. And it must be remembered that individual extreme events can always be assigned a proximate "cause" in terms of the antecedent global distribution of climate parameters, and thus individual events cannot be definitely attributed to the greenhouse effect. Therefore, to detect greenhouse impacts it is important to have long records covering large areas.

The testimony to Senator Gore's committee appeared to provide an opportunity for public discussion of man's influence on climate extremes. There was national news coverage because I had complained about changes inserted in my written testimony by the White House Office of Management and Budget. In my judgment, I should be able to say exactly what I believed because I had prefaced my testimony with a statement that it did not represent government policy or a consensus of the scientific community. I was more concerned about opposition from the scientific community because some of our results were new, and at best it would take many years to get any scientific consensus.

In fact, the publicity did not lead to discussion of the climate science. Photographs of me holding a 1-watt Christmas tree bulb appeared in a few newspapers but with no discussion of what I was trying to explain. Instead, the focus was on politics. *Newsweek* juxtaposed photos of John Sununu and me as apparent antagonists. If there was any positive result from my testimony it was a slight alteration in the administration's willingness to participate in international discussions about goals for greenhouse gas emissions, but this was not based on an improved understanding of the science.

If anything, the kind of experience I had in Washington, D.C., could make working scientists even less eager to participate in public discussion of a politically sensitive topic. In a *USA Today* story, a scientific colleague stated that "Hansen's political tangles are puzzling. He's rather apolitical, but he believes in what he's doing." I was lucky to escape with my job. I don't know exactly what happened behind the scenes, but I received a phone call at home one evening from Senator John Heinz III of Pennsylvania, informing me that he had spent some time defending me in a discussion with Sununu. He read a letter that he had written to Sununu, in which he argued that my statements were reasonable and that it was within my rights to make them.

In my opinion, there is a self-imposed reticence of scientists that reduces communication with the public. This is illustrated by an article that appeared in *Science* in May 1989 entitled "Hansen vs. the World on the Greenhouse Threat," which described a meeting of a group of climate researchers who appeared to condemn my testimony that the world was getting warmer and that the warming was probably due to the greenhouse effect. But the article quotes the participants as saying, "If there were a secret ballot at this meeting on the question, most people would say the greenhouse warming is probably there" and "What bothers a lot of us is that we have a scientist telling Congress things we are reluctant to say ourselves."

Another factor contributing to our reticence is the fact that we scientists tend to be poor communicators. In research it is important to include all necessary caveats and qualifiers, but when speaking to a lay audience these can also function to bury important conclusions. We need to communicate better with the public, without compromising the integrity of the science. Although the world now may be well aware of the greenhouse issue, the urgency of the need to communicate about climate change is just beginning.

How has the greenhouse story evolved since the media blitz of the late 1980s? First, there has been the rise of the issue in international circles, including assessments of the state of scientific understanding. Second, there is a remarkable change in the growth rate of greenhouse gas climate forcing and complications caused by changing tropospheric aerosols. Third, there is the observed climate change of the past several years and the expectation that climate changes over the next several years could illuminate the most fundamental science issues. Fourth, there is the need for improved science education and better public understanding of how research works, which may be necessary to achieve prudent public policy.

The increased prominence of the greenhouse issue internationally has been spectacular, culminating in an Earth Summit in Rio de Janeiro in 1992 and a global treaty that has been signed by about 165 nations. The first major goal set by the convention, to reduce carbon dioxide emissions to 1990 levels by the year 2000, probably will not be fully met, but there has been a remarkable decrease in the rate of growth of anthropogenic greenhouse gases. Procedures have been set up for further discussions and for periodic assessments of scientific understanding of climate change.

Scientific assessments are carried out by an Intergovernmental Panel on Climate Change (IPCC), formally set up by the World Meteorological Organization and the U.N. Environmental Program. Principal IPCC reports, expected to appear every five years (the first was in 1990 and the 1995 report is now undergoing peer review), involve the participation of several hundred scientists, and criticisms are sought during an extensive peer review process. Inevitably, some scientists will criticize any scientific review process, but the intense interest of the media and affected parties assures that all viewpoints are publicly aired.

The scientific process thrives on criticism and repeated reexamination of assumptions and conclusions, so true scientific critics represent an asset to the assessment process. However, those who simply hammer on model or data deficiencies, rather than finding ways to use existing capabilities insightfully, are of little value to the process. The number of nonproductive critics seems to have increased in the past several years, in some cases with support from economically interested parties. This impedes public understanding since the media often focuses on the extreme points of view.

The fundamental problem faced in the assessment process is the great difficulty in quantitatively extrapolating climate change and social impacts several decades ahead on the basis of current understanding. A good example is provided by the effect of global warming on ice sheets and thus on sea level. Ten years ago there was the fear that global warming of, say, 4° C could cause a sea level rise of 1 to 5 meters in the next century. More recent estimates tend to be in the range of 30 to 70 centimeters by the end of the next century. Still these estimates are strongly influenced by the sea level change observed in this century, which is about 15 centimeters, and has accompanied an 0.5° C global warming.

The truth is we simply do not know how ice sheets will respond to a global warming of several degrees. Over the past several decades, mountain glaciers around the world have been melting at remarkable rates, but mountain glaciers are too small to contribute much to sea level. Antarctica and Greenland contain enough ice to raise the sea level 70 meters if it melted entirely. Presently, most of the ice in Antarctica and Greenland is too cold to melt, but a warming of several degrees would make much of Greenland and the edges of Antarctica subject to possible summer melt. Once a melting starts it may increase with temperature in a nonlinear way, as, for example, summer precipitation and a freeze/thaw cycle can speed breakup of the ice.

If we estimate a global warming of 4° to 5° C, I suspect that we will be writing off–not immediately but in the next one to two centuries–not only island nation's such as the Maldives and Marshall Island, but much of Bangladesh, the Nile delta of Egypt, and even large parts of Louisiana, Florida, and New Jersey. This issue is complicated by the ocean's long response time, which assures that a large fraction of the warming due to existing greenhouse gases is still in the making. Given the large uncertainties in present projections, a sensible strategy would be to try to slow down the anthropogenic climate experiment.

Life on Earth is expected to be altered considerably by climate change, but our understanding is not adequate for specific reliable predictions. It is likely that agriculture, the managed biosphere, can adapt to changing climate in the developed world, but the most detrimental climate impacts are projected for low latitudes, where many developing countries may be ill-prepared for adaptations. Much of the natural biosphere, including forests and wildlife, may have great difficulty in migration or other adaptation to rapid climate change, because the habitats have been confined by human expansion into these areas. Increasing climate change combined with other stresses, may greatly accelerate the loss of plant and animal species.

Overall, because people and the biosphere are adapted to the climate that has existed in recent centuries, it is probable that large rapid global climate change will be very detrimental. Unfortunately, we cannot predict reliably the global distribution and effects of climate change. Some regions, especially at high latitudes, may benefit from it, which complicates international considerations.

A remarkable change in the growth rates of anthropogenic greenhouse gases has occurred recently. The greatest change has involved chlorofluorocarbons (CFCs), which represented 25 percent of the anthropogenic increase of greenhouse climate forcing during the 1980s. The growth rate of the principal CFCs has slowed dramatically in the 1990s as a consequence of the Montreal Protocol, which aimed at reversing ozone depletion, and these CFCs should begin to decline within the next several years. The increase of methane emissions, the third most important man-made greenhouse gas after carbon dioxide and CFCs, has fallen by half, from about 1 percent a year to about 0.5 percent a year. Even the growth rate of carbon dioxide has slowed from its maximum rate in 1988, though this is probably only a temporary respite, as total fossil fuel use has continued to rise slowly.

Our climate simulations in the late 1980s used three scenarios for trace gas growth rates: "business-as-usual," with continued exponentially increasing growth rates; "slow growth," with constant linear increases; and "draconian emission cuts," as required to stabilize atmospheric greenhouse gas amounts. IPCC has considered qualitatively similar scenarios. Observed trace gas growth rates since 1988 fall below the "slow growth" scenario, yet attention often remains focused on the "business-as-usual" case. There are good reasons to consider cases that bracket the plausible range, and recent slower growth rates may not be maintained, but these changes provide a basis for optimism that worst-case scenarios can be avoided. The principal factor determining long-term greenhouse forcing is whether coal will become the dominant energy source as oil and gas are depleted.

Tropospheric aerosols are the greatest source of uncertainty about current anthropogenic climate forcing. The predominant man-made aerosols are sulfates, arising from the burning of fossil fuels. Although carbon dioxide is the main product of combustion, coal and oil generally contain small amounts of sulfur. The sulfur dioxide gas produced from the burning of coal and oil is oxidized further in the atmosphere to form sulfates, which condense into fine droplets. These droplets scatter sunlight to space, and also alter cloud properties, before eventually being removed from the air as acid rain.

Aerosols have been recognized as an important climate forcing factor for many years, but only in the past few years has the modeling of their effects on the Earth's radiation balance become sufficiently realistic to allow useful comparison with greenhouse gases. The direct effect of the aerosols in scattering and absorbing sunlight is calculated to cause a negative forcing, that is, a cooling, of a few tenths of a watt per square meter, averaged over the Earth. The indirect effect of aerosols on cloud cover and cloud properties is very difficult to estimate but could be as much as about 1-watt per square meter. Unlike carbon dioxide, aerosols are distributed very unevenly over the Earth because their lifetime is only a few days. Thus, their climate forcing is not homogeneously distributed and does not cause a simple reduction of the greenhouse forcing.

A strong clue about the magnitude of the total aerosol climate forcing is provided by observations of changes in the diurnal cycle of temperature. Specifically, it has been found that over the past 40 years nighttime temperature increased much more than daytime temperature in most areas in the world. The only known mechanism that is capable of causing this phenomenon on a global basis is an increase of aerosols and associated cloud cover changes, in combination with an increasing greenhouse effect. The added aerosols and clouds reduce solar heating of the Earth's surface in the daytime and reduce thermal cooling at night. The aerosol and cloud increase required to match the observed change in the diurnal cycle yields a climate forcing of 1-watt per square meter, which is enough to reduce the global average greenhouse effect almost by half.

It is probably not coincidental that this aerosol forcing is just the amount required to bring calculated global warming of the past century into close agreement with observations. If climate sensitivity is 3° C for doubled carbon dioxide, as indicated by paleoclimate data, then the global warming estimated for the past century, due to increasing greenhouse gases, is about 1° C, when the delaying effects of the ocean's thermal inertia are taken into account. This is almost twice the observed warming. However, when the cooling effect of aerosols is included, the observed warming and the best estimates for climate sensitivity and climate forcing are all mutually consistent.

Although this explanation makes quantitative sense, it is unsatisfactory because the aerosol forcing has been estimated circuitously. The aerosol forcing needs to be measured not only to verify this interpretation but so that future changes of climate forcing can be estimated. Aerosol climate forcings, especially the indirect effects on clouds, are not simply proportional to sulfur emissions, and they vary with location. Satisfactory measurements will require both the global view of a satellite and detailed sampling of aerosol properties at representative sites. At present, there are no plans for satellite measurements with precision sufficient to track aerosol trends.

How has climate changed since the late 1980s? In 1990 the global average surface air temperature was the highest in the period of instrumental records, adding to concerns about global warming. In June 1991, Mount Pinatubo in the Philippines erupted, blasting about 20 million tons of sulfur dioxide into the stratosphere, where it formed a layer of sulfate aerosols that was spread globally by the winds. These aerosols reflected back to space almost 2 percent of the solar radiation reaching the Earth. At their maximum amount, the Mount Pinatubo aerosols caused a climate forcing of about 3.5 watts per square meter, briefly exceeding the total forcing by all man-made greenhouse gases. By the end of 1994, the stratospheric aerosol forcing had declined to about 0.4 watts per square meter. As expected, global temperatures cooled by several tenths of a degree in 1992 but by 1994 had rebounded more than half way to preeruption levels.

At this point, we are on the verge of being able to provide information on the most fundamental aspects of the climate system: the present amount of "unrealized warming" and all the implications which that has about climate forcings, climate sensitivity, and the response time of the climate system. It is commonly assumed, because of the large natural variability of climate, that it is not possible to predict short-term climate trends. However, if the world is substantially out of radiative equilibrium with space because of past growth of greenhouse gases to which the climate system has only partly responded, then the forcing associated with this unrealized warming potentially can overcome both the cooling remaining from Mount Pinatubo's eruption and natural climate variability.

The specific test is whether or not new global temperatures records will be obtained during the remainder of the 1990s. It has been shown that because the Mount Pinatubo cooling moved global temperature well away from the record level of 1990, it is very unlikely that natural variability could lead to new records within the next several years. Thus, a new record would imply the existence of a substantial positive climate forcing. In the absence of a measurable change of other forcings, such as solar irradiance, the plausible cause of such a forcing is a planetary radiation imbalance arising from unrealized greenhouse warming. Therefore, a new record global temperature would also support the high climate sensitivity and long climate response time required for the existence of substantial unrealized warming.

Recently, considering that it might be useful to draw attention to this potential information about near-term future global temperatures, I offered Richard Lindzen, a well-known "greenhouse skeptic," a friendly wager: specifically, that a new global temperature record would be set in the remainder of the 1990s. But even when I offered to make $1,000 if he won and a penalty of $10 if he lost, he declined, suggesting an alternative wager in which I would win only if the observed rate of warming in the 1990s exceeded 0.25° C per decade. This represented a way to avoid any wager because all of our model simulations published since 1981 show warming rates of 0.15° to 0.20° C per decade in the late twentieth century. Greenhouse skeptics like to set up a strawman warming rate of 0.3° to 0.4° C per decade knowing that such a rate occurs in our models only in the twenty-first century and only with the "business-as-usual" scenario.

The debate about climate change will not disappear, even if the observational evidence becomes noticeably stronger. This was demonstrated when observed ozone loss exceeded the levels predicted by models, yet some books and some radio talk-show hosts declared to wide audiences that the ozone warnings were a hoax. Also to convince the public about the climate issue will be far more difficult because it may be a long time before the observational evidence for anthropogenic change is as convincing and because the economic interests involved are far greater and more widespread.

Ultimately, at least in the United States, it will be the public that decides what actions are taken, or not taken, to deal with global warming. This emphasizes the need for our citizenry to be educated and informed in scientific topics that are inherently complex. Yet science curricula and instruction are not keeping pace with scientific and technical advances. Students are not being prepared to effectively participate in public debate about science issues.

Public education is also hampered by the fact that many scientists are reluctant to communicate with the public. There are many reasons for this: uneasiness about the nature of reporting that may oversimplify or misrepresent the science; concern that colleagues may be hard on scientists who appear in the media; and, probably most important, the amount of time and effort required to deal with the public and the media. Still balanced against these issues is a single overwhelming reason why we must vigorously pursue this communication: The public has the need and right to know the status of research, and, ultimately, it is the taxpayer who funds most research.

The best way scientists can aid communication, I believe, is by helping to improve science education in our schools. All of our students, both science and nonscience students, need to better understand how science research works. Science cannot be understood simply by looking up the right answer in the back of the book. In research, the "answers" are usually multifaceted, and as we learn, each thing raises new questions.

The most effective way, perhaps the only way, to teach students about research is to get them involved in it. In the next several years, as our schools are connected by the internet and information highway, we have the opportunity to open the door of science research to all students. This will require developing curricula around real ongoing research, in such a way that the process can be understood by all students, with the most precocious or hardworking ones having possibilities for original contributions.

I like to imagine the possibility of launching a small, inexpensive satellite to measure precisely the spectra of reflected solar radiation and emitted heat leaving the Earth. Such data, transmitted to classrooms, could serve not only to inform students about the most basic physical processes determining the Earth's climate, but to help construct maps showing how the global distributions of clouds, aerosols, sea ice, vegetation cover, and other climate-related quantities change from month to month and year to year.

Bridging the gap between the scientific and education communities, scientists and teachers could work together to design courses for teaching about climate, seasonal climate change, and natural variability of climate. Exactly the same data could be used by the scientists in joint research projects with the educational community. Together they could search for long-term climate change and the mechanisms for that change because all climate forcings and feedbacks operate by altering the spectra of reflected solar and emitted thermal radiation. If that cooperative effort is achieved, I would predict with great confidence that students would make some of the most interesting discoveries that lie ahead.

22

PRESERVING THE EARTH'S BIOLOGICAL RESOURCES

THOMAS LOVEJOY
is Counselor to the Secretary of the Smithsonian Institution. From 1973 to 1987,
he directed the program of the World Wildlife Fund–United States and was
responsible for its scientific, Western Hemisphere, and tropical forest orientation.
He is generally credited with having brought the tropical forest problem to the
fore as a public issue and is one of the main protagonists in the science and conservation of biological diversity. For his many conservation initiatives in Brazil,
he was decorated by the Brazilian government in 1988, becoming the first envi-
ronmentalist to receive the Order of Rio Branco. Dr. Lovejoy is the originator of
the concept of debt-for-nature swaps, which have been initiated in Bolivia, Costa
Rica, Ecuador, the Philippines, Madagascar, Jamaica, and Zambia, among other
countries, and is the founder of the PBS series "Nature," the most
popular long-term series on public television.

THE UNITED NATIONS CONVENTION on Biological Diversity, launched at the U.N. Conference on Environment and Development in 1992, constitutes a historic recognition of the crisis in biological resource conservation. It is perhaps most popularly understood in terms of attractive vertebrate endangered species or the rapid rates of tropical deforestation. The best estimates of rates of species loss are on the order of 1,000 to 10,000 times normal. It is not easy to be precise, because life on earth is so poorly explored: perhaps one species in ten has been described by science. Nonetheless, while biologists argue about the precise rate of extinction engendered by human activity, all agree that there is a problem and that it is a serious one.

This presents various consequences for human health. There are numerous examples of environmental disturbance leading to disease. The classic example is how the sylvan cycle of yellow fever spills over into human populations, which Colombian epidemiologist Jorge Boshell revealed after he observed woodsmen who had downed a rain forest tree surrounded by the little blue *Haemagogus* mosquitoes which were the vectors of the howler monkey sylvan cycle. It is likely that Lyme disease is at least partly the consequence of major land use change in the eastern United States, and there are major implications for changes in vector distributions and associated epidemiological cycles inherent in global climate change.

The variety of plants, animals, and microorganisms extant constitutes the most sensitive set of indicators to environmental change. Thus, it was a whelk experiencing the condition of imposex (wherein a female whelk grows a penis) that provided one of the first signals that the use of tributyltin (TBT) as an antifouling compound in nautical paints might be problematic for human health. Current reproductive problems in wild species, such as the American alligator, have raised serious questions about many human-created molecules acting as endocrine disrupters. Basically, the staggering variety of biological systems in biological diversity provides an early warning system about potential human health problems.

Of course, biological diversity has provided a major source of medicines for millennia. This is a story older than aspirin, and its origin begins in Hippocratic times and earlier, as an infusion of willow bark being used as an analgesic. Various figures are given as to the percent of medicines having plant origin; the lowest seems to be about 25 percent. Penicillin and streptomycin, with broad-spectrum antibiotic activity deriving from molds, digitalis from foxglove for heart conditions, taxol from the Pacific yew for breast cancer, quinine for malaria, airare (an arrow poison) used as a muscle relaxant, and Mexican yams as precursors for cortisone and oral contraceptives are all well-known examples.

The exploration of nature for medicinals somewhat fell from fashion in recent decades as pharmaceutical chemists found easy ways to create potentially useful new molecules in the laboratory. Interestingly, the same advances in laboratory biochemistry have now made it much more efficient to screen samples from wild sources, and pharmaceutical companies are turning once again to such sources. Rapid screening of many samples is being used in a number of exercises in biochemical prospecting. The most advanced and best known of institutions undertaking these practices is Costa Rica's Instituto Nacional de Biodiversidad (INBio), which currently is working with Merck and Bristol Myers. A number of joint ventures with those and other companies are under way, under the auspices of the National Cancer Institute, in a number of countries. INBio is currently doing some biochemical prospecting with insects that promise to have more complex and interesting molecules.

In the end, one of the most powerful contributions biological diversity has to make to human health and well-being is at the level of the molecule. The most dramatic current example is the polymerase chain reaction (PCR) that multiplies genetic material a billion times in just a couple of hours. This is now fundamental to diagnostic medicine, to forensic medicine, and to the entire human genome project. PCR works because of a heat-resistant enzyme from a bacterium, *Thermus aquaticus*, known as Taq polymerase, found in a Yellowstone hot spring. PCR alone is at the core of multibillions of dollars of economic activity annually. It is no wonder that the Japanese are currently investing $25 million in search of heat-resistant enzymes in organisms associated with the thermal rifts on the bottom of the sea.

Indeed, as one explores the potential for biotechnology and molecular biology to contribute to human health and well-being, it is apparent that that potential is based squarely on being able to draw on biological diversity. Genetic engineering does not make new genes; rather, it rearranges existing ones. The endonucleases that molecular biologists use to cut a DNA strand at precise places are molecules drawn from nature in places as disparate as New Guinea, Minnesota, and the sea floor.

Perhaps even more important is the contribution biological diversity makes as the fundamental library for the life sciences. The life sciences progress in significant degree through research about species other than ourselves and our disease organisms and their vectors. Often fundamental advances in life sciences are made by studies, which then have enormous import for human health, of nonhuman organisms. Vaccinations and antibiotics responsible for hundreds of millions of lives saved or lived more healthfully are paramount examples of concepts derived from studies involving other species–cows, cowpox, and humans in the one instance and accidental contamination of laboratory culture by mold form from a cantaloupe in the other. The angiotensin system of regulation of blood pressure (and the hypertension drugs that work on it) was discovered by studying the mechanism and its effect on the venom of a South American viper.

The foregoing makes a strong case for conservation and for avoiding what most knowledgeable biologists project will be one of the major extinction spasms in the history of life on Earth. A thorough review of the situation, the Global Biodiversity Assessment, is currently under way under the auspices of the U.N. Environment Program (UNEP). It will assess the respective contributions to biodiversity loss of habitat destruction, habitat fragmentation, introduction of exotic species (e.g., Dutch elm disease in the United Kingdom, the brown tree snake in Guam), and pollution. All of those factors leading to biotic impoverishment as well as potential global warming are driven by human population growth and patterns of technology and consumption. Increasingly, what biodiversity remains is sequestered in isolated reserves surrounded by highly converted landscapes. When natural or unnatural climate change occurs (and the former or both *inevitably* will), it will be difficult for species to track their required conditions as they were able to do during past climate changes. Unless there is a major modification in the way we relate to the land, so that we restore connectivity between natural areas, the consequences will be a major biotic disaster.

The solution that seems to be emerging revolves around the concept of ecosystem management. The notion is relatively simple: starting with a relatively large ecological unit of landscape (as has been done in South Florida), to move from thinking of nature as something that exists (survives) in a small piece of human-dominated landscape to thinking of human aspiration being conducted within a natural (ecosystem) one. If the unit is large and the various interests within succeed in voluntarily sharing information and decision-making, there should be multiple options and flexibility–although the greater the population density and the less surviving nature, the harder it will be to maintain ecosystem function and characteristic biodiversity. By definition, ecosystem management requires taking into account all factors intrinsic and extrinsic that will bear upon the particular ecosystem. This provides an operational definition of sustainable development. If such sustainable ecosystem management is practiced for all ecosystems in the world, however delineated, the sum would be sustainable development at the global scale.

Much as this century has been dominated by the physics and information revolutions, the next and those to follow will be the centuries of biology. Already we can perceive the outline: biotechnology, genetic engineering, bioindustry, nanotechnology, bioremediation. To reap the benefits, and for a healthy and productive society, we will need biodiversity.

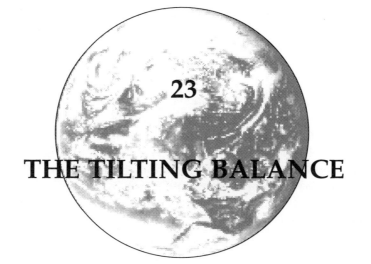

23

THE TILTING BALANCE

PAUL JOHNSTON, RUTH STRINGER, AND DAVID SANTILLO
are with the Greenpeace University of Exeter Research Laboratory, Greenpeace
International. Greenpeace was conceived in 1971 when members of the Don't
Make a Wave Committee in Vancouver, Canada, renamed their organization the
better to proclaim their purpose: to create a green and peaceful world. The
organization's remarkable growth reflects the strength of the conviction that
the planet's very survival depends on defending the natural system
of which we humans are but one element.

THE POPULATION OF THE WORLD is expected to reach some 7 billion by the year 2010, double that of the 1960s. Moreover, by the year 2050 it is projected that some 12 billion human beings will be living in the world. Yet already the natural ecology of 70 percent of the total habitable area of the planet is significantly disturbed.

Much of this increase in population will take place in coastal regions that are currently not heavily industrialized, and there will be a concomitant intensification of agricultural and industrial activity. Inevitably, human pressures on the environment also will increase. The changes are likely to be most marked in those regions within 60 kilometers of the sea. This is an obvious characteristic, for example, of the burgeoning industrial development taking place in the countries bordering the Pacific region. In such coastal areas, degradation of many critical marine and terrestrial environments is already well advanced.

A degraded environment is not simply a matter of aesthetics or conservation, although, of course, these are fundamentally important aspects to consider. Questions also arise about the quality of human life resulting from such changes. Currently, the true costs of many modern environmental impacts are hidden and externalized upon the environment itself. The economic costs of protective measures are rarely examined in the light of the growing societal costs of failing to formulate, adopt, and implement them. These costs manifest in a number of ways. Direct loss of livelihood is often obvious and relatively easy to quantify in fiscal terms. Impacts upon human health and welfare, by contrast, are often more subtle and more difficult to recognize. They involve a formidable array of practical, philosophical, and ethical issues. Nonetheless, the impact of toxic exposure on a human quality of life is a clear and increasing problem, and one that is beginning to be understood as such.

TOXIC EXPOSURES DEFINED

Toxic Metals

Early references to the harmful effects of toxic metals upon human and animal health can be found in the classical works of Xenophon, Lucretius and Pliny. Indeed, chronic lead contamination is widely believed to be linked to the decline of the Roman Empire. Analysis of peat cores dating to the 17th century has shown that the increasing scale of metallurgical processes in Europe was already being reflected by this time in increased metal levels in remote regions of Scandinavia. Other historical records, such as of ice cores and sediments, document increasingly severe toxic metal pollution from the Industrial Revolution to the present day. Once dispersed, these metals are not degraded, nor does technology exist to recover them. The environmental impacts of metals tend to be permanent even though they occur naturally, undergo natural cycling in the environment, and, indeed, may be vital components of biochemical pathways. For elements such as copper, zinc and selenium the balance between the essential amounts required for normal functioning of the body and the amounts producing toxic effects is an extremely fine one. Others, such as lead, cadmium, and mercury, have no known biological function and the ability of many organisms (including humans) to regulate body levels of these is very limited.

Metals are naturally released from the weathering of rocks and from volcanoes and forest fires. Prior to industrialization metal inputs cycled in a steady state, and these processes controlled and restricted metal distributions in natural systems. These sources, though, are now equaled or exceeded by the amounts currently being released from mining, smelting, and industrial processes, including oil and coal combustion. In urban areas, natural sources are now insignificant in amounts being released when compared with amounts released by human activity. Globally and regionally, the ambient levels in the environment reflect proximity to industry. Levels in the atmosphere above the South Pacific Ocean, for example, are much lower than those above the North Atlantic while these levels in turn are exceeded substantially in the air above the Mediterranean and North seas. These balances have been inexorably and unfavorably tilted within a comparatively short space of time.

Much of the focus upon the human health effects of this insidious increase in environmental metal levels has centered upon acute poisoning incidents. The Minimata incident, involving mercury in Japan, affected many hundreds of people directly and effects were carried across into the next generation. Cadmium was responsible for Itai-Itai disease in another area of Japan. What is not clear, however, is the degree to which chronic exposures may be taking place and what the effects of this may be. Impacts are likely to be subclinical in many cases, and any overt clinical disease is likely to have poorly characterized symptoms. Current clinical tests are too insensitive to detect important but subtle changes in biochemistry. Indeed, metal-mediated changes in vital signs may not become evident until toxicological processes are well advanced. Bodily mechanisms capable of compensating for metal exposures may be overwhelmed before the damage becomes obvious.

All the evidence points to a substantial global problem affecting human health.

Exposure to toxic metals has been implicated variously in the etiology of cardiovascular disease, reproductive disorder, allergy, and some cancerous diseases. It has been estimated that between a quarter and a half million people worldwide may suffer renal dysfunction due to cadmium poisoning. Up to 80,000 people dependent on fishing may be suffering from the effects of mercury poisoning due to ingestion of contaminated seafood. Another quarter of a million people are believed to be suffering from skin cancers caused by arsenic exposure. In laboratory studies, at least eighteen metals have been implicated in cancerous diseases.

The numbers of people actually at risk are inevitably much higher than estimates indicate. In the case of lead, for example, between 130 and 200 million people worldwide are estimated to be at risk of poisoning, as gauged from their blood lead concentrations. Although hard data was lacking, it seems that at least a billion people are unwittingly exposed to elevated levels of metals in the environment.

These problems are likely to increase in scale and scope. Consumption of metals and the products made from them is linked to, and fueled by, increase in population and rising gross national products. Initial markets in durable metal items expand to embrace less durable products, more frequently discarded and replaced. Rising energy consumption based upon fossil fuels also adds to the environmental burden. Moreover, observers have noted a growing trend for metal wastes and scraps to be exported from industrialized nations to those striving to develop their industrial base. They are variously disposed of or used as marginal resources, employing methods that would certainly not meet environmental regulations in their country of origin. The burgeoning trade in used vehicle batteries is a well-known example; the significant trade in mixed metal compounds and metal-rich residues is less recognized. Some gold wastes can contain 40 percent by weight of arsenic. There are significant gaps, too, in the international regulations governing the trade in such wastes. The current situation has already been described as a "Silent Epidemic of Environmental Metal Poisoning." If metals consumption continues to grow in line with the increasing global population, this epidemic will surely grow to pandemic proportions.

Organic Chemicals

Of the chemicals in common industrial use, the greatest proportion are organic chemicals. Used as solvents, raw materials, chemical intermediates, and as final products in their own right, these substances are manufactured from petroleum. Some idea of the scale of the problem facing the industrial hygienists and environmental toxicologists can be gauged from the fact that an estimated 63,000 chemicals are in common use worldwide; that about 3,000 account for 90 percent of the total production; and that anywhere between 200 and 1000 new synthetic chemicals enter the market each year. The properties of those organic chemicals of greatest concern are their toxicity, coupled with their persistence in the environment and a tendency to accumulate in the fatty tissue of organisms exposed to them.

To a very large extent, studies on the effects of these chemicals have concentrated upon their ability to cause cancer. This represents a convenient point of reference both for the public (who justifiably fears such diseases) and the medical profession (who is well aware of the difficulty of treating them). Some cancers have been found to be associated with particular exposures. Indeed, cancer of the scrotum in chimney sweeps in Victorian England was the first identified cancer resulting from toxic exposure. Since then, other links have been found. Some are specific, other less so. Agricultural workers are a high-risk group, presumably due to their exposure to agrochemicals. Industrial workers involved in producing vinyl chloride used to make PVC (polyvinyl chloride) are at risk of contracting liver cancer. It would be wrong, of course, to ignore these signs of extreme disturbance of body systems. As largely incurable diseases, they represent an ultimate threat to the life of individual humans. Arguably, though, the investigation of cancer-causing properties has tended to divert attention from other effects of toxic exposure. Although at first sight these may not seem to be as severe, their effects extend beyond the individual to embrace the whole human population.

Levels of persistent organic pollutants (POPs) in the environment have increased markedly since the Industrial Revolution. Some, such as the polynuclear aromatic hydrocarbons (PAHs), are released predominantly from combustion processes. Increases in levels have been traced through archived samples of soils and cores of peat, ice, and sediment. Some of these chemicals are highly potent carcinogens. The most important group of these persistent chemicals, however, contain chlorine, and for the most part these have no counterparts in nature. Members of this group include the pesticides DDT, dieldrin, chlordane, toxaphene and lindane, the polychlorinated biphenyls (PCBs), and the chlorinated dioxins and dibenzofurans. Many other organochlorines are used as bulk industrial and consumer chemicals. In general, increases in environmental levels of these chemicals are easy to measure. Quite simply, prior to their industrial production from the 1920's onward, they did not exist in the natural environment.

Organochlorine Pesticides and PCBs: Organochlorine chemicals were eventually recognized as ubiquitous global pollutants, and restrictions on their manufacture and use were emplaced in many national legislatures. Still international legislation has been slow in coming. Restrictions followed after they were found to build up in the tissues of birds and animals. Severe reproductive and infertility problems were found in species at the top of the food chain. Fish-eating birds and mammals were found to be most badly affected, but humans too, accumulated these chemicals from their food. Most, if not all, humans, now have residues of these chlorinated pesticides and industrial chemicals in their body fat.

Paradoxically, populations in some of the most remote regions of earth may eventually become the most severely affected. In many cases, chlorinated pesticides that are banned or severely restricted in industrialized nations remain in intensive use elsewhere. As agricultural systems also intensify to feed the growing population, so this balance of toxic exposure will tilt inexorably towards the nations of the Southern Hemisphere.

One very recent discovery is that persistent organic pollutants can also be transported in the atmosphere over long distances. Their physical properties mean that they tend to "condense" out at cold, high latitudes. This means that Arctic ecosystems are particularly vulnerable, but temperate areas will also be affected. This transport is a progressive process. Before ending in the remote cold areas, these chemicals will pass through the more temperate regions of the Northern Hemisphere where population densities are highest.

The various regulations put in place initially appeared to restrict growing environmental levels of some persistent organic chemicals. Bald eagles, a national symbol of the United States, together with a host of less well known wildlife species, appeared to have been saved from terminal decline. After an initial sharp fall in the level of these chemicals, though, the downward trend leveled off. Even after a decade of regulating PCBs and other organochlorines, they were implicated as toxic contributors to the mass mortality of seals in the North Sea in 1988, when 18,000 animals died from a viral infection, and in the die-offs of dolphin species in the Mediterranean Sea and North Atlantic Ocean, which seem to be still continuing. Fish from the Baltic Sea contaminated with organochlorines were fed to seals. The immune systems of the animals quickly became suppressed, endangering their defense against infection.

It was thought initially that the organochlorine pesticides and the PCBs were relatively nontoxic to humans. True, there had been at least two direct poisonings due to contamination of rice oil with PCBs, one in Japan (the Yusho incident) and one in Taiwan (Yu-cheng disease). In addition, in the U.S. there were widespread toxicity problems in livestock due to contamination of animal feed with a fire retardant similar to PCBs. While these events were closely studied, they were regarded as exceptional. Chronic problems with wildlife, attributed to toxic exposures, were regarded as a peculiar consequence of their feeding exclusively on contaminated fish. Humans, it was reasoned, were only exposed to contaminated fish under exceptional circumstances, and these exposures could be controlled. This assumption has proven to be ill-founded. Although the amounts required to produce a lethal response in humans are relatively high, the more subtle effects have only become evident after much closer scrutiny. For example, extensive studies were made of children born to mothers who consumed organochlorine-contaminated fish from the Great Lakes only twice a month. These children were smaller at birth and showed poorer cognitive development, indicating prenatal neurological damage.

As a result of the poleward migration of persistent chemicals, dangerous levels have been found in the bodies of indigenous populations in the north of Alaska who depend upon marine resources. In some cases, Faroe Islanders who consume blubber from pilot whales caught in the supposedly clean waters of the North Atlantic are exposed to levels of organochlorines that exceed international advised daily intakes. Toxaphene, more dangerous than the PCBs, is found in fish and porpoises in the North Sea and is thought to originate from Caribbean cotton fields where it is used in pest control. Traces of many organochlorines can also be found in fish oils produced from fish taken in waters far distant from industry. Given that organochlorine pesticides are still being produced and used, that PCBs are still being released to the environment, and that PAH emissions are increasing from our consumption of fossil fuels, these findings do not auger well for the future.

The Chlorinated Dioxins: The chlorinated dioxins and dibenzofurans, known collectively as "dioxins," were only identified as important environmental contaminants in the early 1980s although their toxic properties had been made evident before that time. The Seveso accident in 1976 released large quantities of the highly toxic chemical known as 2,3,7,8-TCDD, and they were recognized as contaminants in Agent Orange, to which many Americans were exposed in Southeast Asia. The regulatory issues attached to this group of 210 individual chemicals are complex since they are not deliberately produced but appear as by-products in industrial processes, particularly the manufacture of other organochlorines, and through the combustion of chlorine-containing wastes. Waste incineration is an important source, as is the production of steel, nonferrous metals, and the plastic PVC. The dioxin group of chemicals also build up in the food chain and can be transported for great distances. Greater human exposure to these compounds will inevitably follow from increasing industrialization. Again, the balance of these increasing exposures will tilt toward the developing countries.

Unsurprisingly, much effort has been directed toward investigating the toxic properties of dioxins. For many years, it was believed that the only real effect was a disfiguring skin disease known as "chloracne." More in-depth research, however, has shown that they can affect the immune system. Indeed, such interferences may be taking place at the levels according to which people already have been exposed to these chemicals. They can be passed on in breast milk to nursing infants and may cause interference with the function of the thyroid gland and vitamin K metabolism, producing a life-threatening syndrome. They are carcinogenic and there does not appear to be a threshold for their effects. Any exposure could, therefore, cause cancers to appear many years later. These effects can be identified when levels of chlorinated dioxins in the blood and body fat reach part per trillion levels. There is now also strong evidence that dioxins and other organochlorines, together with some of the PAHs, may interfere with estrogen and other hormonal pathways at extremely low concentrations.

Hormonal Effects

Of all the subtle deleterious effects of toxic exposures, chemical interference with body hormones is, with hindsight, an effect that should have been foreseen. It is the effect with the most profound implications. For instance, some years ago this property of the pesticide DDT was identified in the laboratory, yet the significance of this finding was not applied, despite the fact that the most frequently observed effect in wildlife populations was reproductive failure. The implications for human populations are now becoming clear. In areas of Europe, research has shown that sperm counts have been declining at around 2 percent per year over the last 20 years, a trend that can be traced back over at least the last 50 years. The most likely cause is thought to be exposure to toxic chemicals.

Plausible links have made between low-level exposure to organochlorine chemicals and cancers of the reproductive tract in humans of both sexes. Exposure of unborn children at critical prenatal stages may have repercussions of equal importance to the intellectual disadvantage already identified in the Great Lakes studies. Genital abnormalities may occur, as may lowered fertility in adult life. It is, of course, not simply the POPs that could be responsible for these effects. Breakdown products of commercial detergents, for example, are suspected of causing male fish to develop female characteristics when discharged in rivers in sewage. Nonetheless, the majority of chemicals exhibiting these properties are persistent organic pollutants that can be transported by natural process across the globe. The greatest proportion of these is the group of organic chemicals containing chlorine.

As scientists have come to appreciate the power of these chemicals to interfere with the systems that crucially support the workings of the body, so have they realized that the science of toxicology now requires a fundamental reappraisal. No longer can threats to the quality of human life be understood exclusively in terms of the risk of contracting cancer. The problems must now be investigated on a broader base. If it is true that the survival of vulnerable nonhuman species is at stake, that the world faces a series of chemical extinctions due to toxic exposure, why should these predictions not extend to humans?

TILTING BALANCE: AN ALTERNATIVE?

Human exposures to toxicity depend upon a series of balances. As the industrial base broadens and deepens in the developing world, so increases the exposure of the population to metals through contamination of natural systems. Equally, increased use of agrochemicals and control agents in health programs is likely both to increase toxic exposures on a local basis and to extend the areas affected through the transport of chemicals in the atmosphere. The potential magnitude of the effects of chemicals on hormone systems are as yet unknown.

The problems produced by many groups of chemicals could grow substantially. Emissions of PCBs, for example, are widely perceived to be under control and a problem of the past. Yet even in the case of this well-studied group it is possible that emissions, and hence human exposure, will increase despite the current regulations and controls. Total world production figures for PCBs are estimated at between 1 and 2 million tons since they went into production in 1929. It is estimated that around 35 percent of these have escaped into the environment while only 4 percent have been destroyed. The balance, some 60 percent, is in dumps and landfills or still being used in electrical transformers and capacitors the world over. Most of the equipment containing PCBs will reach the end of its useful life by the year 2005.

Hence, the scope of problems involving PCBs, one of many chemicals of concern, could well double or triple unless concerted efforts are made to prevent this happening. These chemicals need to be systematically collected and detoxified, using an environmentally benign technology. More radical measures are required to control levels of PAHs reaching the environment. A substantial decrease of human dependence upon and consumptions of fossil fuels is required. Similarly, control of chlorinated dioxins can only take place by decreasing human dependence upon the diverse processes, including primary chlorine production, which generate them.

Obviously, the problems cannot be allowed to grow and intensify. Equally, no one measure will suffice to address these problems of toxic exposures. What is needed is a profound adjustment of philosophy. Instead of only regulating chemicals when their ill effects become obvious, a preventive approach is required, one that gives human and environmental health the positive benefit of any doubts that may exist. We must come to regard regulations as staging posts on the road to zero emissions and develop alternative clean technologies for both industrialized and nonindustrialized nations. Agricultural practices must move toward an ideal of ecological agriculture that utilizes ways of minimizing and eliminating the use of agrochemicals. Health programs will need to be supplied with alternatives to persistent organochlorines. Economic concerns also must be considered. A global effort is required.

The alternative is grim: to allow the balance of pollution to tilt further, to permit toxic exposures to increase, to watch the environment continue to degrade, and to let the human race collectively bear increasing chemical compromises to its health and its future.

24

TOXIC EXPOSURE AND HEALTH:
Perspective of the U.S.
Environmental Protection Agency

LYNN GOLDMAN
is Assistant Administrator, Office of Prevention, Pesticides, and Toxic Substances,
and Spokesperson for the U.S. Environmental Protection Agency. The EPA was
created in 1970 in response to the growing awareness of ecological concerns, and
is charged with the preservation of a clean environment and the protection of
public health from exposure to environmental insults. Despite intense resistance
from industry and what has often been a very adversarial process, the EPA has
dramatically improved the environment in the United States. The land, air, and
water have become cleaner. In fact, some rivers and lakes, once so contaminated
they were flammable, have now been reopened to fishing and swimming.

THE ESTABLISHMENT of the U.S. Environmental Protection Agency (EPA) was preceded by a decade of increasing concern about environmental pollution. In 1962, Rachel Carson's *Silent Spring* was a call to alert the public to the hazards of pesticides. Photochemical smog had been identified in the Los Angeles Basin and was increasing in metropolitan areas throughout the world. Water pollution was an enormous problem, with untreated sewage discharge from many large cities and little if any control in place of chemical pollutants.

Because of how U.S. environmental laws evolved over the last 25 years, the EPA's organization reflects statutes that address separate environmental media: pesticides, toxic substances, air, radiation, water, drinking water, solid wastes, and toxic waste sites. This arrangement, while segmented, has resulted in remarkable improvements in environmental quality in the United States: cleaner air; safer drinking water; safer food; more lakes, rivers, and streams that are fishable and swimmable; and more responsible handling of wastes.

Yet the environment continues to pose potential health threats, particularly to those living in urban areas where air pollution exceeds standards set to protect the public's health. The incidence and mortality of asthma–on the rise in the United States–have prompted a renewed search for causative factors. With continued ozone exceedences and smog alerts, we have not yet assured clean air for all communities in the U.S. Similarly, too many rivers, lakes, and streams are still highly polluted. Contamination of coastal waters is also a problem in many areas. Despite the progress in cleaning up abandoned and uncontrolled toxic waste sites, many of these Superfund sites still await completion of cleanup. Problems with drinking water contamination continue to occur in many areas. In 1993, for example, there was a major bacterial (cryptosporidiosis) outbreak in Milwaukee, Wisconsin. In addition, we have a greater appreciation today of risks from indoor exposures to pollutants. Studies show that persons in industrialized nations spend more than 90 percent of their time indoors. For infants, the elderly, persons with chronic diseases, and most urban residents the proportion is probably higher. Indoor risks include, but are not limited to, environmental tobacco smoke, emissions from stoves, furnaces, and fireplaces, pesticides, solvents, cleaning solvents, asbestos, radon, and the whole complex of exposures for which we use the term "sick building" syndrome.

An important consideration underlying future efforts to reduce toxic exposures is the compelling logic of sustainable development. This principle recognizes the interdependence of environmental protection and economic growth. Development that is sustainable will provide the resources for environmental protection, and environmental protection will provide the resources for economic growth and the well-being of generations to come. Clean air, water, and land are vital for expansion and for a viable quality of life. Countries that compromise the environment for immediate economic gain ultimately pay–in diminished health conditions, fewer usable resources, and higher costs to solve pollution problems retroactively. Prevention is more cost-effective than remediation.

What follows is a general overview of how the U.S. has controlled toxic exposures over the last 25 years and of newer approaches to deal with these problems today. The problems that we all face in 1995 are more complex and difficult than those that confronted the EPA when it began in 1970. These more challenging problems require new tools to better address toxic exposures: right-to-know measures, pollution prevention, the agency's Common Sense Initiative, and market incentives. Importantly, the newer tools do not replace traditional "command and control" approaches; strong standards will continue to undergird our efforts. These tools offer more effective, less costly control strategies that deliver greater environmental protections. Solutions to address the more complex problems we face in 1995 also require strengthening the scientific basis for assessment of toxic exposure and risk.

EXPOSURES TO TOXIC CHEMICALS

In the United States, there are more than 70,000 chemicals on EPA's inventory of toxic chemicals. Of these, there are some 16,000 nonpolymers that are produced at levels of more than 10,000 pounds per year and to which workers and citizens may be exposed. Additionally, there are approximately 2,000 new chemicals submitted to EPA each year by U.S. industry for premanufacture approval. The volume of pesticides being used in the United States is also large. In 1993, for instance, pesticide use totaled more than 4 billion pounds, based on the amount of active ingredients. This included conventional pesticides, wood preservatives, disinfectants and sterilants, and water treatment and swimming pool chemicals.

The large number of chemicals in use at high quantity underscores the need for setting priorities so that exposures of most concern receive attention first. The cases of pesticides, lead, and environmental tobacco smoke are useful examples of assessing and managing toxic exposures.

Pesticides

When the EPA was created in 1970, one of the first problems to be addressed was to ban or severely restrict a number of persistent and bioaccumulative pesticides: aldrin, amitrole, BHC, chlordane, and DDT, to name a few. Although most of the legal cases developed to control these pesticides relied on cancer-testing data, there were also concerns about serious ecosystem effects. For example, many reasoned that if exposure to DDT caused a disruption in the reproduction of birds, then there might be similar effects in humans. While many other industrialized nations have also banned or severely restricted these so-called "organochlorine" pesticides, international use of some of these persistent chemicals continues to add to the earth's burden: long-range transport of these pesticides pose a threat everywhere.

Today's pesticide control efforts are more complex and challenging. One result of the banning of persistent toxic pesticides was a sharp increase in the use of pesticides that are acutely toxic to farmworkers–the organophosphate and carbamate pesticides. These pesticides inhibit the enzyme acetylcholinesterase, causing illness with acute overexposure. In the U.S., we are moving to carry out new farmworker protection regulations. The primary aim is to prevent or reduce exposure, using a combination of engineering controls such as enclosing tractor cabs, clothing, posting of warning signs, and training of pesticide applicators and farmworkers to ensure that they are aware of the hazards and can adequately protect themselves. However, these pesticides are used with very little restriction in developing countries, where challenges exist to managing occupational risk: for example, limited access to engineering controls and infeasibility of certain types of protective clothing in hot and/or humid climates.

Keeping the food supply safe and making it healthier still are also important, particularly where infants and children are concerned, because diet is a major route of exposure to pesticides for children. In 1993, the U.S. National Academy of Sciences published a report entitled *Pesticides in the Diets of Infants and Children*, which emphasized that children may be both more exposed and more vulnerable to pesticide residues on food. In response to this report, we are evaluating ways to improve our ability to assess exposure and risk to infants and children. It is clear that we need to improve food consumption data for children and pesticide residue data for the foods most frequently eaten by children. With increased international commerce, issues of differential standard-setting for pesticide residues in food will become more important to resolve.

Another challenge is the more recent recognition of exposures to pesticides used on lawns and in homes and offices. We are conducting research to develop improved techniques to evaluate skin and hand or object-to-mouth exposure of young children, which occurs following the application of pesticides on residential lawns and in homes. Only by better understanding the sources, routes, and pathways of exposure will it be possible to reduce or eliminate toxic exposures from household products.

Lead

One of the most successful examples of toxic-exposure reduction is the case of lead. As with organochlorine pesticides, the EPA early in its history recognized that lead poses high risks to the population because it bioaccumulates. Epidemiologic studies in the late 1970s demonstrated adverse health effects to children at lower and lower levels. Between 1977 and 1981, U.S. government agencies acted vigorously to regulate lead exposures, including those from gasoline, plumbing materials, house paint, and consumer products. The sources of lead targeted for action were those that are most likely to expose children to potential risk–lead in the air, drinking water, house dust, and consumer products and toys. The national effort has paid off. Data from the recently released National Health and Nutrition Examination Surveys show that average blood-lead levels in the United States have fallen by almost 80 percent since the mid-1970s.

Children, for whom lead is one of the gravest environmental health threats, have benefited to some extent from this trend, but the same report also shows differential lead exposures of very young children, minorities, and the poor. From 1988 to 1991, 11.5 percent of children between the ages of one and two had blood-lead levels above our current level of concern, compared to only 4.4 percent of the U.S. population. Exposure is greatest for minority children–10.2 percent of Latino children and 21.7 percent of African-American children. It is greatest as well for low-income children, especially those living in large urban areas.

We are now working to deal with these residual exposures to lead, which are mostly due to deteriorating lead-based paint in pre-1950 housing. Recent efforts to reduce lead exposures include proposals to ensure that individuals engaged in lead-based paint activities are properly trained, that training programs are accredited, and that lead-abatement contractors are certified. Once made final, these rules will ensure that lead-paint abatement activities reduce rather than increase lead exposures. U.S. rules proposed in 1994 would require disclosure of lead hazards during real estate transactions and bring about protective measures in renovating older homes.

These measures illustrate a pivotal shift in U.S. policy to address environmental justice and, therefore, environmental health protection for all Americans. In the U.S., as elsewhere around the world, it is typically the disadvantaged areas that frequently incur a greater share of toxic exposure. This is the case with lead. It is also frequently the case with unhealthy air in large urban areas. One of our targeted responses is to provide as much information as possible to local communities in the U.S., to empower them to know what potential exposures they face, and to encourage them to participate in decision-making. Information is a powerful tool to enable and motivate the private and public sectors to take action to reduce toxic exposure and resulting risk.

Internationally, much more work needs to be done, especially with regard to the continued use of leaded gasoline in many developing countries, leading to elevated air levels. Products in commerce that contain lead provide the potential of transboundary movement; some, such as cookware, dishes, and children's toys, can pose significant risks.

Environmental Tobacco Smoke

One particularly critical indoor exposure is to environmental tobacco smoke. Research conducted in the early 1990s indicated that it is responsible for both cancer and child health risks. It has been estimated to cause approximately 3,000 lung cancer deaths in nonsmokers each year in the U.S. The risk for infants and young children whose parents smoke is also very serious. It has been estimated that environmental tobacco smoke is responsible for between 150,000 and 300,000 lower respiratory tract infections annually in infants and children under 18 months of age, resulting in 7,500 to 15,000 hospitalizations each year. In terms of asthma, our estimates indicate that exposure to secondhand smoke causes an increase in the number of episodes and severity of symptoms in a 200,000 to 1 million children each year; it may also cause thousands of children to become asthmatic.

The U.S. does not strictly regulate household exposures. However, the federal government's role in controlling exposure to secondhand smoke has been to assess the potential hazards and risks and to provide information to local and state governments, which regulate smoking in public buildings, and to members of the general public, who may wish to avoid exposing their children and family members. Thus, information about exposures and risks can help empower others to make decisions to prevent exposures. For example, smoking has been banned on domestic U.S. air flights, and some airlines are moving toward bans on international flights as well, while there has been consideration of regulations to control smoking in workplaces.

RIGHT TO KNOW

The environmental information now available to the American public is unprecedented in the world, in terms of specificity and scope. Manufacturing companies must annually report to both federal and state governments their environmental releases of certain toxic pollutants to the water, air, and land. The initial number of toxic chemicals subject to the reporting requirements was more than 300. In 1994, the list of chemicals was expanded to include nearly 600 chemicals. There has been demonstrable progress in voluntary efforts to reduce release of these toxic chemicals. In 1992, reported releases of toxic chemicals into the U.S. environment totalled 3.2 billion pounds, a decline of 6.6 percent since 1991 and 35 percent since 1988. The sheer volume of releases was surprising to all involved–government, communities, and industry–and this has led to many changes.

One important result is the "33/50" program. To date, some 1,200 companies, including a high percentage of the top 600 firms in the United States, are participating on a voluntary basis in programs to reduce the release and transfer of 17 high-priority toxic chemicals. National goals of the 33/50 program are to reduce the releases and transfers of these priority chemicals 33 percent by 1992 and 50 percent by 1995. This voluntary pollution-prevention program achieved a 40 percent cut in released pollutants by 1992–a total of nearly 600 million pounds. The program is on track for meeting the 1995 goal of a 50 percent reduction. Companies benefit as well: by saving materials, avoiding potential cleanup and liability costs, and improving their image as socially responsible citizens.

The Toxic Release Inventory empowers states and local communities by making information publicly available. Currently, the information on TRI is widely available in various forms, including viamodem. Information in the database includes facility identification, geographic location, quantities of chemical releases, type of release, and pollution prevention activities. As a result, communities can not only access summary data but also obtain data to help them determine which chemicals may potentially be present in their communities and so to set priorities. Chemical summary sheets will be added to the Toxic Release Inventory to make the information more easily interpreted and used. Since chemicals on the Toxic Release Inventory pose different types of hazards and vary in potency, this kind of information is necessary to help ensure its proper use.

POLLUTION PREVENTION

Traditional regulatory approaches for controlling toxic exposures have been effective in reducing pollution levels in U.S. air and water, providing safer food and drinking water, and assuring more prudent handling of wastes. But these approaches also have certain limits. The U.S. experience shows that the cost of environmental cleanup and retrofitting of equipment can be prohibitively expensive. Common sense dictates that we pursue pollution prevention strategies whenever possible. By preventing pollution in the first instance, we also prevent exposures and subsequent risks.

An innovative pollution prevention effort now under way is the EPA's Design for the Environment Program, which works with large and small businesses on a voluntary basis to foster information exchange and research on pollution prevention. For example, the screen printing industry is participating to help better understand environmental problems and to identify environmentally preferable materials and measures. With approximately 40,000 commercial shops nationwide, screen printers represent an important group of chemical users. The partnership between the government and the screen printing industry is a real success story in voluntary pollution prevention activities.

The Green Chemistry Program is another noteworthy example of the pollution prevention approach. The U.S. government has provided grants for research to identify safer ways of synthesizing chemicals and so preclude the creation and release of toxic chemicals and toxic waste in the first place. We are now incorporating green chemistry principles in the process of reviewing new chemicals. Our aim is to work with industry to identify the safest synthetic pathway before construction of manufacturing facilities even begins.

We also are now taking a "use cluster analysis" approach to setting priorities for risk management of existing chemicals. This strategy involves ranking chemicals available for a particular use, such as paint strippers, based on relative risk to human health and the environment and potential for exposure potential, to identify risk reduction opportunities. By taking into account exposure as well as risk, this tool will help set the agenda for other activities, such as testing, pollution prevention, product labeling, and banning of the riskiest uses.

Pollution prevention also can be instrumental in reducing exposure and risk in the area of agricultural pesticides. We are committed to ensuring that American food is the safest in the world by encouraging farmers and others, through better understanding of the amount needed for efficacy, to reduce the amount of pesticides put into the environment; by offering guidance on labeling and use; and by safer alternatives. We have established a number of "stewardship partnerships" with pesticide user groups to encourage strategies to make pesticide use less wasteful; safer methods of pest and crop management; and decreased reliance on toxic, persistent pesticides. Participants so far include the National Potato Council, the American Corn Growers Association, the International Apple Institute, and the California Pear Advisory Board. The result will be greater protection from exposure to pesticides and lower expenditures for pesticides.

COMMON SENSE INITIATIVE

Today, the EPA is moving toward a more holistic approach to environmental protection by developing solutions to environmental problems on an industry-wide rather than pollutant-by-pollutant basis. We are working with six industry sectors to revolutionize the traditional approach to environmental protection. They are: iron and steel; metal plating and finishing; automobile assembly; printing; oil refining; and electronics and computers. Together, they make up nearly 15 percent of the U.S. gross domestic product and account for some 345 million pounds of toxic releases–one-eighth of all toxic emissions reported–and employ 4 million people. Each of the six sectors has a team composed of EPA and state officials, industry representatives, environmental organizations, labor unions, environmental justice groups, and others. The charge is to develop a blueprint for future environmental protection. The result should be a more rational, less expensive regulatory system that also will deliver greater environmental benefits.

MARKET INCENTIVES

Another approach to controlling chemical exposures in the United States involves using market incentives. An often cited example is the air pollution trading that is allowed under our regulatory scheme for hazardous air pollutants. Many other efforts are under way.

For the pesticide industry, the emphasis is on creating incentives for developing and commercializing safer products. One available tool is the registration process; a speedy registration is worth a great deal of money to the pesticide industry. Because lower risk pesticides have a smaller niche in the marketplace, creating incentives for research and development and registration applications makes environmental and economic sense. Another thrust is the "reduced risk" pesticide registration program, established in 1993. Although registering a conventional pesticide typically takes three to five years, many pesticides that meet the "reduced risk" standard can be registered in less than a year. These types of changes are helping bring biopesticide products on the market sooner: for example, 31 new pesticide active ingredients were registered in 1994. A high proportion–15, or nearly half–were biologically based pesticides.

CONCLUSION

To deal with the issues of the twenty-first century, the international regulatory community must develop new tools for assessing and managing toxic exposures. Some of these new strategies are scientific: undertaking basic research to understand possible new environmental concerns; conducting targeted research to improve testing protocols; and improving models and risk assessment methodology. Some strategies involve policy changes: setting national and international environmental goals; improving the quality of our risk assessments; using risk tools to set priorities for regulatory action; and harmonizing approaches among countries. We can also improve risk management by developing environmental management approaches that address industrial sectors as a whole and that protect entire ecosystems rather than one species at a time; by promoting pollution prevention strategies; by empowering the public and others by providing information about releases from facilities and use and toxicity of chemicals; by considering the impact on children; and by addressing environmental justice concerns. With incorporation of these important policy directions, we will be well-positioned to work with industry and the public in reducing exposure to toxics, in increasing protection for public health and the environment, and in contributing to a sustainable future for generations to come.

25

ENVIRONMENT AND DEVELOPMENT

THE HONORABLE MAURICE STRONG
is Chairman of the Earth Council and Chairman and Chief Executive Officer
of Ontario Hydro, North America's largest utility. He was Secretary-General of
the 1992 U.N. Conference on Environment and Development (the Earth Summit)
and served as Under-Secretary-General of the United Nations from 1985 to 1992.
Mr. Strong has also served as Executive Coordinator of the United Nations Office
for Emergency Operations in Africa, Secretary-General of the U.N. Conference
on Human Environment, Director of the Rockefeller Foundation, Chairman
of the World Resources Institute, and Chairman and Foundation Director
of the World Economic Forum, Geneva, Switzerland.

AFTER THE LAST GAVEL signaled the end of the Earth Summit in Rio de Janeiro in June 1992, the unprecedented attention it had focused on tomorrow's prospects for our planet rapidly became yesterday's news. Predictably, the media turned its attention to here-and-now issues, such as Bosnia and Somalia and the latest political and economic crises. To be fair, so did many others, including most of the world's political leaders. But this should not obscure the fact that for the two weeks of the Earth Summit and several weeks preceding it, the Earth's future dominated the headlines and prime-time news.

Even three years later, it is still too early to tell what the ultimate results of Rio will be. It was clearly a historic event, bringing together as it did the largest number of nations and world leaders that has ever been assembled, as well as a record number of representatives of media and of civil society.

While the agreements reached in Rio had some significant shortcomings, they nevertheless constitute the most comprehensive and far-reaching measures to secure the future of the earth on which governments ever have agreed. The fact that these were agreed, by virtually all the nations of the world at the highest political level gives them a unique political authority, but, as I cautioned in my final remarks to the conference, this in no way guarantees their implementation.

All who participated in the conference would agree it was a memorable experience, but they are far from unanimous in their judgments as to what it achieved. Those who expected it to yield a quick fix for all the planet's ills were predictably disappointed. So were those who insisted that because the agreements did not meet all needs and expectations they should be entirely discounted. It would be as wrong to accept these pessimistic assumptions as it would be to contend that the principal risks of the future of our planet were resolved at Rio. If there is no cause for complacency neither is there for despair.

It should be no surprise that the kind of fundamental changes in economic behavior and in our industrial system called for at Rio do not come quickly or easily. But the agreements reached there provide the foundations for the new global partnership that can launch the world community onto a new pathway to a more secure and sustainable future.

The blueprint is there–and the bricks and mortar. What is still in doubt is whether the governments of the world will muster the political will and the continuing commitment to build on these foundations the sustainable mode of life that is essential to the future of our species. The short-term signs have not been very encouraging. There clearly has been a tendency to lapse back to business as usual, particularly in light of the pressing political and economic concerns with which virtually all governments are preoccupied. The substantial commitment of new financial resources required to enable developing countries to implement the summit's action plan has not been forthcoming. Indeed, even some of the traditionally most generous donors have cut back on their development assistance. Unfortunately, the replenishment of the Global Environmental Facility was at a much lower level than expected.

The needed increases in resource flows to developing countries will not come in response to pleas in traditional terms for more "foreign aid." What is required is a redeployment of existing resources in both developing and industrialized countries. The resources are clearly there, as evidenced by the vast amounts of money now being used to subsidize unsustainable practices. What is required is a reorientation of our priorities in utilizing them. We must be prepared to give the same kind of priority to securing the future of our planet as a sustainable home for present and future generations as we have always been willing to accord to military security. Also many of the best investments we can make in global environmental security will be in developing countries, helping them to revitalize their economies on an environmentally sound and sustainable basis.

One of the more intractable myths surrounding debates over sustainable development is the stubborn notion that integration into our economy of measures to protect the environment would be a recipe for slow growth or no growth. The evidence assembled for the Earth Summit, particularly the report "Changing Course" by the Swiss industrialist Stephan Schmidheiny and the Business Council for Sustainable Development, made it clear not only that this is incorrect but that clinging to this perverse notion could propel us toward disaster, both environmentally and economically. Indeed, the main message of Rio was that only through the integration of the environmental dimension into our economic policies and practices at every level can we make the transition to a secure and sustainable way of life on our planet. Far from being a drag on the economy, investment in the environment and ecoefficiency must be seen as the primary driving forces of the new economy that is emerging as we move into the twenty first century.

The experience of some industrialized countries–both at the national and industrial levels–has demonstrated that environmental improvement, and efficiency in the use of energy and resources, is fully compatible with, and indeed contributes to, good economic performance. Japan has succeeded during recent years more than any other nation in reducing levels of domestic air and water pollution and the amount of energy and raw materials used to produce a unit of gross domestic product, while continuing for most of this period to lead the world in economic performance. In the course of so doing (*or* doing so) it has created a new generation of competitive advantage for Japanese industry.

Germany, too, has discovered the benefits of the ecorevolution. German companies now account for 21 percent of the world markets for "green" products, compared with 16 percent for the United States. In the Ruhr Valley, the traditional heart of industrial Germany, which has felt the impact of progress more than any region in the country, green industries now employ more people–150,000–than the steel industry.

Perhaps more than any other nations, the Japanese and the Germans have realized that the next generation of economic and industrial opportunity will be environment driven. They are setting an enviable example for the rest of the world, particularly in the area of energy efficiency. Yet the political leaders of other countries have been slow to recognize that this also offers the most promising prospect of revitalizing stagnant economies.

The Commission on Sustainable Development, established by the U.N. General Assembly in December 1992, has the mandate and opportunity to facilitate action by governments and international organizations on these issues and implementation of the other elements of the summit's action plan. As it meets in its first substantive session in New York, its members must know that they have the strongest possible support from all those who are committed to the critical importance of ensuring that the results of Rio are implemented. At the same time, they must also know that much is expected of them. There must be real evidence that governments are indeed committed to carrying out the agreements they made in Rio, and continuing the process of building on those agreements and developing more effective means of enforcing them. They must ensure that these issues remain at the center of the international agenda and on the agendas of all governments.

However, we cannot leave the follow-up of Rio to our political leaders alone. In a very real sense, leadership must come from the people. Theirs will be the primary source of the political will required to induce and support government action in following up and implementing the results of Rio, as it was to the conference itself. I have been profoundly encouraged by the evidence of an explosion of grass-roots initiatives on the part of people throughout the world–by scientists, engineers, architects, industrialists, religious leaders, educators, urban authorities, women, youth, and citizen groups, to name but a few. It is to support and facilitate this process that the Earth Council headquartered in San José, Costa Rica, has been established. It will act as a "people's ombudsman" to monitor implementation of the agreements reached in Rio; to bring to bear objective, expert knowledge and opinion in the public dialogue on these issues; and help to amplify the voices of grass-roots people, ensuring that their concerns, interest, and experience are fully expressed and taken into account in the policy- and decision-making processes that affect them. I am confident that this kind of people-based action will infuse the political process with new energies and provide a continuing basis for mobilizing the political will required to ensure governmental action on the Rio agreements.

The industrialized countries must take the lead in the transition to sustainable development mandated by the Earth Summit, the basis for which is set out in its action plan. They must reduce the environmental impacts of their own economies, leaving space for developing countries to grow and helping them to do so in ways that minimize their environmental impacts. They must find new and innovative means of providing developing countries with the additional resources they require to deal with the continuing problems of proliferating population growth and pervasive poverty, which place intolerable pressures on their environment and resources and undermine the prospects of improved conditions of life for their people.

It would be unrealistic to expect the agreements reached at the Earth Summit to be implemented immediately. They comprise, after all, an extensive program that could only be carried out over time. But it is imperative that it be given early and decisive impetus. The evidence of this must be forthcoming at this first meeting of the Commission on Sustainable Development. Governments should confirm that they will, as some already have done, reexamine and reorient their own policies and practices around the summit's action plan while developing their own national plans. I am encouraged by the initiative of more than 80 countries in establishing National Councils for Sustainable Development or similar bodies. These new species of organization are valuable multistakeholder forums, in which representatives of government and various key sectors of the civil society can consult and advise on the development and implementation of the action plan at the national level and provide guidance and support for similar initiatives in local communities.

In addition, industrial countries must make clear in specific terms their commitment to higher levels of support for the Global Environmental Facility, and to such important initiatives as UNDP's Capacity 21 and Sustainable Development Network programs, as concrete evidence of their willingness to begin the process of providing the additional resources required by developing countries for their implementation of the summit's action plan. The commission must also mandate a fast tract for negotiation of the protocols necessary to strengthen the Conventions on Climate Change and biodiversity and lend strong support and impetus to negotiations on the Desertification Convention. Finally, it must establish the modalities for a much closer and continuing interaction and cooperation with non-governmental organizations and citizen groups that proved to be such an invaluable feature of the Rio experience.

Only time will tell whether the Earth Summit will be seen in the perspective of history as a historic turning point onto a pathway to a more secure and sustainable future for the human community, or as a tragic lost, perhaps last, opportunity. What we do or fail to do in this immediate post-Rio period will make the critical difference. We cannot afford to let the promise of Rio remain unfulfilled.

26

POPULATION AND DEVELOPMENT

NAFIS SADIK
is the Executive Director of the United Nations Population Fund and
holds the rank of Under-Secretary-General. She is the first woman ever selected
in the history of the United Nations to head one of its major voluntary-funded
programs. As chief executive of the U.N. Population Fund, the world's largest
source of multilateral assistance to population programs with a program level
of approximately $250 million in 1994, Dr. Sadik directs a worldwide staff of
about 800. In 1990, the Secretary-General of the United Nations appointed Dr.
Sadik Secretary-General of the International Conference on Population and
Development for 1994. Dr. Sadik is known as an advocate for improving
the status of women, especially through programs aimed at addressing
population problems, alleviating poverty, and promoting development.

IN 1994, the U.N. International Conference on Population and Development concluded its deliberations in Cairo with the adoption of a comprehensive and far-reaching Program of Action. This program is viewed by many–especially women's groups–as a major breakthrough in thinking on population and development. The international community has for the first time gone beyond numbers and placed human beings at the center of all population and development activities. It has acknowledged that investing in people, in their health and education, is the key to sustained economic growth and development. What is being emphasized in this Program of Action is an approach that attacks problems at the local level, taking into account individual perspectives and needs.

The Population Conference's Program of Action is a very comprehensive document. Population is no longer seen in isolation but in conjunction with overall development strategies, in particular the eradication of poverty, the need for sustained economic growth and development in developing countries, and the imperative need to empower women. As such, the Cairo agreements provide a framework of action for the entire international community.

POPULATION-DEVELOPMENT NEXUS

While the debate on population and development has been going on for some time, the focus has been concentrated on what happens in the South in the light of structural adjustment programs; how countries adapt to the changing conditions of democratization and government decentralization; and how they can best plan for the future.

Of particular importance are health, maternal mortality, education, food supply, poverty, and the environment, issues inextricably bound to the population-development relationship.

Health

The *Independent Inquiry Report into Population and Development* found that high rates of fertility are negatively associated with health status and that, specifically, "delaying first pregnancy, reducing the total number of births, and spacing births at least two years apart would improve the health of women and children." The report argues that in families with many children, children have to compete with each other for "health resources" (that is to say, money, time, and parents' physiological and nutritional resources), resulting in a negative effect on mortality and morbidity. In addition, due to these resource constraints, allocation issues (often gender-based) arise that favor some children over others. In the developing countries examined, the infant mortality risk for babies born less than 18 months after their next oldest sibling is at least double that of when they are born more than 24 months later. While family size can also affect survival, the effect appears to be highly varied across cultures and is seemingly the least detrimental in sub-Saharan Africa, where children are a shared responsibility throughout a larger family network.

Maternal Mortality

Correlations between high fertility and maternal morbidity and mortality are also positive. In fact, maternal mortality is the largest single cause of death among women in the reproductive age group. Women who become pregnant in developing regions face a risk of death due to pregnancy that is 80 to 600 times higher than women in developed regions. For example, in southern Asian countries that have the highest maternal mortality rates, there are 650 maternal deaths per 100,000 births. In Bhutan alone, this rate is 1,700 per 100,000.

Education

The traditional assumption about the effect of a rapidly growing population on education is that the educational status of individuals will suffer if the resources a government spends on education are fixed. As more children are born, parents have to decide whether they can afford to have their children attend school, and/or choose which child(ren) to send to school. Depending on their perception of the benefits of their children receiving an education, schooling may or may not be considered desirable.

At the community level, one effect, in its most dramatic extreme, is the flooding of a school system with more children enrolled than it can successfully educate and, therefore, fewer individuals receiving adequate levels of education. The scenario, however, does not take into account possible increased efficiencies in the system that might come about with larger numbers of school-age children entering the education sector. In any case, the effect of rapid population growth on education depends largely on the development status of the country, the "culture" of the family and the importance they place on education, as well as the state's investment in education subsidies.

Obviously, while the effects of rapid population growth on education are not unambiguous, a slower population growth should allow governments a chance to improve their educational system.

Food Supply

While forecasts of consumption surpassing agricultural productivity have been challenged by increasing yields and decreasing prices in some regions, overall the situation appears precarious. It has been noted that food production in the developing world rose by an average of 117 percent between 1965 and 1990, but that the majority of this gain took place in Asia. With the subsequent rapid increase in population growth, the actual number of people with deficient diets in Latin America, the Near East and Africa actually rose during this same time period. The earlier assumptions, therefore, may prove more accurate as population growth continues and opportunities for raising agricultural productivity diminish.

There are three categories of constraints to future increases in food production. In the first category lies the possibility of scientific and technical expertise reaching its limit as herbicides, pesticides, and fertilizers reach a threshold in their ability to raise crop yields. Secondly, resource and environmental constraints are well on their way toward reducing capacity for irrigation and increasing erosion of topsoil. The inability to manage toxic effects of agricultural waste constitutes a core part of the third, health-related category. One outcome of these failures to raise agricultural productivity is a strong push factor for farmers to migrate. A still more serious outcome is the failure to reduce or even stabilize the incidence of malnourishment.

While a more optimistic forecast suggests that increases in cultivation still might be possible if past rates of growth can be achieved, there will undoubtedly be more malnourished people, in terms of absolute numbers, in the year 2000 than there are now.

Poverty

While conventional wisdom suggests that rapid population growth and poverty are closely correlated, surprisingly little research has been done on the impact of population growth on poverty. It is generally recognized, though, that while poverty is widespread, it is not evenly distributed across the developing world. The number of people living in poverty has been growing at the same rate as the aggregate population of the South (about 2 percent yearly), but with an increasing incidence of poverty in Africa and Latin America, accompanied by a decreasing incidence in Asia.

The National Research Council report, *Population Growth and Economic Development: Policy Questions*, suggests that maldistribution of income is an important variable related to poverty and rapid population growth. The authors note that given a certain level of per capita income, a greater variation in the distribution of income generally results in a larger percentage of people living below the poverty line. Thus, a reduction of income differences has become a widely espoused developmental goal. Moreover, to the extent that income generation is separate from fertility, fertility change can have positive or negative effects on income distribution, depending largely on how fertility change is distributed by socioeconomic class–for example, if fertility decline happens predominantly among higher income groups, income distribution may become more unequal. Longer term effects, however, suggest that a slower population growth rate will diminish income inequality by raising the rate of return to labor in relationship to other production factors.

Recognizing that it is difficult to track the linkages between population and poverty, the World Bank focuses, instead, on how detrimental rapid population growth is to the possibility of overcoming poverty. In a review of human resource needs, using Malawi as a case study, the bank notes that in the absence of fertility decline, it is "unlikely that the country could increase the amount of capital per worker enough to produce significant improvements in productivity, wages, and living standards in the foreseeable future." In Colombia, after the rapid population growth slowed, the incidence of poverty was cut in half.

Environment

As with other issues, the linkages between population trends and environmental degradation are complex. High rates of population growth and high densities exacerbate ecologically precarious situations, as evidenced by the growing deterioration and decreasing availability of land and water in many parts of the developing world.

Rapidly increasing population growth plays a substantial part in land degradation. Southern Asia, Sub-Saharan Africa, and the Andean countries (all with dramatically growing populations) have had to cope with rapidly deteriorating agricultural land and, not coincidentally, rates of food production. The Worldwatch Institute estimates that if the rate of land degradation continues at the current pace, by the year 2000 there will be only half the amount of productive land available that there was in 1950. Worst of all, the situation will continue to deteriorate as population pressures increase.

Access to safe, clean water is equally threatened in many parts of the developing world, where an estimated 2 billion people live in areas with chronic water shortages. The U.N. Population Fund estimates that between 1970 and 1984 the number of people living in the developing world without access to safe drinking water (or adequate sanitation) rose by 135 million, almost entirely because of population growth.

Research Gaps

While much attention has been given to the relationship between population and development, important research gaps remain. With the exception of the topics outlined above, data have not been collected in critical areas. Little is known, for example, about the effects of rapidly growing populations on health and education resources. The relationship between rapid population growth, savings, and investment remain unclear, as do the full effects of large family size on child welfare. In addition, larger questions, including the impact of population growth on economies and the causal links between rapid population growth and poverty, need to be explored.

Changing Perceptions

The linkages between population and development have been challenging development experts for years. While there has been much argument about various causal pathways, no common answers have been found across all countries and regions. Indeed, it seems that there might not be one "right answer" but rather that multiple perceptions of the situation might be accurate in various settings.

While one school of thought has argued that increasing rates of development will cause population growth to slow, such a linkage has not been borne out in places such as Brazil and Kerala, where, in spite of severe and widespread economic trouble, fertility rates have declined dramatically. The reverse, in fact, appears to be the case in Mauritius, where fertility declined rapidly and economic development followed.

Others argue that population growth is part of a natural self-regulating mechanism: that high rates of growth put pressure on parts of the economy, causing prices to shift and large families simply to become less attractive, a perception that ultimately leads to a drop in fertility rates. Again, this hypothesis has been challenged in the past 15 years, as countries have demonstrated fertility trends that diverge widely from economic trends. In some countries (e.g. Peru, Colombia, Bangladesh) the rapidity with which fertility declines have taken place cannot be explained by gradual shifts in the market, pointing to the fact that economic trends are not the sole nor even the principal determinants of fertility decline. Pent-up demand for reproductive health, including family planning services, appears to be a strong independent variable.

Many factors have to be recognized to understand the true linkages between population and development: namely, that fertility, mortality, and migration probably each have different economic implications; that any interactions between population and economic variables potentially go both ways; and that there are a host of other important components of economic growth, including government policy, political stability, and investments in human resource development.

Unmet Need for Reproductive Health, Including Family Planning

Parallel to the evolution of development paradigms, the aims of population policy are changing. Importantly, the economic/demographic rationale for reproductive health and family planning is increasingly being replaced by a human rights approach, largely characterized by considerations of the unmet need for reproductive health/family planning. This approach was prominent at the Population Conference, which is discussed in more detail in the last section of this chapter. As it was originally conceptualized, "unmet need" refers to the number of women (and couples) wanting to postpone or avoid future pregnancies, but not currently using modern methods of contraception. The recent recasting of the phenomenon of unmet need has focused on creating universal access to high-quality, client-appropriate family-planning services across all categories of women and men. The contention of this perspective is that the traditional categories need to be expanded to include the needs of unmarried women; women whose methods are unsafe, ineffective, or unsuitable; and women whose pregnancies are not wanted but who lack access to safe, legal abortion. Whatever the numerical measurement of unmet need, however, universal access has one simple goal: that of the creation of an environment in which everyone has the right, the information, and the ability to obtain contraceptives.

POLICY IMPLEMENTATION: INFLUENCE ON POPULATION GROWTH AND DISTRIBUTION

The implementation of policies meant to affect population trends has usually involved a small set of concerns. In this section three areas where experience in the implementation of policy has accumulated are examined: changing population age structures, population redistribution and migration, and changing access to reproductive health and family planning programs.

Changing Population Age Structures

The changing age structure in populations across the world presents a challenge to the formulation of population policies. Because the age structures of populations affect social and economic development conditions to such a broad extent, dramatic changes in the number of people in any given age category require ongoing re-evaluation of policies. Moreover, the point at which countries go through a general demographic transition is usually closely correlated to their development status, so the implications for population policy are crucial at this point.

Currently, the general demographic picture is characterized by wide divergence in the developing world, both within and between countries. In some countries, the most advanced in their demographic transition, levels of fertility, and life expectancy are approaching those of the developed world. Others, at an earlier phase in the demographic transition, have large, young populations, with little improvement in life expectancy to date. Others fall somewhere between these two categories. The global estimate of the proportion of the population under 15 is around 32 percent, suggesting that one out of three people on the planet is a child (while only one out of 16 is older than 65).

While the situation varies widely across countries and regions, the youngest populations are currently found in East and West Africa, where the proportion under the age of 15 approaches 50 percent. Projections of the largest regional variations for the year 2015 are found in Asia, where the proportion under 15 is expected to range from 18 percent in Eastern Asia to 34 percent in Western Asia. As the AIDS epidemic sweeps across Africa and Asia, the number of "AIDS orphans" is expected to increase dramatically and thus change still more radically the relative proportion of young dependents in these regions.

The numbers of people who fall into the category of "dependents" (i.e., younger than 15 or older than 65) are not only important for policy concerns relating to labor force participation and demand for goods and services; they also are the basis of more specific needs for nutrition, education, and special health care. This situation will grow more acute as more countries pass through the demographic transition, and aging becomes a primary global concern. For these reasons, special attention must be given to age-distribution patterns in the formulation of population policies.

Changing Conditions of Migration

While migration has always played a key part in the population-development debate, prescriptions have never been entirely clear. Now, however, new phenomena are arising that link migration to population growth and pressure-areas of obvious concern in policy-making, especially in the formulation of population and development strategies.

Environmental factors are increasingly responsible for mass migrations and redistributions of people. The Population Institute reports that despite the world's plethora of examples over time of migrations linked to environmental conditions, "environmental disruptions . . . are happening with greater frequency and severity than ever before; the contemporary crises offer tangible evidence of the devastating impact of pollution and despoliation on the suitability for human habitation of increasing portions of the earth." Sadako Ogato, the U.N. High Commissioner for Refugees, has noted that "environmental degradation has increasingly become both a cause and symptom of population movements" and that the bulk of "environmental refugees" are currently living in arid and semiarid areas of the poorest countries in the world, thus putting additional strain on fragile ecosystems and meager resources. Moreover, these poor living conditions usually have an adverse effect on the health of refugees. As poor environmental conditions cause people to leave their homelands, the lure of more favorable conditions becomes greater and the very core of what once made these areas attractive becomes threatened by increasing population pressure.

Economic factors are also substantial. Across the developing world, as rural-urban migration becomes still more intense, millions of "refugees" find themselves in cities ill-equipped to deal with their needs. Burgeoning urban growth reinforces the urban bias of policymakers, causing the rural dwellers more hardship and more reason to move to cities, continuing the cycle.

Changing Access to Reproductive Health and Family Planning

As mentioned previously, a current priority of those working in reproductive health and family planning is devising the means to ensure universal access to contraception in a human rights framework. In reformulating ideas about access and usage, though, several concepts have emerged that challenge traditional assumptions.

In the early days of family planning assistance, user fees were, for the most part, considered a potential obstacle to acceptance of family planning services. There was widespread feeling that the provision of contraceptives should be free or, at the very least, low cost. However, as the number of family planning programs in the developing world grew in the 1980s, and the funds to pay for them decreased, there was increasing pressure placed on service providers to charge fees for contraceptives. As a result, social marketing projects flourished, supported by research indicating that moderate price increases did not result in decreased numbers of "acceptors."

Still, it has been noted that in the developing world the correlation between consumer prices for condoms and usage is stronger than many had been led to believe. The findings suggest that the price of contraceptives, particularly condoms, must be kept well below the equivalent of 1 percent of per capita gross national product for a year's supply, in order to achieve satisfactory use of condoms in either a family planning or an AIDS prevention context. Given these findings, country-specific research is needed to determine the cost for maximizing usage of contraceptives and program sustainability for various population groups.

SIGNIFICANCE OF THE U.N. POPULATION CONFERENCE

The Population Conference, which took place in Cairo, was a landmark event for population-development issues. More than 180 countries took part in the conference and adopted by consensus the Program of Action, which presents a far-reaching strategy for addressing population-related problems into the twenty-first century.

Of major significance was the agreement that population issues are not isolated from other problems of development: How populations grow and change in composition are intimately affected by the socioeconomic development of countries. This, of course, has been appreciated by scholars for many years, but knowledge had not been translated into policy decisions in many cases. At the conference, a profound global consensus was reached that should see policies modified to reflect the holistic reality of population-development interrelationships. These changes will be seen–if the momentum generated at Cairo can be sustained–at the national level, at the level of donor agencies, and at the international level by closer cooperation among multilateral development agencies.

Another strong conviction coming out of the conference is that the empowerment of women is an indispensable element for achieving development. Reproductive rights and reproductive health, areas where women in developing countries tend to be at a particular disadvantage, are important features in any strategy for improving the position of women in society. The Program of Action therefore gave great emphasis to the need to make reproductive rights and reproductive health integral parts of development strategies. The linkage between these elements and lower fertility and slower population growth was abundantly clear to the policymakers gathered in Cairo.

The Population Conference was a turning point in understanding the essential need for strong involvement of nongovernmental organizations. In its recommendations, the international community strongly endorsed the need for the further strengthening of nongovernmental organizations and called for their effective partnership with governments in the formulation, implementation, and evaluation of population–and development–related programs.

The conference also set some specific goals for countries to aim for over the next 20 years, that cover those vital aspects of social development to which population issues are most profoundly linked. These include goals for lowering infant and maternal mortality, increasing female education, and making reproductive health/family planning services widely accessible. The expectation is that countries will now integrate these concerns into their overall development plans in the conviction that a more rapid socioeconomic development will thereby be achieved.

Delegates came home from Cairo filled with optimism. Although the challenges remain enormous, given the progress achieved in the last two decades and the innovative and forward-looking agreements reached at the conference, participants could feel confident about the future, provided that the financial resources were made available. The conference was specific in spelling out the quantum of future resources needed to implement the Program of Action. Compared to other expenditures–for instance, defense budgets–the amounts required are indeed modest. The program of action presents a coherent plan that holds out real hope for genuine progress in an interrelated set of social concerns and that would do much to energize rapid development across a wide range of socioeconomic dimensions. The world will do well to listen to the message from Cairo and to make its program of action a centerpiece for development efforts in the coming years.

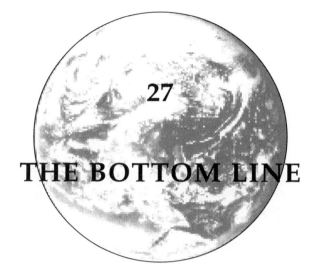

THE BOTTOM LINE

27

W. HARDING LE RICHE
is Emeritus Professor of Epidemiology at the University of Toronto, Canada.
Dr. Le Riche is a recipient of the R. D. Defries Award, the highest honor accorded
by the Canadian Public Health Association.

As Jeremy Rifkin has pointed out, every worldview has its architects. The architects of the present machine age are Francis Bacon (1561-1626) who published his book *Novum Organum* in 1620, René Descartes (1596-1650), and Isaac Newton (1642-1727). We are still living off their ideas, which together comprise the mechanical worldview. John Locke explained government and society in terms of the world-machine model and Adam Smith did the same with the economy. Locke assessed the ownership of property as the prime duty of the citizen. The individual in this system is reduced to the hedonistic activities of production and consumption to find meaning and purpose. The assumptions of these thinkers are that there is a precise mathematical order to the universe, but, as most matters on earth are chaotic, these should be rearranged. The logical conclusion to this is that the more material well-being we amass, the more ordered the world will become.

With the publication of Charles Darwin's *On the Origin of Species* in 1859 we come upon the theory of biological evolution. The system became a part of the Newtonian world-machine. Survival of the fittest was interpreted to mean that in the state of nature each organism is engaged in a relentless battle with all other creatures. The fact that this is not true has not penetrated the consciousness of many people. What we should remember, and what many of us probably have not thought of, is that the mechanical worldview–the world of mathematics, science and technology, the world of materialism and progress–is beginning to lose its vitality, because the energy environment upon which it grew is running down. This result obviously will not be immediate, but it is lurking in the background.

As Rifkin points out, both laws of thermodynamics can be stated in one small sentence: "The total energy content of the universe is constant, and total entropy is continually increasing." In simple terms, entropy is a measure of the amount of energy no longer capable of conversion into work. This means that as entropy increases there is a commensurate decrease in available energy. Pollution represents some of the energy in the world that has been transformed into unavailable energy: in our increasingly mechanistic society, our high energy-consuming society entropy is increasing all the time. We see this in the waste and ruin around us, from decay of agricultural land to the developing world's plethora of disused and misused machines. Large areas of the world are becoming cesspits. We are in a state of imbalance with nature, and this imbalance is particularly expressed by vast population growth and by destruction of the earth–both its land surface and beneath.

What has this to do with medicine and science? This has everything to do with medicine and science. Many of us have accepted the mechanistic view of the world, confidently believing that through the application of these principles the world will become better and that more and more people will survive happily. We have forgotten about the tremendous waste of energy that is, in the end, self-defeating.

Obviously, we should continue to use scientific methods but with humility; we should try to look at the total picture. This brings us to the ecological point of view. The medical profession should try to take an ecological view of the human condition. It should try to see the total picture–to see humankind in relation to the environment, and to see the interactions among human beings, the other animals, and the environment. Many younger scientists have developed tunnel vision, and they are obsessed with statistics and methodology–good things in themselves, but even a good thing can be overdone. The entropy law mentioned above is basic to the concept of ecology. There cannot be an infinite use of energy, whether it be in terms of food or in its production. There cannot be infinite development and growth of human or any other populations. These are limited, the limits having been set by the extremely complicated ecological balance of nature, now often forgotten.

The assumption that "science" can solve all human problems is plainly an illusion that dazzles intellectuals, politicians, and many others. Human nature and motivations are incredibly complex, and the assumption that we behave rationally is in itself a gross oversimplification. We are rationalizing rather than rational creatures. We are obviously capable of rational and logical thought, but this takes place only in special situations and circumstances. In our arrogance and increasing dominance, we believe fully that we are always rational and almost omnipotent. This attitude of mind is, again, both humanity's strength and its weakness, which leads it both to great heights of achievement and to depths of cruelty and injustice. We must rescue our scientists from this type of arrogance, who often forget the base from which they operate. This base is the earth on which we live. This base is the land and the food and the energy that we use. This base is the wealth we produce. Without these there will be no life.

In a recent CIBA Foundation symposium, Peter Hjort pointed out that it is useful to divide medical research into three areas: biomedical, clinical, and health services research. I would suggest that added to this should be the whole question of the environment of humankind, which increasingly concerns all of us. This is the environment with which we interact. This is the environment we change, and this is the environment we damage. When we think of medical and scientific research, we should always think of them in ecological terms; we should get away from our technologically induced narrow vision. Medicine and science are so interesting that people who become involved in one aspect of them tend to become obsessive, and they forget why they are doing whatever they are doing. The objective of medicine is to make the world a better place for people to live in, but the world cannot be made a better place for people to live in if there are vast numbers of people multiplying like cancer cells all over the world. The world cannot be made a better place if the land has been destroyed by bad farming practice and if the land, the air, and the water have been poisoned by the chemicals we produce in our industrial processes. And the world cannot survive if there is not enough food for its people.

However, let us consider in detail harmful environmental effects on the health of the people. These environmental effects have not been sufficiently studied by medical scientists. In fact, they have not been sufficiently studied by anyone. The realization of their noxious actions is only slowly dawning in the developed world. In the developing world, unfortunately, where the urge toward industrialization follows the model of the developed world, there is but little perception of the effects of the deleterious environments created by human beings.

In the following table, which was developed some years ago by Daniel Cappon of York University, the items are arranged systematically and in an interesting fashion. The table deals with humans as workers; the population dynamics of humans as builders; humans as herd animals; as oral consumers; as inventors; and with interactions between humans and the communicative environment, the genetic constitutional environment, and the biopathological environment. Finally, humans are examined as targets, that is, of the microbiological environment and, of course, as targets of the natural hazards created by humanity itself.

SUMMARY INVENTORY OF ENVIRONMENTAL
HAZARDS TO HEALTH

MAN AS PRIMARY PATHOGEN

Man the Worker
> Air, water, and soil pollution
> Air, water, and soil deprivation
> Energy depletion
> Meteorological change

Population Dynamics
> Population explosion
> Spatial congestion

Man the Builder
> Built environment pressures
> Siting
> Architectural spaces and shelters
> Transportation

Man the Herd Animal
 Operational, attitudinal, and public behavior
Man the Oral Consumer
 Nutritional effects of ingestion
 Toxic drugs intentionally and unintentionally consumed
 Inhalation and orally transmitted infections
Man the Inventor
 Man/machine

MAN AS TRANSMITTER

Communicative Environment (Sentient Man)
 Sensory disequilibria
 Psychosocial under- and overstimulation
 Emotional and psychosomatic disorders
Genetic Constitutional Environment
 Genetic constitutional environment general
 Hereditary and constitutional predisposition
Biopathological Environment (Defective Man)
 Biopathologies (unknown etiologies)

MAN AS TARGET

Microbiological Environment (Man as Target)
 Microbiological environments
Natural Hazards
 Atmospheric, temperature, solar radiation,
 geologic, hydrologic, altitudes

In considering the first broad category in the table, humans as the world's primary pathogen, humans as workers are also seen to be involved. We have made machines, which, in turn, have created the hazards of the industry, great engineering works, urban concentration, and the effects of war. When we move to the more specific area of air pollution, a subject that is receiving increasing attention, we talk about gaseous chemicals, ozone, sulphur dioxide, sulphuric acid and nitrous oxides, which together make up acid rain—a problem of growing importance all over the developed world and increasingly in the developing world. There is a lot of talk going on about acid rain throughout the world, but action is slow. Obviously people will only start acting when their forests really do start to die, as they did in Czechoslovakia. We are the chemical particulates, cadmium or lead, organic compounds, rubber, PCBs, other hydrocarbons, carcinogenetic particulates, asbestos; radioactive fallout; allergens, humanly induced or produced, and temperature changes; and the increase of carbon dioxide in the atmosphere. Certain chlorine-containing chemicals are destroying the ozone layer, leading to increased ultraviolet radiation, which may destroy crops, damage eyes, and cause skin cancer. The greenhouse effect is said to be producing a global temperature increase. This will have substantial effects–including the melting of polar ice, which may lead to flooding in certain ports. Also, of course, in considering air pollution, we must include cigarette smoke and airborne infections.

Moving on to water pollutants, obviously these consist of chemicals and organic waste, such as phosphates and nitrates; there are radioactive materials, metals, lead, mercury; there are temperature effects in Canada and the United States. (The cooling towers one sees in Great Britain are not often used.) There is the effect of eutrophication–the excess fertilization of bodies of water leading to overgrowth of plants in the water. These plants then kill the fish or they rot. We have waterborne infections that used to, and in many parts of the world still do, kill many people, with the sentinel disease here being cholera.

Coming to the question of soil pollution, we must consider inorganic soil and organic chemicals; organic solid waste, which we put into landfill sites; rubber and plastics; these inorganic solid wastes and the vast amounts of garbage produced by our cities, which we are only slowly learning to recycle. We should also remember that there is a great deal of soil lost due to roads and buildings.

Moving down the table to the next environmental hazard, we come to water deprivation. It is clear that this is the final stage in limiting population growth, and in many parts of the world this point has already been reached. There are limits to growth, and medical research should be cognizant of this. Water deprivation is one such limit. This ensures loss of fisheries, deprived agriculture, and the loss of the ability to fight fires. Soil deprivation involves the loss of arable land and forests, overcultivation, poor resource management, and interactions with natural hazards such as droughts and flooding. All these things are becoming matters of common interest in the news media.

The next extremely important hazard category is that of the depletion and loss of natural resources–the overuse of sources of energy such as wood, fossil fuels, petroleum, and coal. Then, there are problems in connection with nuclear energy, solar energy, wind, and geothermal and tidal energies. There may be a decline in the availability of metals for our use. It is incredible how much material we use. If we misuse water, there may be reduction of hydroelectric power. The last hazard in this section of the table is also of considerable importance to the environment, namely, meteorological changes. Cutting down the forests may affect rainfall, as may diversion of water.

As to the old question of population explosion, there are increasing absolute numbers, questions of migration, and extraneous geopolitical pressures from migration of peoples. There also is the question of population pressures in apartment complexes. Concerns mentioned in this category include the siting of cities and the importance of architectural spaces in shelter and transportation. Then there is the vast area of social and psychological effects of overpopulation. In terms of occupation and organization, public behavior in societies where there is discrimination or intolerance of certain groups or peoples must be considered. From these come threats of war.

Next, we address the matter of nutrition–the availability of food and its production–and then the question (*or* subject) of the toxic effects of drugs, intentionally and unintentionally (for example, herbicides and pesticides) consumed. We should consider the question of orally transmitted infections and noxious materials. We think of humans, the inventors, and the effects of their inventions; we think also of humans as transmitters of information; we think of psychosocial understimulation or deprivation; we think of sensory overstimulation. We then consider the whole area of emotional and psychosomatic disorders, which are insufficiently considered in the mechanistic explanation of human behavior. This is an area that is considerably neglected in the training of most medical students. From here, we get into the question of genetic constitutional environments, an area in which there is increasing interest; we think of hereditary effects. These are all part of the environment. If we go on to consider defective individuals we think of biopathologies, and we think of microbiological environments when considering humanity as a target.

Last, there is the whole area of natural hazards in the atmosphere in terms of temperature, solar radiation, earthquakes, floods, tidal waves, and ice, and we think in terms of altitudes. Theses are some of the things that are considered in the table's three broad categories: humans as primary pathogens, transmitters, and targets. Many of these elements are frequently not considered in discussions of medical research.

Let us look more closely at the question of world population growth. We know that population growth rates have doubled and redoubled from one billion in 1830 to two billion in 1930 to four billion in 1975 to more than five-and-a-half billion at the present time, and that world population will possibly reach six billion in the year 2000. In the meanwhile, the area of the Earth has remained the same. More land has been used and built upon, but the area in which this has occurred remains the same. A great deal of this area has been destroyed, not only by noxious agricultural practices, but by the building of cities and roads in the developed world and the growth of deserts in many parts of the developing world. A great deal of land has been irretrievably damaged by the senseless cutting down of forests, particularly in the tropical and subtropical countries.

If we look at the largest metropolitan area populations predicted for the year 2000, the biggest city will be Mexico City, with close to 30 million people, followed by Shanghai with more than 25 million people, Tokyo with just under 25 million people, Beijing with about 22 million people, São Paulo with about 20 million people, New York with about 16 million people, Greater Bombay with 17 million people, Calcutta with 15 million people, and Jakarta with 13 million people. These are enormous masses of people. One should consider here the effects on the health of these populations, the stress not only of overcrowding, but as a result of the congestion of transportation and hence the inability to remove the waste produced by these cities, in addition to the tremendous difficulties that will be developing (and have already developed in some areas) in bringing food into these cities. And where will this food come from–a question especially perplexing in light of the knowledge that in many parts of the world the rural areas are becoming depopulated, bringing on a decline in food production.

At present, in the developed world, there are approximately 35 million unemployed people. Most of these people want to work, and the most serious element of this unemployment is that a disproportionate number of the unemployed are young people starting out their lives. One can imagine the horrendous psychological and social effects on all these people. These are problems before which science and medical science research cowers in impotence. What can medicine and science do about these enormous social cataclysms?

It is startling to know that many developing countries, especially those with newfound wealth, are attempting to industrialize their economies along the same lines as the Western world. Their economic policies in many cases can only lead to tragedy. At a time when the world is running short of nonrenewable resources, it is unwise to develop an economic infrastructure based on a high energy flow of nonrenewable resources. Developing nations such as Brazil and Nigeria will have built an enormous industrial infrastructure by the year 2000. Then, at least one of them will find that it no longer has adequate amounts of nonrenewable energy to keep the economic machinery running. Brazil will try to base its industry on lumber and alcohol from sugarcane.

At present there is enormous industrial development in southern China, which has become one vast city. Where will the raw materials come from for all this building?

Time is running out in regard to the equation of populations versus the environment. For the fourth time in 10 years, parts of northern India were devastated by floods when the monsoon rains came in August. This is largely a man-made calamity. The cutting of the forests in the foothills of the Himalayas has removed the vegetation that used to absorb the first rainfall. Now, in many places, runoff rushes across the land, destroys the soil, and enters the rivers. Not very long ago a dust cloud settled over parts of Malaysia. Where did it come from? Was there a volcanic eruption? No. A more likely explanation was that it was a smoke pall from the burning of forest areas by slash-and-burn cultivation methods.

We should remember that humanly engineered environmental disasters are not new. The ancient Greeks and their goats stripped the hills of forests and vegetation, and erosion set in: "All the rich soil has melted away," wrote Plato, "leaving a country of skin and bone." In ancient Rome, the Tiber was so foul that only eels could survive in it. So, too, fish disappeared from the London reaches of the Thames in more recent times. This environmental destruction is now spreading all over the world. As the developing world adopts the Western model for industrialization, the horrors increase. The axe has been replaced by the chain saw, the ox-drawn plow by the tractor, the pick and shovel by mechanical diggers.

We should remember that the people of the industrialized countries, amounting to about a quarter of the world's population, use or consume about two-thirds of the world's resources. We cut down tropical hardwood in the forests of the Amazon and West Africa to make furniture for North America and Europe. Great forests are cleared and sometimes burned in Central and South America to provide grazing land to supply meat for the United States and Europe. Soviet and Japanese factory fishing ships scour the oceans of the world, including the east and west coasts of Canada. In per capita terms, world forest wood production peaked in 1964, the world fish catch in 1970, and meat from world grasslands in 1961 for mutton and in 1976 for beef. In many places, grazing land is being lost to desert, soil is lost to erosion by wind and water, forests have been cut faster than they can be replanted, and fisheries are being overfished. In Canada, by 1994, the fishing industry in Newfoundland and the Maritime provinces had collapsed. The salmon fishing in British Columbia is in serious trouble, also the result of overfishing.

As a result of tremendous population increases in many parts of the world, there is a growing legion of the landless. This situation is well known in India and Pakistan, but it is probably the most advanced in Kenya. In that country, the population growth is 4.1 percent per annum. It will double in 17 years. The population is outpacing the expansion of crop area, which increased only 12 percent between early 1960 and 1975. It cannot increase more because there is no more land. Increasing land scarcity and competition are inevitable. In the absence of national policies to control private land accumulation and tenancy practices, as well as to slow population growth, Africa will develop the same land-based social conflicts that have long been apparent in Latin America and in Asia. In the semiarid zones of Africa and Asia, land-hungry farmers plant in low rainfall areas. When the inevitable drought comes, these turn into dust bowls. In the 1930s, this happened in the United States and it also happened in Canada. There is no doubt that questions of land availability and distribution are at the heart of the continuing political violence in Central America. Giving more guns to these people will not help. If they use more contraceptives, their population problems will decrease, but they will only learn to use more contraceptives if they can be educated. How is this to happen? In addition to deforestation and soil erosion, there is the formation of new deserts. The Sahel remains the world's terrible example of the growth of deserts. This desert is caused by deforestation, overgrazing, and overcultivation. There are too many people pressing too hard on a fragile environment, and the fact that drought is normal in Africa has completely escaped notice by interested observers in North America and Europe. Drought in the Sahel is normal, rain is exceptional. Aid money has had very little effect on the Sahara. Observations grow faster than food production. Like leprosy, the bare sandy blotches of deserts creep across the land. In the eight Sahelian countries, Chad, Niger, Mali, Upper Volta, Mauritania, Senegal, Gambia, and Cape Verde, the population is growing at a steady 2.5 percent per annum while food production grows at 1 percent. And the cities in this area are growing much more rapidly than either food production or total population growth.

The camel trains loaded with firewood that cross the President Kennedy Bridge into Niamey, the capital of Niger, every morning, city and village alike, are surrounded by growing circles of deforestation. A decade ago, kerosene was an alternative fuel. At present, high oil prices rule it out for all but the relatively rich. When we come to the topic of the enormous destruction of forest, Duncan Poore, Director of the Commonwealth Forestry Institute at Oxford University, says that in 1980 more than 1.2 billion Third World people were able to meet their wood fuel needs, but only by using their wood faster than it was being replaced. He explains that until recently there have been wildly conflicting judgments–estimates of the rate of destruction of tropical forests have varied from about 6 million to 25 million hectares a year. The reasons for this destruction are known–shifting cultivation, settlement, agricultural development, overcutting for fuel, overgrazing, fire, commercial logging, urbanization, and the North American meat trade. Meat comes to the United States from developing world countries in South America, where splendid forests have been cut down to provide pasture for cattle to feed less than needy North Americans. Professor Poore concludes by saying that taking the countries and tropics as a whole, deforestation as a result of overpopulation causes problems on a scale that so far is beyond the capacity of governments to resolve. The point about destruction of forests is that in many developing countries the politicians who run the countries do not know that there is a problem, and this is perhaps the most serious aspect of the situation. Because the ruling elites do not know that a problem exists, they do not know that their country is being destroyed, and those who do know are not sure what to do about it. People need wood with which to cook their porridge; and if populations are vastly increasing (as they are), they will need more wood. The only solution is to practice more birth control–a very complex subject.

We should realize that cities destroy not only the land on which they are built but vast areas of land and fresh water often long distances away. Cities pollute fresh air, and their physical growth takes up land. Furthermore, they need great amounts of food. Deforestation is widening in swathes around the world's cities. Providing metropolitan areas such as Mexico City itself and São Paolo with water already presents huge problems. In most Third World countries there are two cities–cities of the elite, where Western standards are evident, and the largely self-built cities of the poor, the shantytowns. It is the shantytowns that lack drinking water, sewage connections, and other systems to safely dispose of human wastes and garbage collection and that lack preventive and curative health services. This ensures that many diseases are endemic–diarrhea, dysentery, and typhoid.

Let us for a moment consider the Communist world, specifically, the People's Republic of China. Have they done any better in regard to the environment and population matters? There is no doubt that the Chinese have understood that their population is growing too fast, and they certainly are doing something about that aspect of this particular equation. However, according to Professor Vaclav Smil of the University of Manitoba, almost all of China's major cities are heavily polluted because China is largely dependent on coal. I have visited Beijing in the winter-time, and it is extremely polluted. Not only is there air pollution in Beijing but there is a great deal of soil erosion. Shanghai is contaminated by acid rain. A great deal of industrial waste is put into the rivers or dumped by the wayside, and 90 percent of the country's urban sewage goes untreated. Enormous areas of forest have been destroyed in China. Many of that country's environmental problems result from its drive to increase grain production and to industrialize.

Clearly, the Chinese, like the Russians, have not devoted enough time, effort, or money to agricultural research. China has been using increasing amounts of fertilizers and pesticides on its crops. This has generated more ecological problems. Many of the chemicals have been improperly applied or overused. The soil and water supplies have been contaminated. In the Shanghai River delta, 95 percent of the industrial and domestic sewage is released directly into the waterway. In Nanjing, a plant producing aniline dumped into the waterways 9,000 tons of sludge and 20,000 tons of soil contaminated with this poisonous organic chemical, and there is a high frequency of illness among the workers at the plant. In 1978, pollution controls were installed so that the situation might improve. The Chinese are taking some steps to stop pollution, but they are not very effective.

The environmental practices of the former Soviet Union are as unsatisfactory as in many parts of the rest of the world. Since the 1930s, Russian bloc policies in favor of reservoir construction on rivers in the plains to generate hydroelectric energy have led to rapid depletion of water sources and serious pollution. Intense water deficits threaten to curtail economic activities in the most productive southern regions and force the Russian leaders to further restructure the river network. The

Black Sea estuaries, including the Azov Sea, will be blocked by dams, and the Danube flow will be diverted northward to alleviate the water shortages in the Ukraine. The gigantic constructions of the Baltic-White Sea, the Moskva-Volga, and Lenin's Volga-Don canals have been environmentally damaging, extremely costly in operation, and play a very small role in overall traffic. These were political decisions that took heavy tolls in human lives. The Russian area people are splendid inheritors of the mechanistic view of life. The environmental degradation continues in the Russian sphere at an ever-increasing pace. In seven decades, the Soviet system was not able to develop an efficient economic mechanism to ration scarce water resources among the competing users. It has also been unable to control environmental pollution.

If we return to North America and look at the water supply, we notice that in spite of the relatively good supplies of water, we face a need to curb our insatiable thirst. The U.S. high plains states, including New Mexico, Texas, Wyoming, Colorado, Oklahoma, and Kansas, have been turned into lush farmlands by 50 years of using the great underground water system, the Ogallala Aquifer. Now, a growing number of wells in Texas are producing sand, and desperate farmers say only massive water diversions can revive their land. These diversions presumably will have to come from Canada. In the western part of Canada, there is increasing lack of water. At the root of this problem, quite apart from industrial pollution that is increasing in the Great Lakes, both in Canada and the United States, there is the overriding factor of population increase. In both countries it should be obvious that immigration should stop or be greatly reduced, and clearly the population itself in these countries is heading toward zero population growth. Ordinary people are limiting their numbers; governments still bring in immigrants.

Let us look briefly at the picture of health in the world because this has obvious important relationships to the types of medical research that are needed. In the affluent world, mortality from infectious diseases is low. There are two disease categories that are overwhelming, cardiovascular ailments and cancer. Obviously, as far as cardiovascular ailments are concerned, all our hearts must ultimately stop. Cardiovascular disease is the most important disease in the affluent world. However, looking at this disease during the last 20 years or so, the death rate from ischemic heart disease in Canada and the United States is going down. Cancer, which takes about one-fifth of the lives in industrial countries, ranks second as a health challenge. We should remember, though, that most of the people who die of cancer are old.

In the Third World, the cause of most diseases is malnutrition, a fact that tends to be forgotten when people do medical research. The main killers in poor countries are infectious diseases, which include dysentery, pneumonia, tuberculosis, bronchitis, influenza, and measles. This is the situation that existed in Europe and in North America 100 years ago.

Quick gains in the reduction of death rates in the developing world are now rapidly coming to an end. In the developing world, water supplies are becoming increasingly more polluted, and malnutrition is likewise increasing.

The problem of human waste is monumental. The careless handling of human waste spreads debilitating parasites. Diseases that are now extremely important in tropical countries include malaria, schistosomiasis, filariasis, trypanosomiasis, leprosy, and leishmaniasis. These are the targets of new international programs of research and control. We should note that large sums of money are being spent on research into heart disease and cancer but very small sums of money on research into tropical diseases. The reasons for this are obvious–in the rich world, the old men are afraid of dying, and in the poor world, there is not enough money to spend on tropical diseases.

By 1994 the situation in regard to infectious diseases had changed. AIDS delivered a serious blow to the complacent, who claimed in the 1970s that infectious diseases had been conquered. This disease syndrome was reported in 1981, first in the United States but also in Europe, Africa, throughout the Americas, and increasingly in Asia. It is transmitted by sexual contact, sharing of unclean intravenous needles, and through blood transfusions and blood products. Transplacental transfer may occur. Opportunistic infections associated with AIDS are pneumocystis, carinii pneumonia, cryptosporidiosis, dissemenated strongyloidiasis, toxoplasmosis, tuberculosis, and candidiasis. Some individuals develop Kaposi's sarcoma. Most of these conditions can be treated, but there is no adequate treatment for AIDS itself. Thus far, there are only palliative drugs, such as AZT.

In 1994, there was an outbreak of cholera in refugee camps in Rwanda. It was brought under control by providing clean water and treatment of the sick with rehydration and, if necessary, tetracycline or doxycycline, if available.

In 1994, there was an outbreak of pneumonic plague in Surat and elsewhere in India. It was controlled by the use of tetracycline.

There is a deterioration of health in the former Soviet Union, with outbreaks of cholera in Ukraine. In the United States, tuberculosis is increasing among certain sections of the population, so we cannot be complacent about infectious diseases. Tuberculosis kills three million people worldwide each year.

We also must not lose sight of a clamant need for considerably better research in regard to birth control. It is interesting that during the last 10 or 15 years, there has been a campaign against Depoprovera, which is a good, although not perfect, injectable long-acting contraceptive. The most recently developed long-acting contraceptive is Norplant.

The question of food security remains urgent. As Lester Brown has pointed out, per capita grain production worldwide climbed 14 percent during the 1950s, 8 percent during the 1960s, and only 5 percent during the 1970s. In Africa, with population growth during the 1970s being the fastest ever recorded for any continent, the food safety margin disappeared entirely as growth in food production fell below that of population growth. The 14 percent decline in per capita grain production during the decade was the first sustained continentwide decline since World War II. In many African countries, food production has declined considerably during the last 20 years.

Another source of world food insecurity is the dependence of the entire world on North America for food supplies. Prior to World War II, Western Europe was the only grain-importing region. North America was not the only exporter nor even the leading one. During the late 1930s, Latin American grain exports were nearly double that of North America while Eastern Europe, including the former Soviet Union, was exporting 5 million tons annually, the same amount as North America.

The situation has now changed beyond recognition. Asia has developed a massive deficit. Africa, Latin America, and Eastern Europe all import food. Western Europe, consistently importing 15 to 30 million tons, has been the most stable element throughout the period. North America's emergence as the world's bread basket occured in the 1940s. There is no doubt, though, that the time will come when American food production, in spite of current optimism, will start to decline as a result of land and water depletion. Cropland loss is serious all over the world; we cannot say that it is not happening in North America.

The enormous world population increase since 1945, particularly in the developing world, has come about mainly because of the availability of more food. This food has been produced because of cheap energy. At the beginning of this period food production increased because of the increased availability of land. The cost of energy has now risen enormously, and there is not much land left for agricultural use. It is possible to make more land available for agriculture, but at the cost of destroying wetlands and other small areas of land still available for the survival of other animals.

Obviously, medical science has contributed to population growth, especially since the advent of sulfonamides, antibiotics, and immunization.

It is interesting to learn that only recently have some medical schools begun to teach their students about the importance of nutrition. It took many years for the advances in this important field to penetrate into the schools. Doctors seemed to assume that everybody was well nourished, and only a few in medical faculties were interested in malnutrition. Fortunately, in many parts of North America at least, nutrition is now being studied by medical students. Though, the subject is still somewhat foreign to the medical mind.

As Bruce Ames has pointed out, there are many natural mutagens and carcinogens in food, a fact that is not generally known. He has also noted that there is no convincing evidence of a generalized increase in the cancer rates in the United States or the United Kingdom, other than what could be ascribed to the possible effects of previous increases in tobacco usage. If we subtract the effects of tobacco from cancer, we will find that there is actually a decline in cancer death rates. One mentions cancer because, increasingly, chemicals–whether they are in foods or additives–are being implicated in the disease. We now know that there also are anticarcinogens in foods; among these are vitamin E, beta-carotene, selenium, glutathione, ascorbic acid, and other substances. There is evidence that cabbage may inhibit carcinogenesis in experimental animals. These are some of the exciting relationships between nutrition and diseases that in the past were misunderstood.

As a background to medical research, thinking people in the world and thinking politicians must come to the following realizations:

1. There is a shocking deterioration of the resource base of the world: seafood, beef, grain, lumber, oil, soil, forests and water.
2. Stronger efforts must be made to stabilize world populations, especially in Africa, the Indian subcontinent, most of South and Central America, the Arab countries, Indonesia, and the Philippines. Good progress in this is being made in the People's Republic of China, Taiwan, South Korea, Barbados, Cuba, Hong Kong, Singapore, and Thailand.
3. We must protect croplands by limiting loss of topsoil and erosion. We must support farmers all over the world.
4. We must reforest the earth, including the United States and Canada, where there has been much destruction.
5. We must move beyond the throwaway society; we must recycle raw materials.
6. We must conserve energy more efficiently.
7. We must develop renewable energy: wind, solar, biomass, geothermal, and small hydroelectric systems. We must promote better use of remaining stocks of oil, coal, and natural gas and reexamine nuclear power sources. Some countries will use nuclear power.

And while we are doing these things, we should try to use some balance in worldwide medical research. Obviously, this balance will be far from perfect because most research money will come from the West and from Japan, much dominated by cardiovascular disease, cancer, and the diseases associated with old age.

From a world stage, the areas of considerable concern are:

1. Better methods of birth control for men and women. Better methods of convincing people that if they have fewer children, more will survive. At the

same time there must be more effective social and economic development to support people in their old age, a very difficult problem in poor countries. These are social aspects of medical research.

2. More research on the control and treatment of AIDS.

3. More action, all over the world, to improve the health, social, and educational status of women.

4. The whole range of nutritional research, ranging from food production to clinical nutrition. Closely related to this is research into naturally occurring mutagens, teratogens, and carcinogens and the effects on humans of pesticides.

5. All tropical diseases, but especially malaria, schistosomiasis, filariasis, trypanosomiasis, leprosy, and leishmaniasis.

6. The effects on man and beast of the toxicants and dangerous situations generated by our industrial society.

7. The diseases and disabilities of old age.

In conclusion, may I note that we already know how to prevent the common conditions from which infants and small children die in the developing world, but if we save lives, there must be food for them to eat.

28

THE WAY FORWARD:
HEALTH AND HUMAN RIGHTS

FRANCISCO AYALA
is the Donald Bren Professor of Biological Sciences and Professor of Philosophy
at the University of California, Irvine. He is Retiring President and Chairman
of the Board of Directors of the American Association for the Advancement
of Science (the AAAS publishes the prestigious journal *Science*).

AUDREY CHAPMAN
is Director of the Science and Human Rights Program of the American
Association for the Advancement of Science. Formerly the World Issues Secretary
of the United Church Board for World Ministries, she coordinated justice, peace,
and human rights programs for the international agency of the United Church
of Christ. She was also Chairman of the National Council of Churches
Human Rights Committee.

HALF A CENTURY AGO, the United Nations Charter affirmed "faith in fundamental human rights, in the dignity and worth of the human person, in the equal rights of men and women and of nations large and small" as a foundation of the postwar international order. Forged in the cauldron of World War II, contemporary standards of human rights embody a commitment to protecting and promoting human dignity. Human rights express the claims or entitlement each person possesses to specific goods, services, and liberties by virtue of being human. The Universal Declaration of Human Rights, the principal standard by which human rights are identified today, enumerates nearly two dozen specific rights, including traditional civil and political rights, as well as social and economic or welfare rights.

Human rights are inalienable attributes that all persons hold, independently of recognition by governments. In order to make the implementation of human rights more effective, the United Nations and some regional bodies have formulated human rights conventions based on the Universal Declaration. The provisions of these instruments are legally binding on the governments that ratify or accede to them and on the states ("states parties") that these governments represent.

Recognizing the intrinsic relationship between health and human dignity, many major human rights documents specify rights relevant to the protection and promotion of health. The most expansive vision appears not in any human rights instrument but in the constitution of the World Health Organization. WHO links the right to health with a definition of health as a "state of complete physical, mental and social well-being and not merely the absence of disease or infirmity."

Rights relevant to the protection and promotion of human dignity in relationship to personal health that are enumerated in various international instruments include the following:

- Respect for human dignity and worth (Universal Declaration and all subsequent human rights instruments);

- right to equality before the law (International Covenants on Civil and Political Rights and Economic, Social, and Cultural Rights);

- protection of the rights of vulnerable individuals and communities (Universal Declaration and all subsequent human rights instruments);

- nondiscrimination (International Covenants on Civil and Political Rights and Economic, Social and Cultural Rights; International Convention on the Elimination of All Forms of Racial Discrimination; and International Convention on the Elimination of All Forms of Discrimination Against Women);

- right to life/right to life, liberty, and security of the person (Universal Declaration and virtually all subsequent instruments);

- protection against torture and other cruel punishment and treatment (International Covenant on Civil and Political Rights and the Convention Against Torture and Other Cruel, Inhuman, or Degrading Treatment or Punishment);

- right not to be subjected without free consent to medical and scientific experimentation (International Covenant on Civil and Political Rights);

- right to protection against arbitrary interference with privacy, family, home, or correspondence (International Covenant on Civil and Political Rights and the Convention on the Rights of the Child);

- right to marry and found a family (International Covenants on Civil and Political Rights and Economic, Social, and Cultural Rights);

- right to enjoy the benefits of scientific progress and its applications (International Covenants on Civil and Political Rights and Economic, Social, and Cultural Rights);

- right to freedom for scientific research and creative activity (International Covenant on Economic, Social, and Cultural Rights); and

- right of everyone to the highest attainable standard of physical and mental health; to that end it is specified that states parties undertake: (a) provision for the reduction of the stillbirth rate and infant mortality and for the healthy development of the child; (b) improvement of all aspects of environmental and industrial hygiene; (c) prevention, treatment, and control of epidemic, endemic, occupational, and other diseases; and (d) creation of conditions that would assure for all individuals medical services and medical attention in the event of sickness (International Covenant on Economic, Social, and Cultural Rights).

During the past fifty years, Western democracies and many other states, with the notable exception of the United States, have ratified or acceded to most of the international human rights instruments. As of June 1994, the two major international covenants based on the Universal Declaration, the International Covenant on Civil and Political Rights and the International Covenant on Economic, Social, and Cultural Rights, had respectively 127 and 129 states parties. The Convention on the Rights of the Child has been ratified by a larger number, a total of 160 countries.

The United States has only ratified four of the seven major conventions and those very recently. In contrast with other industrialized countries, health and medical sciences in the United States have been informed by ethical rather than human rights norms. Bioethics has been dominated by philosophers working on ethical issues, who have tended to draw on moral philosophy and theory, disciplines that have implicit commitments to protecting individuals from abuses but do not incorporate human rights as a central and explicit commitment.

Medical researchers and practitioners in the United States have been primarily concerned with protecting the autonomy of patients by requiring informed consent for treatment. This constitutes a much narrower standard than the human rights framework outlined above. It is noteworthy, nevertheless, that representatives of major professional organizations in the life and medical sciences, participating in a March 1994 consultation organized by the American Association for the Advancement of Science (AAAS), affirmed the universality of human rights standards and their applicability to the life and health sciences in all countries, including the United States.

The U.S. Commission on Human Rights, "recognizing the need for international cooperation in order to ensure that mankind as a whole benefits from the life sciences and to prevent them from being used for any purpose other than the good of mankind," adopted a resolution in March 1993 entitled "Human Rights and Bioethics." In that resolution, the commission invited governments, the specialized agencies and other organizations of the United Nations, and nongovernmental organizations to identify the key issues that need to be addressed and activities being carried out in order to ensure that the life sciences develop in a manner respectful of human rights.

What has been learned from the past half-century's experience? What kind of initiatives would facilitate a more effective implementation of human rights in the health sector?

OBSTACLES TO THE IMPLEMENTATION OF HUMAN RIGHTS IN THE HEALTH SECTOR

Scientists and health professionals have been victims as well as accomplices, albeit often coerced, of human rights violations. Scientists and health professionals can arouse the suspicion of repressive governments, precisely because they maintain professional relationships with colleagues outside their countries and have considerable respect and status in their own society. They have been persecuted for their work, for the peaceful expression of their opinions or beliefs, and for their efforts to oppose human rights violations in their countries. AAAS's 1994 *Directory of Persecuted Scientists, Health Professionals, and Engineers* documents 468 current cases, which represent only a portion of all violations. Health professionals constitute the group with the second or third largest number of cases each year.

Medical personnel have particular problems when participating in situations of conflict. Some governments do not respect principles of medical neutrality in regions of armed conflict. Although provisions of international humanitarian law and professional ethics require health personnel to care without discrimination for all who are sick or wounded, governments have punished individual physicians and health workers who treat adversaries, even when the doctors were unaware of the identity of the patient. Governments have, on occasion, arrested groups of health workers located in areas of conflict or opposition strongholds so as to intimidate their colleagues and deprive rebels from receiving medical care.

In contravention to a health professional's paramount responsibility to "do no harm," physicians, nurses, and other health-care providers have been implicated in serious human rights violations. It has often been difficult to ascertain whether these health professionals were willing accomplices or were threatened and coerced by governments. Most serious violations are cases where physicians have been accessories in the practice of governmental torture. Investigations in several countries have revealed that physicians have examined detainees to determine whether they could tolerate torture, monitored the torture of individuals, developed or refined techniques of torture, falsified or omitted medical information from the medical records of detainees and prisoners, and falsified death certificates.

Another documented type of human rights violation is the involvement of physicians in the political use of psychiatry, committing political dissidents to psychiatric hospitals and forcing them to undergo psychiatric treatment. Governments that impose cruel and unusual punishment, like the amputation of limbs, ears, or eyes for crimes, have required health professionals to carry out their sentences.

Even in societies that generally respect human rights, the rapid development of the life and health sciences poses challenges to preserving and promoting human dignity. New discoveries and technologies may offer great promise to improve human welfare but often raise ethical and human rights dilemmas for which no adequate guidelines or precedents exist. Technologies for extending human life, for example, have raised the question whether there is a right to die as well as a right to live. The ability to create human preembryos in the laboratory demands the clarification of their status and the determination whether it is permissible to create or use preembryos for research purposes. Transnational research projects may involve researchers and subjects in societies with different standards, which raises issues such as the meaning of informed consent in diverse cultural settings.

A commitment to human rights requires constant vigilance in order to maximize the benefits to human welfare and protect against unintended human rights violations derived from new technologies and treatments. The U.S. Human Genome Project, which seeks to map and sequence the full human genetic code, is furnishing a plethora of new knowledge and techniques to diagnose and treat many genetic disorders, but it opens up the possibility of many forms of discrimination. A Boston-based 1992 study of patients with five genetic disorders found evidence of genetic discrimination on the part of a wide variety of social institutions. Respondents, including presymptomatic individuals and carriers, reported discriminatory practices by insurance companies (life, health, disability, and mortgage); employers (hiring and promotion); the military; schools and universities; adoption agencies; and health providers.

The potential for genetic discrimination will increase as the vertiginous pace of discovery accelerates through the next decade and beyond. The subtle but greatest danger is that the human body may be completely desacralized and reduced to little more than a machine, with the DNA as the molecular text that defines the individual and determines his or her destiny. The rhetorical excesses of some scientists and social commentators have moved their critics to fear that the *Brave New World* nightmare is all but inevitable and that individual freedoms and all human rights may vanish. The U.S. Human Genome Project includes a component dedicated to investigate the ethical, legal, and social implications, to which some 3 to 5 percent of the project's funds are allocated. Other governments have mandated research and allocated funds to face the same concerns.

The development of new reproductive technologies also raises a host of ethical, legal, and human rights issues, although the debate has focused on abortion. For example, the development of forms of contraception inserted by providers and that women cannot stop using without provider assistance is a technology that has enabled some governments to encourage or even coerce targeted groups, such as poor women. In societies with strong preferences for male children, such as India and China, the diffusion of ultrasound technology that can determine the sex of the fetus has led to the selective abortion of female fetuses and the skewing of the sex ratio in the population. Surrogacy arrangements, where one woman conceives and/or carries to a child for another, have raised concerns about potential economic exploitation, as well as questions about the rights of the "birth mother" vis-à-vis the child.

The escalating cost of modern health care confronts countries that recognize the right to health care with the challenge of how to contain costs while meeting a commitment to universal health care and equitable access to medical diagnosis and treatment. Many of these countries, not including the United States, came to accept in the years following World War II a legal entitlement to health care, which translated an acknowledgment of government responsibility for health services into a legal entitlement. Escalating costs make it increasingly difficult for these governments to provide universal access to a full range of health services. Addressing this issue, a recent Government Committee on Choices in Health Care in the

Netherlands has recommended a new standard based on the provision of "neces-sary care," rather than all health care. Under this formula, every inhabitant would be insured for a broad basic package with an income-related premium. Necessary care covered by universal insurance would be broad, but government controls and restrictions would regulate the introduction of new technologies and restrict access to expensive procedures such as heart surgery and organ transplant. Such controls and other forms of rationing may seem objectionable, but the alternative may be a U.S. style health system that provides unlimited treatment for some while denying basic health care to a significant portion of the population.

A WAY FORWARD

There are no easy answers to promoting implementation of human rights in the health sector. The following steps, however, would improve the protection and promotion of human rights.

(1) The promotion of human rights in the life and health sciences requires that abstract legal standards be translated into concrete guidelines and requirements. This can best be undertaken through partnership between health professionals and scientists working together with human rights advocates and experts. Because human rights often develop to protect human subjects from "standard threats," it would be beneficial to pursue in-depth studies that can pinpoint existing human rights violations in the health sector. An appropriate mechanism for this purpose within the U.N. system is the appointment of special rapporteurs. However, academic cen-ters and nongovernmental organizations are generally more competent to under-take this research. In any case, there need to be international mechanisms for the collection and application of the data.

(2) Human rights standards need to be persistently applied to developments in the life and health sciences. An exemplary document is the Council of Europe's recent "Draft Convention for the Protection of Human Rights and Dignity of the Human Being with Regard to the Application of Biology and Medicine." The con-vention embraces professional standards, equitable access, consent, protection of persons lacking capacity, privacy and access of information, research on embryos *in vitro*, the human genome, and other topics. The articles of the convention are fol-lowed by a longer explanatory report that interpret the articles.

(3) It is essential that effective mechanisms be established on international, national, and professional levels for assuring that the life and health sciences remain respectful of human rights, for collecting reliable information to inform pol-icy and practices, and for providing a means for ongoing application of ethical and human rights standards to new issues. The international character of science calls for an international bioethics/human rights commission, established under U.N.

auspices, to monitor scientific and technical advances from a human rights perspective. At a minimum, the international commission would identify issues and formulate recommendations for responding to human rights threats. One role of the international commissions could be to encourage member states to establish national commissions that would report yearly to the international commission and would become vehicles through which the commission could disseminate reports and guidelines.

(4) Fundamental reform of the U.N. system is unlikely to happen any time in the near future, because the ineffectiveness of international human rights oversight mechanisms emanates from a disparity between rhetorical affirmation and commitment to compliance. Still, some measures could improve the effectiveness of current mechanisms and procedures. While it is beyond the scope of this chapter to enter into the details, the measures could include: investing greater resources that would be more commensurate to the tasks; applying scientific methodologies and incorporating scientific expertise; developing information management systems linking monitors in the field with international and regional oversight bodies; developing indicators for assessing compliance with the standards set in international human rights instruments; and systematically publicizing governments' failures to conform with international human rights standards.

(5) Conformity with human rights standards obviously requires that they be adequately understood. Yet few medical schools or universities provide adequate training on matters related to human rights. The exceptions are a few medical schools that offer human rights courses or incorporate human rights into professional ethics courses. This situation needs rectification. Human rights need to be incorporated into the formal curriculum for health professionals and scientists working in the health sector and into continuing education programs.

(6) Human rights standards should also be incorporated explicitly into professional codes of ethics and should inform professional standards of conduct, position papers, and issue statements prepared by professional associations and societies. Professional associations and societies also need to develop systematic programs for monitoring compliance with these codes.

(7) Health professionals and scientists can support beleaguered colleagues in countries where serious violations of human rights occur by engaging in human rights networks. One such network is the AAAS's Human Rights Action Network (AAASHRAN), which circulates information on human rights violations throughout the scientific community. Alerts are sent on electronic mail to AAASHRAN subscribers, along with copies of letters of inquiry or appeal. Subscribers are encouraged to spread information about these cases to colleagues and the public and to support efforts to remedy the violations by sending their own appeal letters. Amnesty International maintains a health professionals' human rights network.

29

SCIENCE AND THE HUMANITIES

THOMAS KEMPF
is Secretary of the Conference of the German Academies of Sciences and
Humanities. This is an association of all seven scientific academies in Germany,
which represents the common interests of the academies at home and abroad
and establishes contact with the federal government, federal states, and
international academic organizations.

AIDS, CLIMATE, ENVIRONMENT, ENERGY, POPULATION: the important areas for scientific investigation are quickly listed. They involve problems that are of central significance for the coexistence of human beings and the development of human societies. These are the topics of the future.

International conferences and countless publications and communiqués have addressed each of these problems. Even if the disciplines involved refrained from raising new issues, they would not run out of tasks. But even if science had found an answer to all these questions, the problems would not be solved since other disciplines are involved in the process of solution. These problems would remain unsolved without the support of the sciences, but at the same time they are closely connected with political, social, cultural, religious, and economic questions, whose answers are not within the range of science.

There will not be a solution to the so-called "big topics" without the sciences, even if the sciences do not set the goals. However, our perception of the sciences has changed. Each discipline or field of research is now evaluated by its meaning for our society, our living together, or our welfare system. In a word: it is now important to know whether it is serving a commonly accepted purpose. Politics have discovered the sciences. The sciences–especially in the eyes of the public–have developed a political factor that may be legitimate, sometimes even necessary, and helpful.

It may be useful to explore some features that characterize the independent development, and the identity of the sciences themselves, and three of the tasks whose solution is significant for their success.

A)   The sciences and research have to develop a new time management. This is an old problem, that has been altered under new circumstances. Traditionally defined, it could be phrased as follows: The sciences and research must keep their independence. They must demonstrate that only independently developed scientific projects, performed without interference and driven primarily by the passionate search for knowledge, are the projects upon which the solution of our problems will be based.

This sounds self-evident, but it has become to a high degree not self-evident because in order to reach this goal the sciences now have to fight for what always was at its disposal in former times and now is being challenged from all sides–time.

This chapter on basic and applied research is largely a discussion on the reaction time between the start of a scientific project and the time when its results can be applied. A recent catch–phrase, "sciences as innovation-culture," is based on the comparison of how much time competitive societies require to accelerate the process of modernization and cycles of investment, in which scientific knowledge can favorably affect the economy. According to this point of view, scientific progress stands for the saving of time. Today, discourse on the sciences is a discourse on saving time.

Still, the sciences, especially basic research, need time. *We do not have enough resources to produce quick solutions. Sustainable solutions need reliable research.* This is not done in a day. Not having adequate time at its disposal, research is forced to become old-fashioned to be prepared for the future.

B)   The sciences and research have to develop a new management of information. This is one of the central tasks for the future. In the period of the European development of the sciences between 1750 and 1850, not only were the modern disciplines created but also the still valid shapes and rules of scientific communication. One of the essential rules said: Hearsay stories are not acceptable. A scientific statement has to have an author and the author must be identified. Careers built on the authorship of several accepted scientific statements can be lost in case of proven mistakes. In more than one respect, authorship was and is associated with individual responsibility.

Electronic data networks challenge this basic rule by bypassing authorship. Nobody is able to take responsibility for theses, lab reports, and articles incorporated in those networks. Today, with the help of international data networks, it is possible to enter unidentified hypotheses and assumptions into scientific communications that would never have been accepted in traditional, reviewed journals.

In a period when the sciences are expected to be more and more responsible for global development, they face the danger of being unable to guarantee individually responsible scientific communications.

For the progress of knowledge, an effective management of information as well as the elimination of unimportant information is essential *Sciences have to learn to forget. We have too much information at our disposal and cannot afford to keep everything on hand.* This demand is paradoxical because in order to regard information as unimportant, it has to be noticed. The paradox cannot be solved; the problem behind it has to be solved.

So the question of building "centers of excellence" around central tasks of the sciences will be less a question of the equipment of labs or the regional concentration of scientists. It will much more depend on whether at the right time the exactly correct and suitable quantity of information is available or whether this information is covered by other information and is therefore unable to have an impact.

The problems of changing status of the authorship and the surplus of information–just two examples!–are able to be solved only by the sciences themselves. Even as they are closely connected with other issues, they describe a field for which basically only the sciences or the scientific community is able to develop an approach to solutions. The other issues include jurisdiction, dealing with the question of authorship and copyright in a completely different way; and funding organizations, taking into consideration the electronic transfer of information and having to accept that financial input and results involve totally different issues.

C)   Sciences and research have to develop new models of cultural management. This means that sciences that have advanced to an essential factor for the development of societies have to understand and present themselves as such in an extensive sense: as an integral part of the culture of a society.

The high rank of sciences today is delicate. In order to secure this high rank for the future, sciences have to become a part of our cultural identity. Today the sciences in Europe seem to have political meaning, but it is not object and motive within the process of building a cultural identity. In the so-called developing countries this might be the fact to an even higher degree. At the same time, it makes sense that questions concerning topics like environment or population will not be resolved if the solutions worked out by the sciences are not accepted by indigenous cultures of the societies concerned.

Furthermore, there are two other problematic sectors. First, the sciences have to have a transdisciplinary interest to maintain scientific variety. The more successful sciences are in coping with the mentioned "big topics," the more disciplines that are dealing with "secluded" issues will come under pressure. Also, the ability of a culture to cope with problems of the future are based on its inner variety and its ability to address all people. *The biodiversity of sciences is too important to be exploited.*

Second, there is the external relationship of science. The imparting of scientific knowledge to the public will gain greater importance. This mission is to some degree beyond the scope or ability of scientists, but they must provide advice in order to enable the scientific organizations or journalists to act. As simple as it may sound, public relations of and for the sciences is an essential task for the future, and the sciences themselves have to give. In our media society, the phrase "Do good and talk about it" gains new dimensions.

In this respect, in the more conservative scientific community in Europe, it is significant that the union of the European Academies, "All European Academies" (ALLEA), built a working group under the rubric of "The relevance of basic research in society," which also is dealing with questions concerning the public image of science. *Science can no longer afford to avoid the media.*

It is obvious that in the field of cultural self-portrayal of the sciences not only a cooperation of the natural sciences and humanities is needed. The humanities deserve high recognition for their cultural competence. But whether both "cultures" are ready for a dialogue and for cooperation will be the decisive factor.

The essential factors of time–, information–, and culture-management tasks refer to the "operation of sciences" itself. The sciences will have to solve problems relating to these, if they are not to be dominated by outside forces whose wishes might be legitimate, but will remain unfulfilled if the prerequisites are missing. Only free, effective and culturally accepted sciences will be able to perform according to our expectations.

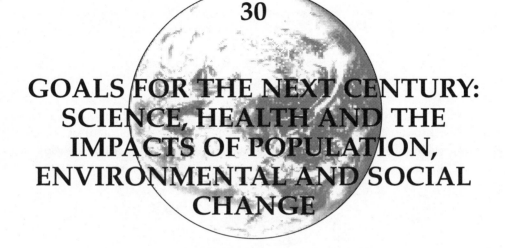

30

GOALS FOR THE NEXT CENTURY: SCIENCE, HEALTH AND THE IMPACTS OF POPULATION, ENVIRONMENTAL AND SOCIAL CHANGE

SIR DAVID PLASTOW
is Chairman of the U.K. Medical Research Council, Chancellor of the University of Luton, and Chairman of Inchcape pic. Sir David is the former Chief Executive of Rolles-Royce Motor Cars, Chairman and Chief Executive of Vickers PLC, and non-executive Governor of BUPA.

SIR DAI REES
is Chief Executive of the U.K. Medical Research Council and President of the European Science Foundation. Sir Dai is the former Director of the National Institute for Medical Research and a member of Council of the Royal Society.

FOR THE MAJOR ORGANIZATIONS responsible for funding medical research, such as the U.K. Medical Research Council, the debate about what we should be aiming for in the next century is far from an indulgence in speculative futurology. It is central to our futures. The future will certainly throw up many new goals–some of which will no doubt be unexpected and indeed surprising–yet to a considerable degree it will also be shaped by the goals we set ourselves now.

Inevitably, national priorities must strongly condition the goals that national organizations set. In the United Kingdom, the Medical Research Council's mission to improve human health is strongly influenced by the goals of the U.K. Health Departments and the National Health Service. Equally important as shaping influences are the dynamics of the research process itself, the opportunities for technology development, the power of public opinion, and international influences.

DRIVES FOR CHANGE

The power of chronology is such that the impending end of the century is provoking much thought and discussion on the nature of things to come. Yet it would be surprising if any dramatic shifts were to occur with the onset of the new millennium. Much more likely is that we in medical research will remain committed to steady development along the lines of present progress, namely, by advancing and promoting strong linkages between parallel strands of research activity–basic, clinical, public health, and health services.

Health Demands

One starting point for our goals is and must be health needs of the population. How will these needs change as a result of changing circumstances in the next century? How can medical research respond to them?

Crucial pressures will arise from the great expansion of the population of the world, at least in the early part of the next century, and from the growth in the number of old people in the developed world–which will continue for at least the same period. Here already are implicit goals for medical research, involving strategies and techniques for the health of mothers and children and for family planning, on the one hand, and for understanding and dealing with the many and diverse health problems of aging on the other.

There are at least two other new determinants for health services, though their scale and intensity in the next century are not yet realistically calculable. These are the health impacts of environmental change, both global and local, and the health impacts of living with the social changes that will continue to occur with increasing pace, often with violent influences on traditional relationships and life-styles.

Progress of Science

To consider the likely development, from the complementary viewpoint, of changes in the state and the possibilities of science, we must make some assumptions, however strange they might turn out to appear with hindsight. The first assumption we would make is that the current run of spectacular research successes in basic cell and molecular biology will continue, to the degree that problems that now seem intractable will be solved. Past experience over many decades has been that the rate of progress in this area has been much faster than foreseen. Almost every week brings startling discoveries that to a previous generation would have seemed almost miraculous. These days, for example–and it really is only comparatively recently–the characterization of disease genes unknown in previous generations has become commonplace. There seems no reason why this progress should not continue.

Our second assumption might be more controversial, among scientists, at least. This is that science will move to what we might call a postreductionist stage: from the characterization of the very small to the characterization of the larger. Before too long, in historical terms, the human genome will have been sequenced in its entirety, along with other genomes. The way the genes express their encoded proteins will have been discovered in great detail. The way these proteins fold–an apparently intractable problem now–will have been solved, so that we will know in three dimensions how the most important proteins are structured and how they interact with other proteins and with nucleic acids. In short, we will know the basic rules according to which molecular components act out their parts in the play of life. When this fundamental achievement in the progress of human knowledge is accomplished, we will have crossed a great mountain barrier to the furtherance of biological science, and yet it will be only to see other barriers raise themselves up, perhaps even higher. Some of these new problems already are visible, and researchers are beginning to tackle them. For example, how is it that life processes can seem to be more than the sum of their molecular parts in the cell, the smallest unit of that very special thing we call life? One key goal for medical research in the next millennium must be the elaboration of a general theory of the cell.

This and other developments that integrate fundamental mechanisms into more quantitative models will require researchers to go beyond biology to draw increasingly on the ideas and techniques of mathematics and physics. Developments in our understanding of macromolecular systems and mechanisms of action will require that we break down the barriers that exist, particularly in the U.K., between the disciplines of chemistry and the physical sciences and mathematics, on the one hand and life sciences and medical research on the other.

Increased effort will also need to be devoted to understanding questions of psychological well-being, of mood, feeling, perception, and reasoning. Buoyed up, perhaps, by the stunning string of advances in the natural sciences toward the end of the last century, pioneers such as Freud and Jung sought to formulate general theories in these areas. Perhaps they were too much in advance of their time. In the century to come, medical research will be aiming at expanding understanding of the brain, the mind, and the emotions-supported by the full armory of recently developed cellular, molecular, and imaging techniques.

IMPACTS OF CHANGE

The three guesses about sources of future health demands identified earlier in this chapter were population change, environmental change, and social change. It is worth looking at each in turn, recognizing that while their relative priorities are likely to change, each will continue to be important.

Population and Demographic Change

The twentieth century expansion of global population might in one sense be said to represent a triumphant success for the human species. A world that could not feed all its citizens 40 years ago now is feeding more than twice as many as the entire world population at that time. It is only too clear that continued growth at the present rate cannot continue if each child is to have an adequate nutrition, let alone the various other opportunities that we associate with civilized societies. Among the many advances so urgently needed from medical science are new, simple, cheap forms of birth control to provide the possibility of choice and control on the part of women over the planning of their families. When this is accomplished, each new child will have a better chance of being born into an environment in which he or she can be well nurtured and provided for. Just how and to what extent any new technologies are employed is for each national society to determine for itself, influenced no doubt by the ethical and religious convictions that prevail.

For science, the goal is twofold. First, it is to increase our understanding of reproductive biology at molecular, cellular, and physiological levels, so that we can deliver increasingly safe, effective, and beneficial influence over conception, fetal development, and birth. Second, recognizing that the paramount objective is to enable human dignity and fulfillment, rather than merely to provide new interventions in personal biology, the medical and social sciences must join forces with each other and the humanities to support and facilitate personal and social aspirations rather than to address only functional approaches to social organization.

Another consequence of a rising population is likely to be an increase in problems from existing and new infectious diseases. These are always exacerbated by crowding and malnutrition and in the future will be further compounded by an increase in population mobility. Medical science will in the next century face both reemerging and new infectious diseases. It is most unlikely that HIV will turn out to be the last of the emerging new plagues to cause suffering and decimation in human populations. Our only protection is to deepen our understanding of the mechanisms of immunity and infection-viral, bacterial, and parasitic. Our goal here must be to put ourselves in a position where we can react to new infections with speed and precision.

Although population growth is a prominent feature of the developing rather than the developed world, where indeed populations are beginning to decline, developing countries will have their own pressing health problems as the proportion of elderly citizens rises sharply to cause increased manifestation of neurological disorders, cancer, and heart disease. The last decade or two has seen spectacular advances in understanding the cellular, genetic, and environmental mechanisms through which these conditions are initiated and developed. Into the next century, it is surely feasible to ensure that the quality and detail of this understanding improve further and are translated into an increasing range of effective interventions for prevention and therapy. To play its full part in this unfolding future, the U.K.'s Medical Research Council must encourage the further application of molecular cell biology and genetics to the understanding of the development and function of the major human organs. This will need to be coupled to increasingly sophisticated clinical and epidemiological studies to characterize function and malfunction in the whole human person and their application to the ways in which these are subject to influence from the physical and social environments. Among the benefits we can expect to flow from these approaches in medical research are an increasing range of technologies for instant diagnosis based on sensors and imaging; even more precise and rapid surgical interventions; and prediction of disease susceptibilities on the basis of individual genetic inheritance, pointing to options for preventive strategies through diet, life-style, and prophylaxis. Medical care will therefore become less dependent on extended hospitalization and more on the delivery of care and intervention by local and community services.

Environmental and Social Change

The extent and influence of global environmental change is more difficult to quantify, and indeed the views of experts on these questions appear to be more disparate. As a result of global warming, we might expect a gradual expansion in the range of diseases now mainly confined to the tropics. Of great concern, too, must be the effects of local environmental change: in areas where the balance between crop failure and a bountiful harvest is on a knife edge, small changes of climate can have a devastating effect on large populations. In the context of international movements, the resulting population migrations can have huge medical implications, both in the short and long term.

Other social changes of our time are driven by forces quite independent of population, demographic, or environmental changes. These include the decline of old industries and the rise of new, the changing relationships between urban and rural communities, altered family structures and altered roles of family members, precocious independence of the young driven by the social environment, and the many and various changes in life-styles delivered by the new communication technologies. It certainly cannot be claimed that social conditions in the past have always been conducive to the good health of our populations. Malnutrition, infections, and death and deformity associated with childbirth, for example, have often owed their prevalence to social deprivation. However, it also could be claimed that any degree of continuity in family structure and social institutions in the past (even if uneven and interrupted) has encouraged a continuity in life-style and habits that drew on past lessons for health consequences. Fluidity in future social structures is likely to be associated with untested behavior patterns, uninformed by health experience. Obvious examples in United Kingdom are the spread of HIV and other infections among drug abusers, the worrying tendency for schizophrenics to join communities of the homeless young, and the plight of the elderly, and of their health-care providers, when they are split from larger family groupings. To what extent medical and social sciences can together develop tools for amelioration presents a major challenge indeed.

SCIENCE AND GOVERNMENT

If there is one important lesson to be drawn from this attempt to see the future challenges to human health, and thus to medical research to develop insights and technologies, it is that health and health research must become increasingly central to the governance of our societies.

Until now, most of science has developed like art and literature, as an independent activity driven by the needs of human creativity. It has been important to maintain the independence to keep up the standards of rigor in enquiry and proof and to remain free to tackle large conceptual problems that, at the time, would not have been chosen primarily for practical reasons. Technology and development have developed in parallel as servants of industry, commerce, the military, and the state. Science, on the one hand, and technology, on the other, have drawn much from each other, and by no means have all the benefits flowed from science to technology. (For example, it has been said that "science owes more to the steam engine than the steam engine does to science.") Yet always, except in times of war and national emergency, there has been a tension between the desire of science to increase understanding of issues that might or might not have practical importance in the future and that of technology for improvement of immediate practical capabilities. As resources for research and technology become more scarce and, indeed, each competes for resources with the other, this tension is turning into a bitter struggle that profits neither.

Political developments also threaten research and technology and any successful partnership between them. In the postwar and post-Cold War periods, which we hope will continue into the next millennium, it is becoming more difficult in the developed world to see the guiding principles around which governments seek to unite their countries and through which political parties seek to win elections. Special interests of particular groups come more into prominence, and small problems for the short term take precedence over large problems for the long term. It can be as important for electoral purposes to generate evidence of an attractive agenda as to deliver real progress on any of its items.

Such trends threaten the forward movement of science, including medical research, in the directions we have described in this chapter. For the improvement of knowledge and the benefit of mankind, the linkages between research investigation, definition of needs, and applications to human health will be possible only by means of effective partnerships between science and technology, on the one hand, and science and government, on the other. Within both partnerships, each side must have a deliberate commitment to the common agenda that is as strong as that to its own immediate agenda. We do not now see such quality of understanding and cooperation in place anywhere in the developed word, and, human nature being as it is, perhaps it is utopian to hope for it. Nevertheless, if perfect partnership is not upheld as the ideal to which we aspire, we will move ever further from it, and the health and well-being of mankind will be the loser.

31

CHARTING THE FUTURE: HEALTH GOALS FOR THE NEXT CENTURY

HIROSHI NAKAJIMA
has been Director-General of the World Health Organization since 1988. Dr. Nakajima has been awarded the Kijima Prize and the Okamoto Award, Japan; the Legion of Honor, France; DATU of the Order of Sikatuna (highest diplomatic merits), Philippines; the Order of Merit of the Republic of Poland; Commandeur de l'Ordre National du Lion du Sénégal; the Order of Health, Bolivia; and Médaille d'Or décernée par Monsieur le Président de la République Tunisienne, among others.

By THE END OF THE TWENTIETH CENTURY, we could be living in a world without poliomyelitis or new cases of leprosy or deaths from measles or cases of guinea worm disease. The world at the end of the century could be one in which infant mortality rates are no higher than 50 per 1000 live births and life expectancy at birth is no lower than 60 years in any country, with many people living healthy and productive lives well into their nineties.

We can predict that new and effective drugs, vaccines, and other technologies will be available to treat major diseases and conditions of ill health. What, though, will be the opportunities missed and problems left untackled? What will be the remaining priorities for international health action, including action by the World Health Organization (WHO)? I see four of them:

- The first priority must be to ensure equitable value for money by refocusing resources on those who need them most.

- The second priority is poverty reduction by investment in the most basic human needs, including food, safe water and sanitation, and access to social services, including health education.

- The third priority is public health and social policy based on democratic involvement of all people–universal health care for all.

- The fourth priority is strengthening national capabilities for humanitarian action and emergency management for sustainable development.

Today, as we approach the twenty-first century, we must continue to bridge the gaps of inequities between nations and population groups. WHO has set for all member states and all partners in international health work ten goals to guide our way.

Ten Goals Toward Health Care for All

1. To increase the span of healthy life for all people in such a way that health disparities between social groups are reduced.

2. To ensure universal access to an agreed upon set of essential health-care services of acceptable quality, comprising at least the eight essential elements

of primary health care.

3.   To ensure survival and healthy development of children.

4.   To improve the health and well-being of women.

5.   To ensure healthy population development.

6.   To eradicate, eliminate, or control major diseases constituting global health problems.

7.   To reduce avoidable disabilities through appropriate preventive and rehabilitative measures.

8.   To ensure continued improvements in nutritional status for all population groups.

9.   To enable universal access to safe and healthy environments and living conditions.

10. To enable all people to adopt and maintain healthy life-styles and healthy behavior.

I recommend to readers interested in pursuing these concepts "The World Health Report 1995–Bridging the Gaps."

Situation in 1990	**WHO targets for the year 2000**

THE FACE OF POVERTY
Health Status

• At least 97 countries (68 percent of the world population) report a figure of 60 years or over	All countries to have a *life expectancy at birth* greater than 60 years
• At least 78 countries (56 percent of the world population) report a figure under 50 per 1000 live births	All countries to have an *infant mortality rate* that will not exceed 50 per 1000 live births
• Global figure is 92 per 100 live births	*Under-5 mortality rate* will not exceed 70 per 1000 live births

Disease Status

• Incidence of poliomyelitis is 116, 000	Eradication of poliomyelitis
• Prevalence of dracunculiasis (adults) is 3.0 million	Eradication of dracunculiasis
• Prevalence of leprosy is 5.5 million	Elimination of leprosy
• Incidence of neonatal tetanus is 0.5 million	Elimination of neonatal tetanus

- Among children there are 350 million Hepatitis-B carriers

  Control of hepatitis-B

- 2.9 million tuberculosis deaths

  Control of tuberculosis

- 2.25 million malaria deaths

  Control of malaria

THE FACE OF INEQUITY
Health Care Coverage (%)

- Diphtheria, pertussis, tetanus third dose   83

  Primary health care available to the whole population

- Polio vaccine third dose   85
- Safe Water   75
- Sanitation   71
- Deliveries of babies by trained personnel 55

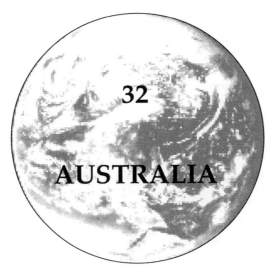

32

AUSTRALIA

THE HONORABLE CARMEN LAWRENCE
is the Minister for Health and the Minister Assisting the Prime Minister for the
Status of Women. Dr. Lawrence was Australia's first woman premier.

AUSTRALIANS ENJOY GOOD HEALTH by world standards. Life expectancy at birth for males is 74.5 years and for females 80.4 years. This places Australia in an intermediate position among Organization for Economic Cooperation and Development countries with respect to life expectancy at birth for both sexes and among one of only 11 countries in the world where women live, on average, to more than 80 years of age.

As in many Western countries, Australian death rates from cardiovascular disease, road traffic trauma, some cancers, and infectious diseases have all declined since the 1960s. However, many Australians still die early or suffer chronic ill health or disability as a result of conditions that are largely preventable.

Despite dramatic declines, cardiovascular disease remains the leading cause of death in Australia. The second highest number of deaths in Australia are attributable to cancers. Although there has been a significant reduction in smoking-related cancers, lung cancer remains the leading cause of cancer deaths overall. Non-melanocytic skin cancer is the most common cancer overall—a legacy of the "bronzed Aussie" image.

Injury and mental health are also major causes of death and disability. Injury is the main cause of death in both males and females between the ages of 1 and 44 and accounts for more years of potential life lost than any other cause of death. Injury also contributes to a substantial amount of disability in the community. With regard to mental health, it is estimated that at least 20 percent of the Australian adult population are affected by mental health problems or mental disorders in any one year.

Although the Australian population overall enjoys good health, there are substantial differentials in life expectancy and health status between various sectors of Australian society. Low socioeconomic status is the primary factor in poor health status. For all age groups, men and women from less advantaged backgrounds have higher death rates and report higher levels of illness than their more affluent counterparts.

It is generally agreed that Australia's indigenous people have the worst health of any identifiable group in Australia. Although available data on Aboriginal and Torres Strait Islander health status is still limited, the latest available evidence shows, for example, that Aboriginal death rates (after standardizing for age) are about three times those of the total Australian population. These high death rates mean that the life expectancy of Aboriginal people at birth is some fifteen to seventeen years less than that for other Australians.

There have been some improvements in Aboriginal and Torres Strait Islander mortality over the past 20 years. For example, infant and maternal death rates have declined by around 60 percent. However, there is growing evidence that these gains have been offset to some degree by a worsening of the non-infectious lifestyle diseases, particularly cardiovascular disease and diabetes mellitus.

Australian authorities are placing greater emphasis in health promotion and disease prevention strategies on modifying social, economic and physical factors in the environment, combined with lifestyle modification, as a means to reduce health differentials and improve the health status of the entire Australian population.

Health promotion and disease prevention are not new to Australia. A significant proportion of health gains in previous years, for example decline in cardiovascular disease mortality since the 1960s, has been attributed to health promotion and disease prevention activities. Gains have been achieved through the implementation of a range of strategies, including individual and community education, mass media information, policy development, legislation, and environmental changes. Australia has received international recognition for its health promotion activities, particularly the National HIV/AIDS Strategy, which is now regarded worldwide as a model participative, community-based preventive public health program.

While the health sector has often been the catalyst for health promotion and disease prevention strategies and policies, much of the successful health promotion action in Australia has involved other public sectors, such as education, agriculture, transport, business, private enterprise, and nongovernment organizations. For instance, Australia's multivariate tobacco harm minimization strategy is characterized by a cooperative approach between governments of all levels and nongovernment organizations. The strategy's integrated and intersectoral approach has resulted in Australia's tobacco control policies and practices being at the forefront of international achievements in this area.

GROWTH AND SUSTAINABILITY OF HEALTH PROMOTION IN AUSTRALIA

The Commonwealth of Australia is a federation of six states and two territories. The state and territory governments fund and manage the public hospital system and a range of other public and community health services. Australians are provided with access to free public hospital care and a variety of primary and secondary health services. The states and territories rely on specific-purpose commonwealth grants to meet a substantial proportion of these costs.

The promotion of health in Australia depends greatly upon government support in respect to infrastructure, funds, and a congenial policy environment.

All levels of government accept that much of the illness and injury evident in the community is potentially preventable and that health gains are not going to be achieved through simply providing health-care services for the diagnosis and treatment of illness and disease.

In recent years, governments have been taking an increasing interest in promoting health, and additional resources have been provided for the measurement of health, the evaluation of health services, the promotion of well-being, and the prevention of illness and disability.

National Health Policy

As a mechanism to reorient Australian health policies and programs toward improving health rather than simply providing health care services, a National Health Policy for Australia has been developed. The policy, which has been agreed upon by commonwealth, state, and territory health ministers, provides a framework for a national approach to improving the health of the population and improving access to health services. The policy aims to ensure that health resources are allocated in such a way as to achieve a proper balance of health promotion, prevention, early intervention, treatment, rehabilitation, palliation, and research.

National Health Goals and Targets

In their move to reorient Australia's health system to one focused more on health outcomes, governments in Australia have determined that a coordinated national effort in a selected range of areas offers the most potential for gain.

National health goals and targets have been formulated as one means of achieving coordinated national effort and increasing the focus on improving population health outcomes.

Four areas have been initially chosen for the goals and targets activity. These are: cardiovascular disease, cancer, injury prevention, and mental health. These four focus areas have been identified as particular priorities that would benefit from additional or better coordinated effort.

Goals, targets and strategies have been developed in each of the four priority areas to encompass the whole spectrum of health care: health promotion and disease prevention; treatment, rehabilitation, and palliative care; research; and the development of data systems.

Responsibility for the implementation of goals and targets in the four existing target areas is being shared between the commonwealth, state and territory governments, and designated peak nongovernment bodies.

Ottawa Charter for Health Promotion

Health promotion in Australia over the last decade has been largely influenced by the Ottawa Charter for Health Promotion developed in 1986 as an outcome of the first International Conference on Health Promotion held in Ottawa, Canada. Australian health promotion initiatives have been guided by the five action areas of the charter: developing healthy public policy, creating supportive environments for health, strengthening community action, developing personal skills, and reorienting health services.

Since the development of the charter there have been significant changes nationally and internationally, including, for example, a widening gap in population health status within and between countries; political changes, particularly in eastern Europe and southern Africa; major development in Southeast Asia; continued world population growth; increasing numbers of disabled and elderly persons worldwide; changes in disease patterns; and technological advances. With such significant changes, it is appropriate, ten years on, to nationally and internationally review the Ottawa Charter, assess its strengths and weaknesses, and, based on the review, set the directions for health promotion over the next decade.

Australia, in contributing to setting the international agenda for health promotion in the twentieth-first century, will undertake a review of health promotion concepts, principles, and practice in Australia.

AUSTRALIA'S INITIATIVES IN ADDRESSING KEY HEALTH ISSUES

National Drug Strategy

The National Drug Strategy recognizes that alcohol and tobacco are most responsible by far for the most widespread public health problems and thus, emphasizes the need to address these issues consistently and comprehensively. Australia has achieved significant gains in the area of tobacco harm minimization in recent years, with smoking rates dropping from 40 percent of the population in 1976 to 24 percent in 1993. However, smoking remains the leading cause of preventable death and disease in Australia, responsible for approximately 19,000 deaths per year, which is 70 percent of all drug-related deaths and 15 percent of total deaths. It is estimated that tobacco use costs the economy $9.25 billion per year in tangible and intangible costs. Thus, Australian governments at all levels are committed to reducing the mortality and morbidity, as well as the economic and social costs associated with tobacco use.

Australia's multivariate approach to tobacco harm minimization is outlined in the National Health Policy on Tobacco. This approach is based on the principle that no single action can address the complex social factors that have enabled tobacco smoking to achieve high levels of participation and acceptance.

The multivariate approach to tobacco control in Australia includes activities in the following areas:

- Marketing (including packaging, labeling, and advertising);
- availability (including limiting access to tobacco products by youth);
- taxation (by both federal and state/territory governments);
- education (in the health effects, cessation options, and reasons behind governments' actions on tobacco control);
- education on the harmful effects of passive smoking;
- cessation services; and
- monitoring and evaluation.

To achieve outcomes in each of these areas, government and nongovernment organizations employ a variety of mechanisms, including research, voluntary agreements, education, and regulation. By working cooperatively to plan interactive and mutually reinforcing activities, jurisdictions ensure that unnecessary duplication does not occur and that resources are used most effectively to meet identified needs.

Examples of these mechanisms include:

- Regulating a national uniform system of health warnings on tobacco products;

- enacting legislation that restricts tobacco companies' capacity for advertising and promotion;

- conducting public education campaigns;

- progressively increasing excise on tobacco products; and

- commissioning research into smoking behavior among target groups, such as young people.

As many tobacco-related diseases occur only after prolonged exposure to tobacco, the success of Australia's tobacco control policies in terms of reduced morbidity and mortality may not be quantifiable for some years. There have been encouraging small reductions in the number of tobacco-related deaths in recent years, which indicate that the reduction in consumption, evident in Australia since the 1960s, is translating into a reduced incidence of tobacco-related diseases.

The most profound indicator of Australia's success in the area of tobacco harm minimization is the change in community attitudes to smoking that have occurred over the last 15 years. Surveys have repeatedly demonstrated that the Australian public is supportive of government policies in this area, including tax increases on tobacco products and the introduction of advertising bans and restrictions on smoking in public places. This strong community support is the most effective indicator of the efficacy of Australia's public health education initiatives and ensures that Australia's successes in the area of tobacco harm minimization will continue well into the future.

National HIV/AIDS Strategy

The cumulative total of people diagnosed HIV positive in Australia as of 30 June 1994 was 18,274. The total number diagnosed with AIDS was 5,075.

Australia is still one of the few countries, even in the developed world, to have developed, implemented, and reviewed a comprehensive national HIV/AIDS strategy.

Australia's National HIV/AIDS Strategy, which commenced in 1989, lays down as its primary goal eliminating the transmission of HIV within the country. While by no means having achieved that goal, which must remain a medium- to long-term aim, Australia can claim that the HIV/AIDS epidemic within the country appears to have stabilized and that it is still mostly confined to the community of homosexual men in which it emerged over a decade ago.

Screening of the blood supply from 1985 effectively ended the risk of HIV acquired through the blood supply, and preventive education from 1984 to 85 limited the rate of transmission to sexual partners in the hemophiliac groups to less than 3 percent (in the United States the comparable rate is 10 to 25 percent).

There has been a strong role played in Australia's HIV/AIDS strategies by community-based organizations. The government dialogue and partnership with the stigmatized and marginalized groups most affected by HIV represented an innovation in public health policy in Australia, one that has been vindicated by the subsequent success of HIV/AIDS prevention efforts in the affected communities.

Since 1987, the rapid implementation of needle and syringe exchange programs and associated educational campaigns in all states and territories have contributed to sustaining a very low infection rate among Australian injecting drug users. The prompt provision of needle and syringe exchange services in Australia was an important preventive measure inhibiting the free spread of the virus beyond the initially affected communities.

Peer education has proved to be a very successful strategy in implementing HIV/AIDS preventive education in Australia.

An important component of Australia's National HIV/AIDS Strategy has been the fostering of a supportive legal and social environment for those with HIV/AIDS, through legislative protection against discrimination, education campaigns, and various social and financial reforms.

The AIDS Matched Funding Program of the strategy is a cost-sharing system under which specific funds provided by the commonwealth for HIV/AIDS education, prevention, treatment and care, and training and evaluation are required to be matched dollar for dollar by the states and territories.

The response to the HIV/AIDS epidemic in Australia is now regarded world-wide as a model participative, community-based preventive public health program.

National Aboriginal Health Strategy

Responsibility for the delivery of health and related services for Australia's Aboriginal and Torres Strait Islander people rests primarily with state and territory governments. However, the commonwealth government has acknowledged the need for a concerted approach to address the continuing poor health of Australia's indigenous people. In June 1990, a Joint Ministerial Forum of Commonwealth, State and Territory Ministers for Health and for Aboriginal Affairs endorsed a National Aboriginal Health Strategy (NAHS).

In December 1990 the Commonwealth confirmed its commitment to the NAHS with substantial funding to lift unacceptable health and infrastructure standards in Aboriginal communities. These funds have been progressively used to address such urgent needs in Aboriginal and Torres Strait Islander communities as housing, water, sewerage, electricity, communications, and roads and to establish new aboriginal community-controlled health services and enable upgrading of existing services.

Recent additional funds will be used to continue and enhance efforts to improve the level of environmental health facilities available in Aboriginal and Torres Strait Islander communities and to further expand the level of available health services.

The funds are administered by the Aboriginal and Torres Strait Islander Commission (ATSIC). The Department of Human Services and Health will work closely with the Commission on efforts to improve the delivery of services for Aboriginal and Torres Strait Islander people, at both commonwealth and state and territory levels.

The evaluation of the first phase of the NAHS was completed at the end of 1994. Based on the evaluation, there will be an increased focus on housing and essential infrastructure services in remote and rural regions in Australia, including the Torres Strait, and improved intersectoral collaboration and increased involvement of Aboriginal and Torres Strait Islander people in the development of health programs, to allow communities and individuals to make informed choices regarding health.

National Mental Health Strategy

Governments in Australia have recognized that many people with mental illness and psychiatric disability are among the most seriously disadvantaged groups in Australia.

Australia is now into its third year of a five-and-a-half-year program, the

National Mental Health Strategy, to improve the quality of life and care that is provided for people with mental illness and psychiatric disability and those at risk of developing a mental illness. The strategy is a cooperative effort between the federal government and the state and territory governments.

It includes initiatives such as major reforms to mental health service delivery, with a much greater focus on integrated community-based care and a much reduced reliance on stand-alone, isolated, large psychiatric institutions; a focus on reducing negative community attitudes to mental illness through a three-year community education and awareness campaign; and the development of a national approach to education and training for the mental health work force.

A key challenge for the future is to give more attention to early intervention, prevention, and promotion of positive mental health.

National Women's Health Program

Australia is one of the few countries to have a National Women's Health Policy. The policy was developed in consultation with organizations and individuals representing the views of more than one million women Australia-wide. The goal of the policy is to improve the health and well-being of women in Australia and to encourage the health system to be more responsive to the needs of women.

As its response to this policy, the commonwealth government established the National Women's Health Program (NWHP) in 1989.

The program has funded over 360 projects throughout Australia, providing innovative women's health services, information, and training, including health promotion, counseling and support services for victims of sexual assault and violence; ethnic liaison services; and Aboriginal and Torres Strait Islander services.

National Healthy Aging Agenda

The proportion of the Australian population aged 65 years or more is projected to grow from around 11 percent in 1991 to more than 19 percent at around 2030. By around 2030 there will be more than five million Australians aged 65 years and over compared to under two million today, representing a growth rate of around double that of the population as a whole. The age profile of the aged population is also increasing–the eighty-plus population at a faster rate than growth in the sixty-five-plus group.

In response to the challenges this progressively aging population poses, the Australian Government has established the Older Australians Advisory Councils to offer people an opportunity to provide direct input into the development of government policies. The councils advise the Federal Minister for Human Services and Health on services for older people and on the roles that older Australians play in family and community life.

The Older Australians Advisory Councils are one component of an overall healthy aging framework to improve access of older people to health services, improve the practices of health professionals in relation to older people, and improve access of older people to preventive services.

The healthy aging agenda includes the commonwealth government and government agencies responsible for program delivery in the arts, sports, communication, education, and veteran affairs. State and local government and community organizations and groups are also engaged in a range of healthy aging activities.

Challenges for Health Promotion in the Future

Australia's commitment to health promotion is evidenced by the infrastructure that currently exists for health promotion within the commonwealth and state/territory health departments, and a number of nongovernment organizations and some areas of the private sector; the allocation of public funds to health promotion programs at national, state, and territory levels; the current emphasis on further improving the infrastructure for health promotion in Australia, including development of the health promotion work force; recognition and support of an intersectoral approach to health promotion; and the development of national health goals and targets encompassing health promotion and disease prevention.

Nevertheless, there are many more challenges ahead for the consolidation and further development of health promotion in Australia.

Addressing these challenges will ensure that health promotion continues to contribute significantly to achieving the health gain desired from the nation's investment in it.

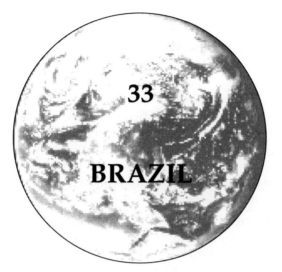

33

BRAZIL

THE HONORABLE ADIB DOMINGOS JATENE
is Minister of Health and Director of the São Paulo University School
of Medicine. He was formerly Secretary of Health of the State of São Paulo,
Director-General of the Hospital of Heart of the Syrain Sanatory Association,
Director-General of the Dante Pazzanese Institute of Cardiology, and President
of the International Society of Cardiovascular Surgery. Dr. Jatene has been
granted 168 titles and honors from more than ten countries.

OVERVIEW OF THE RECENT HISTORY OF BRAZIL

OVER THE LAST DECADES, Brazil has gone through profound and accelerated economic changes during the 1960s to the 1970s, and then through the economic stagnation of the 1980s.

The economic changes experienced during the "miracle years" brought about profound demographic and epidemiological changes. The south and the southeast regions of the country have experienced a massive migration from the countryside to the cities. Between the 1960s and the 1980s the rural population of the southeast region was reduced by 33 percent. Migration from the northeast also has been considerable: in 1960, 32 percent of the Brazilian population was settled in this region; in 1980, 29.5 percent.

The population, facing diverse social and economic circumstances when it migrated, modified its behavior and life-style as a consequence. In 1960, for example, the fecundity rate was approximately 6 percent. In 1980, this figure fell to 4.5 percent and to 3.5 percent in 1985. For the beginning of the 1990s, surveys indicate an average of 2.5 children per woman.

The industrialization and urbanization processes have modified the life-style of the population and the organization of health services as well, as the health risks faced by workers and their families changed. In the 1950s, a typical worker lived in a rural area working in agriculture with a low income. Families suffered from endemic infections. Children died of diarrhea and respiratory infection. Chagas' disease, malaria, and schistosomiasis were the main causes of elevated mortality rates.

In the past year, the Brazilian government has been undertaking many effective remedial efforts. In 1950, life expectancy at birth was 46 years and in 1991 66 years. The mortality rates due to infectious diseases in children under one year of age have decreased in the last three decades. In the period from 1960 to 1980, the ratio of infant mortality decreased from 121 to 83 per 1000 live births.

Special health campaigns, together with regular vaccinations, have reduced the number of cases of immunopreventable diseases. Measles are practically eradicated, and smallpox and poliomyelitis no longer occur.

There have been several improvements in health conditions. Schistosomiasis now is restricted to fewer regions. Chagas' disease is no longer transmitted by vectors throughout the country.

The existing network for the production of health services comprises more than 35,000 health facilities, which have approximately 500,000 beds. Therefore, there are about three beds per 1,000 people. The number of medical doctors is more than 200,000. The use of health services by the population has increased significantly. There are about 15 million hospitalizations, and more than 1.2 million surgical procedures have been performed annually. 360 million medical consultations are provided for the unified health systems each year. Expenditures for medical and hospital assistance are increasing, and, at present, the monthly amount paid by the Ministry of Health is about $600 million U.S. dollars.

What Lessons Have Been Learned?

The success in improvement of health care is due to an increase in income, to improvements in education and in technology, and to the efforts undertaken by the Brazilian government to broaden health services.

All these improvements represent an extension of direct welfare benefits and also reflect a reduction of public investments in the health sector as a consequence of the precarious health of the population.

Outlook for the Future

In 1994, the Brazilian population is approximately 152.8 million people and the country's gross national product is about $530 billion U.S. dollars, which means a GNP per capita of $3,000 U.S. dollars. In the year 2000, with an estimated population of 165.5 million people and a 5 percent annual increase on its GNP between 1994 and 2000, Brazilian GNP will be $613 billion U.S. dollars, which means $3.7 thousand U.S. dollars per capita.

In this period, the number of children aged 14 and under will be relatively constant in absolute numbers (about 49 million). The number of people over 65 years of age will probably increase from 7.3 million to 8.4 milliom, but will remain reduced (4.8 percent and 5.1 percent, respectively, in 1994 and 2000). Thus, the population of active age (15 to 64 years) will be likely to increase the most, especially in absolute numbers (from 96.4 to 108.1 million).

Therefore, Brazil will face, in the coming years, an increase in active population, with the need to generate more jobs and growing urbanization. The population in the active age range will need to be kept in good health in order to fulfill the demands of their jobs.

Now in place are rules stating the prerogatives, responsibilities, and obligations of the state in the health sector. These new responsibilities, set forth in Article 200 of the Brazilian Constitution, are detailed in Laws 9.080/90 and 8.142/90, with a redefinition of duties for the federal, state, and municipal levels of government, based upon decentralization, with social control exercised by the community.

Adequate Use of the Scarce Financial Resources Available

In order to spend well the scare resources available, it will be necessary to develop strategies and programs focused on benefiting the greatest possible portion of the population, with special emphasis on the poor.

Spending well means reducing costs, stimulating scientific and technological developments, seeking new assistance patterns, strengthening nutrition programs, basic sanitation and immunization, and other measures that assist a large portion of the population.

Scientific and technological developments, as well as its marketing and application in the fields of diagnosis and treatment of certain illnesses, especially terminal illnesses, have contributed not only to increasing distinctions among social levels of the population but also to making the present biomedical and health-care systems in many countries fail. Nowadays, not even industrialized countries are able to absorb the growing and uncontrollable costs of intensive technology used in hospital care.

Assistance models are outdated simultaneously with the new technological developments that produce individual miracles and real collective disasters. The benefits of science are not for everybody, but only for those who enjoy privilege, and do not care about the suffering of second-class citizens, disadvantaged by poverty, misery, and illness, and living on the periphery of society. The complexity of procedures to restore health makes therapeutic practices less human since they require incalculable and often unavailable financial resources. Even the richest attempt to improve their rationality to benefit the population as a whole.

The present model, focused on the treatment of diseases and not on prevention, generates artificial demands. It is based on increasingly complex medical and hospital assistance, serving fewer people each day, and provides more expensive treatment with doubtful results, both in terms of quality of life and effective recovery of health. The need for this kind of procedure has become unlimited while financial resources available for its financing are absolutely limited. This incongruence is unbearable and its predictable consequence is a deadlock.

The direction of this process must be inverted. It should focus on across-the-board preventive and educational health measures and be focused on promoting health and preventing illness instead of treating diseases. Brazil experiences intensively the effects of the world crisis on the health sector, and the situation is aggravated by its economic difficulties. The capacity of investment does not provide sufficient resources to apply models of assistance of unlimited costs that are being abandoned even by those countries with strong and stable economics.

In the assistance model based on spontaneous demand, the health system would expect individuals with tuberculosis, for instance, to detect the symptoms of the disease and to look for a service. In assistance models who services would be directed to health needs, problems would be identified within communities by epidemiological studies and sentinels to guide an organized offer of help defined at the local level.

This model, focused on organized offers of services, would redirect health planning for a specific population base, restore epidemiological approaches to control health problems, and also incorporate a constant updating of technical and scientific improvements in the health system. To achieve this goal, the Ministry of Health is supporting its Health Community Agents Programme, which actively undertakes health measures, as opposed to the assistance models of spontaneous demand carried out both by the public and private health assistance network.

Among public health activities, sanitation is the most important tool to prevent diseases. Many diseases are disseminated by a lack of sanitation measures. Lack of good quality water and inadequate or wrong waste disposal are factors that contribute to the spread of diseases.

Improvements in sanitation, applied over wide areas, are needed mainly because of the need to control man's intense interference with the environment. The main sanitation activities concern: water supply, waste removal (sewage system), collection, and final destination of waste, drainage of pluvial water, control of insects and rodents, food sanitation, control of environmental pollution, sanitation of houses, work and recreation places, and sanitation applied to territorial planning.

Actions aimed at increasing and spending well financial resources for the health sector should concentrate on developing new forms of management to set partnerships between the government and society. The state can get together with the community in order to gather experience, as well as technical, financial, and political capabilities, and use them in the process of development to reduce inequities.

State-community partnership arises from the understanding that there are sets of functions of public nature that do not necessarily need to be carried out exclusively by governmental structures. Organizations operating in this domain are not necessarily public (deficient, act at global level) nor private (profitable); they are, rather, social organizations (nonprofitable, not deficient) that act by focusing on segments of the population requiring centralized efforts to reduce social imbalances.

Surely, jobs will be generated in urban areas, but even if jobs are not generated in urban areas, their population will grow and bring about an increase in the numbers of the disadvantaged.

In this context, the job issue is likely to become a central point for the success of the national trajectory toward development, if this process is considered as a global process, incorporating social and political dimensions.

In the past, growth has acted as an element for the reduction of poverty, espe-

cially in urban areas, because of generation of jobs with few qualification requirements. Alternatively, rural poverty has been reduced by migrations to the cities. It
is doubtful, however, if such mechanisms will act with the same effectiveness when
new patterns of growth are considered.

By 2010, if we experience an annual population growth of 6 percent in the first
decade of the next century, and if there are greater national efforts in the fight
against poverty, its incidence will likely be reduced to 14 percent of the population,
but that will still comprise 28 million people.

The main Brazilian social issue is its critical poverty. The priority objective of
Brazilian social politics is to find means to integrate this huge mass of urban and
rural marginal people. They represent our most prominent health, education, and
employment problems.

It is evident that a social strategy focused on the fight against poverty must be
linked to an economic strategy and to the state modernization effort and political
and institutional practices.

One can expect that the country will be able to accelerate toward stable economic and social development through state reform. With the modernization of
public institutions, it should be possible to promote strategic actions in science and
technology, education, health, and the fight against poverty. Thus, it is expected
that three objectives desired by all contemporary society will be achieved: efficiency, understood as the capacity to produce, to ensure at least the minimum
required to provide the essential needs of all; equity, viewed as the capacity to dis-
tribute in a just manner the product of the collective effort; and liberty, viewed as
the capacity to practice a participating democracy and not only a representative
democracy.

CHALLENGES

The complexity of Brazilian health status, both in terms of the population health
problems (epidemiological profile) and those related to the health system (organization of health services), does not mean that it is impossible to amend. The interventions are required to improve health administrative and technical measures but
will require economic, political, and cultural changes. Consequently, sectorial
interventions, are required to improve the organization of services and systems of
the health sector, as well as extra-sectorial interventions involving other sectors,
such as education, work, agriculture, housing, and sanitation.

The present challenge in the health sector is to seek equity and to decrease the
existing inequalities by concrete means and practices toward the improvement of
quality, efficiency, and effectiveness in health care for all. This situation requires
new forms of dealing with health problems based on the causal factors instead of

concentrating on its effects. A new pattern of health promotion *latu sensu*, focused on community, family, and individuals, must be built for the next century. This must be a responsibility of all society: the state, the social and economic sectors, both public and private, and, fundamentally, the people itself.

Containing Disease Impact

Actions should result in the avoidance of early death–the decrease of years of life lost. For this purpose, programs for mother and infant health, children health and women's health will be reviewed and strengthened. The federal government is implementing a plan for reduction of infant mortality within the Program of Solidarity Community.

The mother and infant group encompasses women in reproductive age, children, and teenagers. According to the present definition of adolescence, that includes the age group from 10 to 19 years; the mother and infant group represents two-thirds of the Brazilian population. This group must be treated in a distinctive manner, out of quantitative dimensions, related to its distinctive types of health problems. Its high morbidity and mortality rates, including problems often preventable, and the need for effective health services must be addressed. It also is necessary to study the major problems of children and women. It is necessary to deepen discussion on how and why problems occur to each component of each group, as well as discussion of the main strategies of public health to prevent or control them.

Compliance with Constitutional Principles

Article number 197 of the federal constitution defines health services as a public priority, and assigns to the government the function of regulating, inspecting, and controlling actions and services, apart from its direct implementation. In Article 198, the constitution states that public actions and health services "integrate a regionalized and hierarchic network and constitute a unified system," according to the guidelines for the decentralization of public services, which are centrally directed at each governmental level and are charged with providing integral assistance with community participation.

Comments on the Process of Reform

The cultural, economic, and political changes suggested in this text cannot be accomplished in the short run but must be started as soon as possible, before special interest groups and government bureaucracy prevent this from happening.

Making changes is difficult since it will displace the established power and reorient financial resources. Most changes will take several years to be implemented, since they will involve substantial reallocation of public resources and will require development of a new institutional capacity. Still, changes are possible. It is necessary to direct political motivation toward to the desired goals.

The first question to be raised is: What kind of development do we want?

The model we have followed in Brazil needs to be reviewed. This should not be a task exclusively for economists. Other social actors need to participate in such discussions, particularly those responsible for dealing with the social sectors.

Among the main features of the process of development important to the health sector are the production of growth and also the process for macroeconomic stabilization. Increase in production should be sustainable, requiring serious institutional support and a better integration of the country into the world economy. However, production should contribute to social welfare and equality. Lack of attention to this assumption put Brazil among the most disadvantaged countries in the world, and this lack of equality has had disastrous effects on the economic system. The concentration of income in a small segment of the population defines a type of demand and production that responds to the distribution of purchase power within the marketplace instead of taking into account the basic needs of the majority. But there is not productive investment since economic history has shown that the most equitable systems allow more saving, accumulation, and investment capacities and, therefore, sustained development.

Another feature of the necessary development is that it has to be undertaken with liberty, offering equal opportunity for the economic agents and for the individual to exercise his or her rights of citizenship. Real democracy must be an everyday practice for peaceful solutions of conflicts, not limited to a periodic election of political leaders. This development model also involves concern for the environment, as well as a fair use of the advances of science and technology and effective participation in the global economy.

To be effective, social policies require a reduction of the gap between social rights assured by law and effective capacity of the state to provide public services associated to these rights. Without effective equality before the law, it is useless to produce democratic legislations.

The health sector is important in each of these aspects of development, not only because it is influenced by the model chosen but also as a mechanism to improve development itself. It constitutes a productive sector in itself. Health can be the main parameter to measure the level of democracy and act as a bridge for dialogue and cooperation among countries. It also is related to actions aimed at protecting the environment, whose main purpose is to protect human life. Therefore, in order to correct the health crisis we not only have the right to participate in the process to define development but also the obligation to do so.

Another aspect to solve the crisis refers to the functioning of the health sector itself, which should have equity and universality as its main values. If these objectives cannot be quickly achieved, public financial resources should be redirected toward those who have no alternative to public assistance, ensuring universal access to fulfillment of their basic needs. We have to seek efficiency and effectiveness for health actions but not only at the level of a good administration of production units. The quality of health services should aim at satisfying those who seek the service. This is the main indicator of success and a mobilizing instrument for responsible community and individual participation.

The change requires multi- and intersectorial action, for a well-balanced distribution of promotion and recovery of Health. Health promotion must be seen not only in the context of individual or life-style behavioral changes but also within a perspective of public health policies.

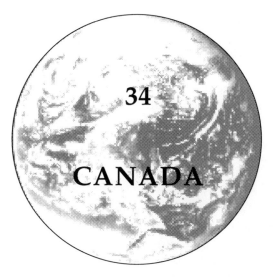

34

CANADA

THE HONORABLE DIANE MARLEAU
is the Minister of National Health and Welfare in the Cabinet of the Right
Honorable Jean Chretien. In this capacity, she is responsible for maintaining a
high-quality health system concerned with protecting and promoting the health
of Canadians. She also has responsibility for the health of groups at risk, such as
seniors and women and children, and for the delivery of health services to First
Nations and the Inuit. Madame Marleau has had a long-standing involvement
in health and women's issues and was the Chairperson of the Canadian
Games for the Physically Disabled.

A COMMON FEATURE OF HEALTH SYSTEMS around the world is that they must remain responsive to the changing and evolving needs of the societies they serve. Health system change is an experience that all countries share. We share many of the same pressures and challenges to which our health systems must adapt and we share a rapid pace of change that is greater today than ever before. The context for health system change is now the world.

In our one world, many of the health issues we face are global. Disease knows no boundaries, demanding that the health systems of all countries cope with existing global diseases, such as AIDS, hepatitis, and tuberculosis. All countries, too, share the same risks as new diseases appear.

We also share the same world environment. The human health impacts of global environmental change are experienced everywhere. No country can escape the health effects associated with such problems as global warming, thinning of the ozone layer, and pollution of our oceans.

Many countries' health systems must deal with the pressures associated with changing demographics. As populations grow older, chronic health problems and conditions become more prevalent. The health needs of an aging population are not well served by health systems that are designed to provide episodic treatment with a focus on cure rather than care. Health systems must develop the capacity to provide continuing care and to improve quality of life.

Other common challenges include lessening the health inequalities that exist within and among nations, keeping our health systems affordable and sustainable in the face of high public expectations, and achieving an appropriate balance or equilibrium among the various determinants of health.

We know that health care is an important factor in determining health status, but it is only one determinant. Genetics, the environment, education, socioeconomic status, and the sense of control one has over one's life are others.

In a world of finite health budgets, where every dollar spent has very real opportunity costs, it is vitally important that we ensure that we invest wisely. The question we must all address is what is the best way to allocate resources among the determinants of health to produce the best health outcomes for our populations.

Because our health systems face so many of the same pressures and challenges, it is important that we take the opportunity to learn from the successes and failures of other countries. Commonality of health issues means that there is tremendous scope for international cooperation and collaboration. Bilaterally and multilaterally, through international health organizations such as the World Health Organization, there is much that can be accomplished.

It is equally important to remember that, while countries may share a world context for health system change, there can be diversity in the way in which we implement change, the processes we use, and the priorities we set. This is because our individual health systems are key social institutions that usually embody the fundamental values of our particular societies.

The Canadian health system, with its single-payer attributes, is often referred to as a model to be emulated because of its success in providing universal access to health care while containing costs. Its economic, competitive, and health advantages have been well-studied and are recognized worldwide.

As a nation, we take a great deal of pride in our health system, which can be best described as an interlocking set of provincial and territorial health insurance plans linked through adherence to national principles. Canadians identify strongly with their system because it exemplifies many of the shared values of our society, such as equity, fairness, compassion, and respect for the dignity of all.

These values underlie the principles that guide the design and operation of our system of national health insurance: namely, universality, accessibility, comprehensiveness, portability, and public administration. The principles are decades old, and adherence to them as our health system adapts and evolves has been an important characteristic of the Canadian health system.

In Canada's experience, maintaining a set of health system principles that reflects the values of Canadians has helped to facilitate the change process. Change is never easy. This is especially true in issues relating to health, where concerns are often expressed in terms of life and death. But health system change is more likely to be accepted and, therefore, successful when a population continues to see itself reflected in its health system. As Canada renews its health system to ensure that it remains effective, affordable, and sustainable, Canadians will continue to see in it the principles that reflect their shared values.

Canada invites its world neighbors to continue to collaborate and cooperate on global health issues and challenges and to share experiences in health system change. In our similarities and our diversities, there is a richness from which we all can benefit, both individually and collectively.

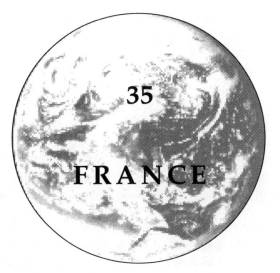

35

FRANCE

THE HONORABLE SIMONE VEIL
is the French Minister of State, and Minister of Social, Health, and Urban
Affairs. From March 1944 to May 1945, she was deported to Auschwitz and
Bergen-Belsen. In 1970, Madame Veil was appointed by the President of the
Republic as Secretary of the Conseil Superieur de la Magistrature (High Council
of Judges). She also has served as Minister of Health, Minister of Health and
Social Security, and as President of the European Parliament.

IN THESE FEW PAGES, I would like to outline what I consider to be the major current health issues from the vantage point of a Minister of Social Affairs in France.

Let me emphasize that France has elevated the Social Affairs Ministry to the status and ranking of a "Ministere D'Etat," a superministry ranking first in the hierarchy of the cabinet, with precedence over both the Ministry of the Army and the Department of State. It has responsibility for social affairs, public health, and urban affairs, as well as social security. If the social security budget is included, the ministry controls the largest budget in the state, about 2000 billion francs ($400 billion U.S. dollars), which is more than the total of the government budget itself.

I had the honor of serving two terms as minister, the first term from 1974 through 1979 and the second from 1993 to 1995. During this period, I have seen a tremendous evolution of the image of health and its social and economic impact in France. Until the end of the 1960s, health care was defined only as an unformalized array of human services. Technology has been the key to transforming health care into a highly organized field of activity, requiring strong government involvement.

The French social system calls for a high degree of common purpose and mutual responsibility. The challenge during times of economic austerity is not to lose this sense of common purpose and to maintain a strong commitment to the alleviation of the tragedies of poverty and inequality.

The means of achieving that goal represents one of the major differences between Europe and the United States. Europe accepts the full meaning of the implication of strong government involvement in public health while Americans are reluctant to see the government play a major role in health matters, which they consider to be primarily the responsibility of the individual. Europeans, though, consider that a proper role of government is to protect them against the vicissitudes of life.

As the preamble of the French Constitution states, "The nation shall guarantee health protection for all." In other words, there is an assumption that the public wants to see the government take strong positions in the health field in Europe while in America there is an assumption that government involvement threatens individual choice and responsibility.

Above and beyond these cultural concerns, technology has transformed health care in the last twenty years. Because technology has high costs and requires special training, there are few instances in which it stays in the hands of individual caretakers, such as physicians in private single offices. Most often, it takes the economies of the scale of large institutions to deliver high-tech care. Thus, in Europe, the relationship between doctors and patients is no longer a transaction binding the consumer and the producer, but is a more subtle bond negotiated between bodies whose concerns are mostly political and budgetary.

This situation has removed responsibility for the cost of service from both the health-care producer and the consumer. Paradoxically, while the cost of health care has risen continuously, the awareness and responsibility for its price have decreased on the part both of the provider and the consumer, who have left the financing of health care up to a third-party payer regarded with suspicion by both sides.

In the late 1970s, at the onset of the discovery of major health technologies, there was little doubt as to the medical benefit of what we all regarded as progress, and there was no reason to question the strong demand for health services. In France, as in the majority of European countries, demand more than exceeded the availability of resources, and there was an absolute need for some sort of planning to regulate an unlimited and generalized quest for new equipment, most of which was imported (mostly from the United States).

The best example of this is the management of costly equipment, such as CAT scanners and NMR (nuclear magnetic resonance) machines. According to a 1970 law, any kind of costly equipment would be submitted to prior assessment of the needs of the population in order to organize more equitable and sufficient distribution of health services. The main instrument of this policy is the *"Carte Sanitaire"* (literally, the "Health Map"), a planning tool that would be an inventory of all health services, including private ones, and that would set norms of facilities and equipment.

According to the law, a proposal for the creation or modification of matters, such as the number of hospital beds or the acquisition of costly equipment (for example, linear accelerators for radiotherapy, renal dialysis machines, nuclear medicine cameras, and ultrasound machines), should be submitted for authorization to the Ministry of Health. According to the law, reimbursement for the medical acts performed with this equipment by the French National Health Insurance (a comprehensive and mandatory plan that makes health care almost free for any French citizen) would be suspended if the equipment was not approved. In fact, there have been only rare examples of violations of this law.

Although this policy has been frequently attacked by all the political forces in France, none of the parties that has come to power in the past 14 years (including the Communist party) has made any major changes in the law. In France we remain committed to a policy that regulates the health-care market primarily through a rigorous control over the supply. This is a second contrast with the United States, where control lies much more in the pressure of demand.

This example of the management of technology represents the first instance of French government involvement in the management of health care back in the 1970s.

Did this involvement improve efficiency in medical care?

The answer would seem to be an unqualified yes. Comparing health-care expenditures in France and in the U.S. as a percent of gross domestic products (GDP), there is no doubt that France has spent less, with 9.2 percent of its GDP devoted to health care in 1993 compared 14 percent of the GDP in the U.S. The rate of growth of the total French health expenditure, which in the early 1980s reached 15 percent per annum, declined steadily after 1985 to stabilize at 8 percent per annum (plus or minus 2 percent). Unfortunately, this rate of growth is still unsustainable, given projected economic growth.

French Social Security is an independent administration, with its own board of administrators, mostly members of the workers' unions and business representatives. However, the government sets the rules, nominates the Director, and has a right to veto the decisions of the board. Every year, the french government has had to take initiatives to avoid a bankruptcy of the social security administration, which had not succeeded in making progress in the control of medical expenditures. It has become clear that the management of technology alone is insufficient to control the increase in medical expenditures.

The social security administration has proven to be quite reluctant to take any decision that would step back from what appears to be sacred social entitlement (*acquis sociaux*). The government has thus found itself alone in insisting that health care is subject to the same discipline as other public expenditures, in a political climate that regards health as a special issue, immune from the restraints of mainstream budget items in the economy as a whole.

In 1992, the French government decided on a major initiative, unprecedented in any country in the world: We offered a deal to the health professionals, including the nurses (here I must pay tribute to the nurses, who were the first to accept the agreement), under which any negotiation to increase professional fees was linked to the economic performances of the branch. Biologists and radiologists signed the deal just after the nurses and the paramedics.

General practitioners, specialists, and the pharmaceutical industry accepted one year later, in late 1993. An important feature of the deal relates to professional guidelines, elaborated by experts and validated by an ad hoc agency (ANDEM–*Agence nationale pour le developpement de l'Evaluation Medicale*).

According to the plan, norms have been established for the different branches and specialties aimed at reducing recourse to the most expensive medical procedures. This system is suggestive and does not bind individual physicians nor is it based on a personal surveillance of each of the 160,000 practitioners in France. It works on a statistical basis, and the entire branch is responsible for respecting the guidelines.

It is meant to create an environment where high technology is used only where absolutely necessary. The global aim is to annually evaluate with the professionals foreseeable trends in the evolution of treatment and prescription, taking into account epidemiological, demographic, technological, and cultural data, and calculate the reasonable evolution of medical expenses in each sector.

When the time comes for the negotiation of fees in the branch (about once a year), the real outcomes of the previous year are brought into the discussion. If the outcome conforms to the forecast, the government is likely to let social security raise the doctors' fees in that branch. Between 1993 and 1994, doctors' fees increased by 3 percent because the rise in doctors' prescriptions did not exceed the limit set by the government.

Conversely, had the government been convinced that there has been excessive prescribing of medical procedures, then there would have been a possibility that the entire branch could be required to reimburse the unjustified expenses. The overall effects on the trend of medical expenditures for the first year of application of the system were very encouraging, and a second set of guidelines was issued in 1995. This year will see the application of the same principle to public hospitals.

I have spent quite a long time in this short paper on managerial and financial issues of public health because these problems are endemic and common to most industrialized countries. Now, however, I would like to mention some specific areas where our ministry has taken a leadership role.

First of all, in AIDS treatment and policy, we organized, under the authority of the prime minister of France, the first World's Summit for the fight against AIDS, which was held in Paris on December 1, 1994. High-ranking ministers (including twelve prime ministers) representing 41 countries, together with AIDS Representatives, intergovernmental organizations, non-governmental organizations, and groups of people living with AIDS, convened to develop a common charter on AIDS research, treatment, and policy. Together we affirmed the need for urgent worldwide mobilization to slow the spread of the HIV / AIDS pandemic and provide care and support to those affected. We affirmed our common political responsibility as leaders to ensure that no continent, no country, no population or group or individual is marginalized or stigmatized, and we emphasized the need to respect human rights and ethics. We affirmed the need to strengthen cooperation with developing countries as only one of the many facets of the common obligations that we have regarding these populations.

The next major issue is drug addiction. My colleagues in the French government and I are determined to tackle the problem of drug addiction. We organized a group of experts who worked for one year to produce a study of all the aspects of this problem. We did not wait for the recommendations of this committee to begin to act, but increased two hundred-fold the number of methadone dispensaries in France.

An important segment of the work performed by my department is urban development. This represents an important change in the traditional handling of such problems. We are convinced that health, housing, and employment are virtually interrelated and that the promotion of health is an excellent–if not the best–justification to care for people. Without health, no durable permanent job is possible; and without a roof over your head, no health is durable.

Health has also to be accepted in its broader sense, including the psychological and social dimension. When we devote our attention to the slums and the violent suburbs, we know that it is not enough to build houses and supermarkets. We have to pay attention to the meaning of life in such settings and to encourage all forms of local action that help our youth to find their real place in our society.

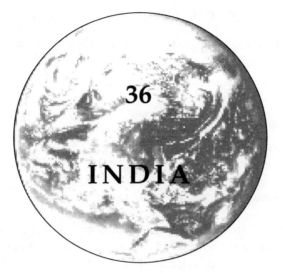

36

INDIA

THE HONORABLE C. SILVERA
is Minister of Health and Family Welfare. He is a Member of Parliament and
the first Mizo M.P. to have been inducted into the Indian Union Council
of Ministers as Minister of State. Dr. Silvera was formerly Medical
Superintendent of Kristian Hospital, Serkawn Lunglei, Mizoram.

GENESIS OF HEALTH POLICY

INDIA ENJOYS THE STATUS of being the world's largest democracy, with a constitution that proclaims the country as a sovereign, secular, democratic republic. It also empowers Indian nationals–constituting almost a sixth of the global population–with the rights of:

> *Justice: social, economic, and political;*
> *Liberty of thought, expression, and belief;*
> *Fraternity assuring the dignity of individuals;*
> *and–above all?*
> *Equity of status and opportunity.*

These provisions are further recapitulated in the constitution by a set of directive principles for the state, which also ensure a development paradigm for the improvement of sociocultural, ethical, moral, and physical conditions of Indian nationals. On issues related to physical betterment, for instance, the constitution stipulates that the state shall regard the raising of the level of nutrition of its people and the improvement of public health as among its primary duties. Similarly, the constitution enjoins the state to protect the health and strength of workers, men and women, and to prevent the abuse of the "tender age of children." Some of these provisions are further reinforced in articles of the Constitution wherein the state is held responsible for maternity aid and similar relief to the needy.

Interestingly, the need for public involvement in the delivery of health-care services was visualized in India long before its constitution came into existence. For example, an important preexisting policy document was the Health and Planning Committee Report, which, while regarding health care as basically a public responsibility, also assigned a role to the community to help meet this responsibility. An important feature of the recommendations of the committee (1943–46)–which also provided a basis for various health policy pronouncements by the Government after Independence–was the emphasis accorded to the primary health unit as the nucleus of an integrated (i.e., preventive, promotive, and curative) health delivery system. A similar approach to health delivery was favored by the Alma Ata Declaration Countries in 1978, in its proposal to reduce the burden of disease and ill health among low-income, underserved rural households. As a signatory to the

Alma Ata Declaration, India has adhered to this approach.

Focal Issues in Planning of Health Services

India relies on planned development, with one of its principal objectives being to minimize social deprivation-especially those that tend to dissipate economic progress. Efforts have been made since the very inception of planning in India to create public health and other medical facilities, including:

- Provision of water supply and sanitation;
- preventive health care of rural population through primary health-care units;
- prevention of food adulteration;
- eradication and control of all vectorborne and other communicable and non-communicable diseases;
- family planning and population control;
- health services for mothers and children; and
- development of medical education and research facilities.

In addition, in successive five-year plans, efforts have been made to meet the training requirements of technical manpower, paramedics, and other health workers.

A more significant emphasis on health-care services was provided during the Fifth Plan period (1974-79), which, *inter alia*, set forth the following goals:

(i)   to integrate health, family planning, nutrition, and other minimum needs programs to improve their utilization and effectiveness; and

(ii) to develop referral services by improving district and subdistrict hospitals, which invariably suffered from overcrowding, leading to inadequate services.

In 1983, the Parliament adopted a National Health Policy to reaffirm public commitment to the "Health for All" objectives by strengthening primary health-care services through organized support from the community, voluntary agencies, auxiliaries, paramedics, and adequately trained, multipurpose health workers of various grades and skills. Other important measures suggested in the National Health Policy to bring about improvements in health-care standards included: restructuring of health service infrastructure, with greater emphasis on control of blindness, tuberculosis, leprosy, and other major diseases; reorientation of the medical and health manpower involvement; and utilization of private medical practitioners and nonprofit voluntary organizations. It also emphasized improving the nutritional level of the low-income population, environmental protection, immunization programs for prevention of major communicable diseases, maternal and child health services, and school health programs.

Considerable strides have been made in the implementation and achievement of these programs, which have helped to bring down the incidence of morbidity and mortality in the country.

The emerging realities over the past few years have opened up considerable scope for reforming India's health sector and its strategies.

India has achieved significant progress in its health status since independence. This is clearly borne out when we look at the inputs into the health system (both public and private) and at various indicators relating to its output. These achievements become far more noteworthy over time. For example, life expectancy, which was barely 32 years at the time of Independence, has now increased to more than 60 years. The infant mortality rate has been brought down to 79 per thousand live births in 1992. The crude death rate had fallen to 9.8 by the end of 1989-90. Similar trends may be noted for most other indicators of health.

Beginning in 1952, India has been able to establish a countrywide network of primary health care in the form of PHCs and subcenters, providing through them basic preventive and curative services, maternal and child health services, family planning, and immunization. Over the period of the last three decades, Government has also demonstrated a strong commitment to population control and has devoted large and steadily increasing financial and human resources for this purpose. Based on the experience gained through these years, emphasis is now on consolidating the gains already achieved and improving the quality of primary health care and family welfare services. Attempts are now being made for improvement in outreach services, initiation of an autonomous medical and health education commission for comprehensive health manpower development, expansion in coverage of a health management information system, greater emphasis on safe motherhood, child survival and integrated child development, universal immunization, prevention of water and environmental pollution, greater involvement of voluntary and charitable organizations in delivery of health services, and involvement of the private sector (including Indian systems of medicine) to enhance the level of health care and its delivery.

While most of these strategies are already at varying stages of implementation, India's health sector is currently at the crossroads, with numerous challenges ahead. These challenges are partly caused by steady shifts in the countries demographic profile. Besides, there is also a sharp rise in incidence of new, nonconventional diseases that have emerged due to major economic transformations in the country followed by changes in life-style and from active to sedentary habits.

Changing Health Scenario and Policy Responses

The changing health scene is influenced by two major developments. One is largely due to the high burden of diseases with the following underlying factors:

i)   Aging and its related diseases in a large segment of the population;

ii) the persistence of traditional (communicable and noncommunicable) diseases; and

iii) the rising incidence of diseases due to stress and changing life style   or working conditions.

Another development basically relates to the structural issues in the health sector and, as such, brings out the need for certain corrective measures in the allocation of public resources to various health-care programs and activities. Fortunately, this aspect has been given serious consideration in India by health planners and policy analysts. Some important studies have already been conducted on health financing issues. These studies should eventually help policymakers in the government to implement necessary changes without affecting the basic objectives of equity and provisions of basic health services as enshrined in the constitution. Attempts are also being made to help secondary and tertiary public hospitals to find avenues for generation of finances through user fees or other similar charges. A health insurance system is also under consideration.

The growing incidence of various diseases in the country are far more challenging, and defy easy solution. While we are still struggling to combat the health hazards of communicable diseases such as tuberculosis, leprosy, and malaria, we also now have to cope with the growing risks of posttransitional diseases such as cataract-induced blindness, diabetes, cancer, and cardiovascular diseases. The threats of new diseases such as AIDS/HIV are further complicating the health scenario in the country.

The government of India is increasingly engaged in creating facilities to combat major communicable and noncommunicable diseases. Several National Health Programs are now directly run as centrally sponsored schemes by the Union Ministry of Health and Family Welfare. There is evidence that these programs have considerable bearing on the reduction of mortality and morbidity caused by these diseases. Some major centrally sponsored schemes include a National Program for Control of Blindness, National Leprosy Eradication Program, National Tuberculosis Control Program, National AIDS Control Program, including Blood Safety Measures and National STD Control Program, National Cancer Control Program, National Malaria Eradication Program, National Iodine Deficiency Disorder Control Program, and the National Mental Health Program.

In addition to these disease eradication and control programs, government has also made attempts to improve the facilities available in the country for medical and paramedical education and research.

Considering the need for greater enforcement of drug and food adulteration laws in the context of health protection, the Union Ministry of Health and Family Welfare has taken initiatives to improve drug control and food standards administration, both in the center and in the states.

The government is also making provisions to improve Indian Systems of Medicine and homeopathy as a viable alternative for many more costly allopathic treatments.

All these measures are expected to achieve better health standards for our people. A role toward the fulfillment of this objective is entrusted in the National Health Policy jointly with the private health-care institutions, voluntary bodies, and individual medical practitioners. Government is keen to provide all necessary facilities for better outreach and efficient services at an affordable price so that the cherished goal of "Health for All" becomes a reality.

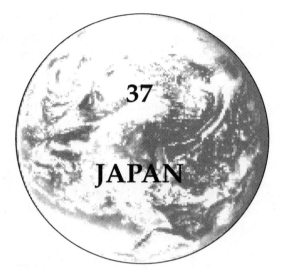

37

JAPAN

THE HONORABLE SHOICHI IDE
is Minister for Health and Welfare, Party Chairman of the House of
Representatives, and Chairman of the General Council of the New Party Sakigake
(NPS). Mr. Ide was also Council Director of the Deliberative Council on Political
Ethics of the House, Director of the Budget of the House, Director of the
Committee on Commerce and Industry of the House, and Director of
the Committee on Judicial Affairs of the House.

As STATED IN THE WORLD HEALTH ORGANIZATION (WHO) report on the current state of primary health care in the world, health care in general is improving. However, the gap in health-care standards between industrialized and developing nations remains vast. We believe that the issue of narrowing the gap is a priority problem not only for developing countries but for advanced nations as well. In Japan, the commitment to health care after World War II helped raise the average life span until it stands today at 76 years for men and 82 years for women. The infant mortality rate has been reduced to 4.4. Thus, a world-class health standard has been achieved in less than 50 years. Unfortunately, these have not solved all health problems. Japan is expected to become a society in which one out of every four persons will be older than 65 by the early twenty-first century. For this reason, it has become very important for Japan to reorganize its social security systems and to raise the efficiency and stability of its pension, medical care, and other social programs.

In late 1994, Japan introduced a comprehensive health-care and social welfare plan, known as the "New Gold Plan," designed to improve nursing care in the twenty-first century. The government is totally committed to enriching health care and welfare to build a society in which people live better and healthier lives.

As a member of the group of industrialized nations, Japan is expected to play a major role in the international community. There are many health issues that nations around the world, including Japan, must work together to resolve–AIDS and other communicable diseases, cancer and other major diseases, population explosion, environmental control, and emergency humanitarian aid. Though AIDS has not been as prevalent in Japan as in other countries, it has become a particularly difficult challenge for the whole world, requiring nations to work together to tackle the problem. To share the experience and know-how that nations have cultivated, we must bolster multilateral cooperation through international organizations and bilateral cooperation chiefly with developing countries. Based on a clear awareness of its position in the global community, Japan is committed to playing an active role in the betterment of health care for people in Japan and the world.

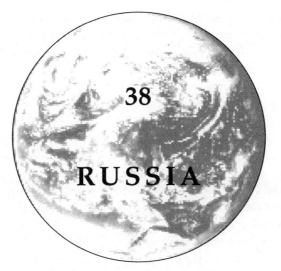

38

RUSSIA

THE HONORABLE EDWARD NECHAEV
is Minister of Health and Medical Industry and Professor of the Russian
Academy of Medical Sciences. Professor Nechaev was formerly Minister
of Health of the Russian Federation, Surgeon-General of the USSR Ministry of
Defence, and Head of the Medical Service of the USSR Army (later confirmed
in this post for the Russian Federation).

THE HEALTH-CARE SYSTEM in the Russian Federation is operating in hard circumstances of continuous economic recession and inflation following the political disintegration process. A recently established system of health financing from what's "left over" has resulted in the fact that the funds allocated to cover health costs at best represent 60 percent of the level of 1991. Funds aligned to health costs in the general budget expenditure on the federal level had decreased to 1.7 percent by 1993. Consistent efforts are being made for a change over to financing per capita in an outpatient hospital and per patient treated in an inpatient hospital. Lack of proper financing has created degraded material facilities in the health care industry and shortages of drugs and medical equipment.

These factors have led to a decreasing level of medical care for the population, limiting the use of advanced technologies in medicine and the eventual deterioration of health of the people.

Measures are being taken to preserve the health and medical science potential gained, the scope of medical care and drug supply, the provision of medical and prophylaxes institutions, and to fulfill state guarantees ensuring accessible and qualitative medical care and vitally essential drugs for the population.

The main health priorities determined are as follows:

- Development of the legislative basis;
- rational management decentralization;
- wide-scale introduction of compulsory medical insurance;
- support and development of the national pharmaceutical industry in order to provide more effective drug supply for the population;
- communicable disease control and prevention; and
- significant improvement of the quality of chronic noncommunicable disease treatment, and prevention of diabetes in particular, as a model for further use in the programs of other socially important disease control.

Considerable efforts have been made to establish an adequate legislative basis for reforming public health in Russia and to provide for the constitutional right of the citizen to accessible and qualitative medical care and drug supply, as well as the protection of their rights and legitimate interests in the provision of such care.

Priority attention is given to the maternity and child health service. Despite the fact that in recent years maternity and child health services have been under permanent and rising pressure from deteriorating maternity and child health quality and an increase in related pathology, we could prevent the total mortality rate in children's hospitals from rising. The mortality rate among children under one year of age has decreased (2.43 in 1992 and 2.29 in 1993), as has the infant mortality rate in obstetric hospitals (4.0 in 1992 and 51.6 in 1993).

The presidential program "Children of Russia" has been formulated and is being implemented. Under this program, activities are taking place to provide maternity and child health services, children's regional hospitals, central district hospitals, centers of family planning, prenatal centers, children resuscitation departments, rehabilitation centers with up-to-date medical equipment, for disabled children, and close monitoring of the health condition of children in the territories involved in the Chernobyl nuclear station accident.

Great efforts are being made to control infectious diseases preventable with immunization. A federal special program, "Vaccinoprophylaxis," is being implemented. In 1994, broad preventive immunization for children under two years of age had increased. According to the data, within the first eight months of 1994, infant mortality has been reduced (18.9 in 1993 and 19.0 in 1994 per one thousand live births). The proportion of child mortality due to infectious diseases, acute respiratory diseases, accidents, poisoning, and injuries has declined.

The number of abortions also has fallen. (The problem of manufacturing homemade intrauterine devices has been solved.) The maternal mortality rate remains stable (50.8 in 1992 and 51.6 in 1993 per 100,000 live births).

Although there has been a reasonable reduction in the number of children's beds in hospitals, the number of pediatric beds for specialized use has been considerably increased. The capabilities of all types of day hospitals are developing. Departments for the treatment of premature neonatals are being opened in the maternity homes. Resuscitation and intensive-care services continue to develop, including that in maternity centers, with up-to-date technology of emergency treatment.

Vigorous action has been taken to establish family planning services, to improve the system of medical care for children in educational institutions, to use the criteria for determining live and still births recommended by the World Health Organization (WHO) to improve the system of medical care for those in babies' homes, and to provide further development of medicogenetic services.

International organizations are making a considerable contribution to the development of maternity and child health programs. Thus, in collaboration with the society "Care–Germany," ten centers for the treatment of children with oncohematologic diseases have been set up in Russia. In collaboration with the United Nations International Children's Emergency Fund (UNICEF), programs for the prevention and treatment of anemia in pregnancy, the treatment of children with viral and bacterial infections, the modernization of vaccine manufacturing, and the development of "cold chain" have been implemented.

Great changes are taking place in the system of curative and preventive care delivery. The reorganization of primary medical and hospital care is carried out on the basis of creative development of our country's traditional medicine practice, and in keeping with the best achievements of the world's public health care and WHO recommendations. Provisions were made for a gradual transition to the general practitioner system and budget insurance forms of financing public health care. A comprehensive infrastructure of obligatory health insurance (OHI), based on the territorial principle, has been established in most territories of Russia. The introduction of OHI and the use of other sources of financing will allow the Russian public health system to maintain the necessary standard of adequate health-care delivery under the existing unfavorable economic conditions.

Infectious diseases morbidity in the country causes great concern. The ministry has formulated, and the government has approved, the state program on prompt action for providing sanitary epidemiologic safety, the prevention of communicable and noncommunicable diseases, and the reduction of the premature mortality rate among the population for the years 1994 to 1996.

The first case of AIDS in Russia was diagnosed in March 1987. At the present time, 831 HIV-infected and 149 sick people have been reported. According to the WHO classification, our country would be classified in the group of low-rate HIV infection countries.

However, the problem of HIV infection for the Russian Federation, as well as for many other countries of the world community, is of great national and social significance. AIDS control is a priority problem that can by solved only by joint and coordinated actions. Today nobody doubts that the prevention of the spread of HIV infection requires appropriate organizational approaches and legislation based on international experience and cooperation.

Our country evaluates the AIDS problem as being of great significance; therefore, AIDS control measures by the legislation have been preventive and effective in many aspects. In the Russian Federation, HIV infection control is an important part of the state policy, a problem that threatens the interests of individuals, the community, and the state. Russia is one of the few countries where not only the AIDS-infected but the HIV-infected people are found and registered. Medical and social aid to these people in the earlier stages of infection is the advantage of this measure.

The preventive measures system provides effective information about AIDS prevention to young people, religious and public organizations, and leaders of the groups most at risk. Extending the network of anonymous and voluntary investigation consulting rooms and providing psychological rehabilitation services are becoming priorities in epidemiological control. The fundamental research foreseen under the State Scientific and Technical Program is being implemented.

The Health Ministry's transformation into the Ministry of Health and Medical Industry has intensified attention to the native pharmaceutical and medical industry development. In spite of our economic situation's complexity, the native medical industry is functioning fully. In 1993 the manufacture of medical products averaged 93 percent of that in 1992. Particular emphasis is given today to the provision of the population with accessible, high-quality medicines. The pharmaceutical market of the country had been oversupplied with foreign medical drugs. During the period from July 1993 to October 1994, more than 10,000 import licenses for medical drugs were issued. Only for the last months, pharmaceuticals valued at $4 billion U.S. dollars have been imported to Russia. High prices and the impossibility of redeeming the drugs from the pharmacy network have resulted in storehouses being overstocked with imported pharmaceuticals.

The territorial health authorities expend considerable financial resources on the centralized purchase of medicines. At the same time, the greater part of these funds is spent for the purchase of expensive foreign drugs, to the detriment of the native manufacturers. The Russian State Program for improving drug provision and the developing pharmaceutical industry represents a 2.9 percent increase in 1995 over that of 1991 and includes a 3.1 percent increase of manufacturing and deliveries of the vital and paramount drugs.

In Russia we have now simplified the registration system of drugs manufactured in countries with developed pharmaceutical industries, which have already been registered in a number of foreign countries and which have been fully tested as regards their efficacy and side effects. A state system of drugs quality control has begun to function. Great attention has been given to drawing foreign investments on the basis of cooperative manufacturing with foreign firms, and some of these joint ventures have already begun to function at this time.

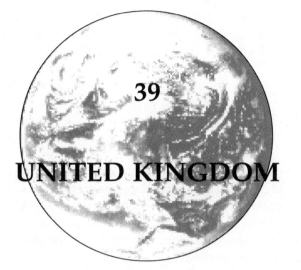

39

UNITED KINGDOM

THE HONORABLE VIRGINIA BOTTOMLEY
is Secretary of State for Health, Freeman of the City of London, and a Governor
of the Ditchley Foundation and of the London School of Economics. She was
previously Minister for Health and Junior Minister at the Department of the
Environment, with responsibility for the Environment, Countryside, Heritage,
and Local Government. Mrs. Bottomley was also Parliamentary Private
Secretary to the Right Honorable Sir Geoffrey Howe, Foreign and
Commonwealth Secretary, and Parliamentary Private Secretary to
the Minister of State for Education and Science and to the Minister
for Overseas Development.

IN THE UNITED KINGDOM, we attach great importance to promoting the health of the population. In England, we have developed a strategy called "The Health of the Nation" which addresses the major causes of ill health and the risk factors associated with them. The strategy adopts targets and It applies across the Government. Action has been outlined to implement it and progress is regularly monitored. It applies only to England. Separate strategies exist in other parts of the United Kingdom which concentrate on the health priorities identified in those areas. There are mechanisms for coordinating activity and exchanging information and ideas.

In June 1991, the government published a consultation document on health in England. It proposed a strategy for health, concentrating on a small number of priorities. These key areas were selected because they are major causes of premature death or avoidable ill health, where effective interventions are possible, and where it is possible to set objectives and targets. Three groups were established to take work forward: one to look at the wide range of interests that could influence the strategy; one to look at target setting, epidemiology, and related matters; and a third to look at the role of the National Health Service in such a strategy.

In response to the document, more than 2,000 submissions were received–from health authorities, local authorities, the professions, special interest groups, and individuals. There were also numerous contacts with other government departments whose work impinges on health. A series of road shows explained the strategy.

The outcome was "The Health of the Nation" White Paper, published in July 1992. The White Paper is a government, not a Department of Health, document. For the first time it set out a number of national priorities for health, with targets and proposals for tackling them.

"The Health of the Nation" White Paper marked a radical shift in thinking about health in England. It has adjusted the emphasis so that health promotion and the prevention of ill health now receive a full share of attention alongside the treatment of disease.

The White Paper sets out five key areas: coronary heart disease and stroke; cancers; mental illness; HIV/AIDS and sexual health; and accidents. Targets have been set in each of the key areas and for the risk factors associated with them–coronary heart disease/stroke, blood pressure, diet and nutrition, cancer, smoking, mental illness, HIV/AIDS and sexual health, and accidents. The White Paper also stresses the importance of continuing work in the area of disease prevention through vaccination and immunization programs.

In England, we have introduced the "purchaser/provider split." We fund health authorities and general practitioners fund holders (general practitioners with their own budgets to purchase a range of services). They secure the health needs of their patients through agreements with providers/hospitals, community units, and voluntary and private sector organizations. Purchasers are required to demonstrate how they are placing "The Health of the Nation" at the center of their strategies and purchasing plans and how they are encouraging providers to improve the service to patients to enable them to meet those targets.

In preparing the White Paper, we needed to consider what targets to set. We had to look for challenging yet achievable targets that could be monitored. It was not an easy task. We looked at recent mortality trends, extrapolation of trends, birth cohort mortality trends, international data, effects of interventions, and recommendations of experts. It should be stressed that target setting is not a pure science-there has to be a certain amount of "art."

Health promotion and the prevention of illness are by nature long term. Results are generally not as swiftly apparent as those for treatment. In view of this, and to make them effective tools, our targets were set to be readily available in almost all areas. The data also highlight those areas where effective effort needs to be concentrated.

We have found that most people have been willing to work toward the objectives identified in the strategy rather than argue about what is not included in it. The point has been accepted that concentrating on the identified priorities is more important than adding others to them and, in effect, diluting them.

For the first time we now have a cabinet-level committee set up to oversee implementation of the White Paper. Its membership covers 11 departments of state. The committee is chaired by a senior minister and receives reports on progress every six months. As well as monitoring progress and development overall, the committee has been looking in turn at each of the key areas. The three groups set up within the Department of Health at the time of the consultation paper continue to meet, with increased representation or closer working relationships with other government departments.

Task forces have been established to carry this work forward. They include an Inter-Departmental Task Force on Smoking; a Nutrition Task Force; an Accident Prevention Task Force; and the Physical Activity Task Force. Task forces have a wide membership, involving a number of government departments, statutory agencies, voluntary bodies, and other special interest groups.

In addition to the key areas, the White Paper identifies a number of different settings where people live and work in which action needs to be taken if the targets are to be achieved. The targets include healthy cities or communities, healthy schools, healthy hospitals, healthy workplaces, healthy homes, healthy prisons, and healthy environments. Many people have little regular contact with health services throughout most of their lives, and delivering health messages has to involve taking them to where people live and work.

An important factor addressed by the White Paper is healthy alliances. A healthy alliance is, in effect, a partnership of individuals and organizations formed to enable people to increase their influence over the factors that affect their health and well-being—physically, mentally, socially, and environmentally. Meeting the targets is everyone's business and will involve alliances between government departments and national agencies, the Confederation of British Industry representing employers and the Trades Union Congress representing employees, and key voluntary bodies. At the local level, too, purchasers need to work with a wide range of players, such as local providers (trusts, private sector), local government, education authorities, environmental health departments, local industry, and voluntary organizations.

Monitoring of the targets is very important. We are monitoring not only the primary targets but also indicators of progress. There are numerous data sources, but one of the most important is the Health Survey for England. A Health Survey was successfully piloted in the spring of 1991, with fieldwork for the main survey carried out between September and December, and will be carried out annually on a national basis. Initially, it has monitored the health of the adult population, concentrating on cardiovascular disease and its related risk factors. The data provided on prevalence and distribution of risk factors are helping to underpin and improve targeting of policies.

The 1991 survey was based on a random sample of adults, aged 16 years and over, living in private households in England. It was undertaken in 90 areas and yielded a response from some 3,100 adults. The survey had three components: a health and socioeconomic questionnaire; physical measurements (height, weight, demispan, waist/hip ratio, and blood pressure); and a blood sample (to be tested for ferritin, cholesterol, and hemoglobin). The findings of this first year of the survey were published in August 1993. The survey was repeated from September to December 1992 on the same basis but with a larger number of people participating-4,000 adults. Agreement has been given to increase the sample numbers. From 1 January 1993, the survey was enlarged to yield a response of some 17,000 adults. It is covering roughly the same ground.

The larger survey will provide sufficient numbers for analysis by regions; it will allow aggregation over the years for the smaller subgroups of interest, such as ethnic minorities; and it will allow a number of aspects of health to be covered over a period of several years, with repetition of major topics at set intervals to enable trend series to be built up. Finally, it will avoid seasonal bias and enable examination of seasonal variation.

"The Health of the Nation" strategy in England involves concentration on five key areas, with numerical targets, driven through the purchaser/provider split and with a strategy for implementation and the ability to monitor progress. It has given England for the first time a coordinated program to tackle the major health problems we face today.

The strategy accords fully with the World Health Organization's (WHO) objective of "health for all by the year 2000," and has been recognized by WHO as an example to other countries in implementing health strategies. Dr. J. E. Asvall, the WHO Regional Director for Europe, has described "The Health of the Nation" as exactly the type of catalyst for action and framework for mobilizing many sectors and groups that is now needed in many other European countries.

I hope that our experience in developing the strategy and setting up the processes to implement it and monitor its progress will be a source of help and inspiration to others. We will continue to work closely with WHO and other international groups to share experiences in health promotion. We intend over time to develop the strategy further. We must first tackle the major problems of avoidable ill health. I am confident that "The Health of the Nation" does that and will continue to do so.

CONCLUDING STATEMENT

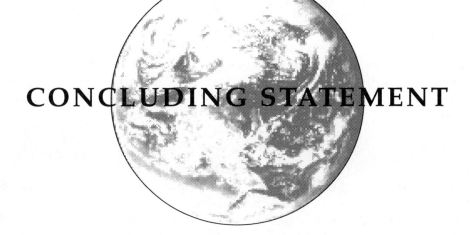

BOUTROS BOUTROS-GHALI
Secretary-General of the United Nations

THE NEXT CENTURY will be the development century. This may seem a bold assertion at a time when the world is learning that the end of the Cold War has led to the proliferation of protracted ethnic conflicts, where the searing horror of genocide, ethnic cleansing, and attacks on civilian populations leaves little room for long-term planning. But these conflicts, characterizing the end of a century of war, can be contained and concluded. Building upon what also has been a century of human achievement, the collective will of the international community, expressed through the United Nations, can deepen the world's realization that the force of arms solves nothing.

It is my firm conviction that the principal task of the United Nations in the coming century is to deal with global issues. The environment, population, human rights, migration, employment and production, the globalization of information and financial flows, and medical crises are the topics that must engage our attention and our resources as the world moves beyond the barbarity of war.

Even after the end of hostilities, we must deal with the heavy legacies of this century's conflicts: Around 150 million land mines, dotted across the countryside of some of the world's poorest countries, pose unacceptable dangers and added burdens on the development effort. Stocks of arms and radioactive material must be controlled and reduced in the interests of future generations.

Today, the United Nations is preparing itself for such a task, even as it must deal with the military crises of the moment. Through a continuum of global conferences and summit meetings, a culture of development is being created out of the diversity of human experience. A global consensus is gradually emerging as to the priorities of the coming century: environmentally sustainable development, responsible population policies, social integration, the promotion of human rights and democracy, the empowerment of women, and the struggle against disease–these are the priorities of international action.

As the twentieth century draws to a close, let us never forget the terrible human suffering in its many wars, but let us retain the inspiration of those who, in the midst of war, saw in collective international action the beginnings of a new world, one world.

–*Boutros Boutros-Ghali*

ABOUT THE EDITOR

ROBERT LANZA, M.D., is currently Director of Transplantation Biology at BioHybrid Technologies, Shrewsbury, Massachusetts, and former Clinical Associate Professor of Surgery at Tufts University. Dr. Lanza graduated from the University of Pennsylvania School of Medicine in 1983, where he was both a University Scholar and a Benjamin Franklin Scholar. As a student, he studied (and coauthored a series of papers) with the noted psychologist B. F. Skinner, with Nobel laureates Gerald Edelman and Rodney Porter, and with medical pioneers Jonas Salk and Christiaan Barnard. A former Fulbright Scholar/ITT International Fellow, he has also done research at Harvard University, MIT, Rockefeller University, Oxford University, and others.

Dr. Lanza has been nominated for a MacArthur Foundation "genius" award and has published extensively in the areas of science and medicine. He is editor (with W.L. Chick) of the *Tissue Engineering/Cell Medicine Intelligence Series* (Landes), the *Pancreatic Islet Transplantation Series* (Landes/CRC Press), and the *Yearbook of Cell and Tissue Transplantation* (Kluwer Academic Publishers). Among his other scientific books, is *Medical Science and the Advancement of World Health* (Praeger/CBS Educational and Professional Publishers), which furnished the inspiration for this book.

Dr. Lanza's scientific articles have appeared in *Science, Nature, Cell, New England Journal of Medicine, Journal of the American Medical Association,* and the *Proceedings of the National Academy of Sciences.* His essays on science and philosophy have appeared in the *New Scientist, Perspectives in Biology and Medicine* (University of Chicago Press), *The Humanist, Pacific Discovery* (California Academy of Sciences), *The World & I,* and in literary magazines, such as *The Ohio Review, Cimarron Review,* and the *High Plains Literary Review.*